Knee
Ligament
Rehabilitation

Knee Ligament Rehabilitation

Edited by
Robert P. Engle, P.T., A.T.C.

Adjunct Professor
Department of Physical Therapy
University of Delaware School of Medicine
Newark, Delaware

Clinical Professor
Department of Physical Therapy
Temple University School of Medicine
Philadelphia, Pennsylvania

Director
Knee Rehabilitation Institute
Berwyn, Pennsylvania

Director
Center for Sports Physical Therapy
Wyomissing and Berwyn, Pennsylvania

Churchill Livingstone
New York, Edinburgh, London, Melbourne, Tokyo

Library of Congress Cataloging-in-Publication Data

Knee ligament rehabilitation / edited by Robert P. Engle.
     p.   cm.
   Includes bibliographical references and index.
   ISBN 0-443-08753-9
    1. Knee—Wounds and injuries. 2. Ligaments—Wounds and injuries.
 I. Engle, Robert P.
   [DNLM: 1. Knee Injuries. 2. Knee Injuries—rehabilitation.
  3. Ligaments—injuries.   WE 870 K674]
   RD561.K576 1991
   617.5'82—dc20
   DNLM/DLC
   for Library of Congress   91-15712
                                            CIP

Distributed in the United Kingdom by Churchill Livingstone, Robert Stevenson House, 1–3 Baxter's Place, Leith Walk, Edinburgh EH1 3AF, and by associated companies, branches, and representatives throughout the world.

Accurate indications, adverse reactions, and dosage schedules for drugs are provided in this book, but it is possible that they may change. The reader is urged to review the package information data of the manufacturers of the medications mentioned.

The Publishers have made every effort to trace the copyright holders for borrowed material. If they have inadvertently overlooked any, they will be pleased to make the necessary arrangements at the first opportunity.

Acquisitions Editor: *Leslie Burgess*
Copy Editor: *Christina Joslin*
Production Designer: *Angela Cirnigliaro*
Production Supervisor: *Sharon Tuder*

Printed in the United States of America

First published in 1991   7 6 5 4 3 2 1

To my wife,
Kerry,
and daughters,
Ashley and Lynsey,
whose love and
support I cherish

Contributors

T.J. Antich, M.S., P.T.
Guest Lecturer, Physical Therapy Program, Temple University College of Allied Health, Philadelphia, Pennsylvania; Director, Newtown Square Sports Physical Therapy, Newtown Square, Pennsylvania; Chief Sports Physical Therapist, Lankenau Sports Medicine Center, Wynnewood, Pennsylvania

Gary C. Canner, M.D.
Staff Physician, Reading Hospital and Medical Center; Team Physician, Reading Phillies Baseball Club, Reading, Pennsylvania

John T. Cavanaugh, P.T., A.T.C.
Senior Physical Therapist and Clinical Coordinator, Sports Medicine, Performance, and Research Center, Hospital for Special Surgery, New York, New York; Director of Rehabilitation, Sportsmedicine/Rehabilitation of Manhasset, Manhasset, New York

Patrick W. Cawley, O.P.A., R.T.
Director of Research, Smith and Nephew DonJoy, Inc., Carlsbad, California

William G. Clancy, Jr., M.D.
Clinical Professor of Orthopaedic Surgery Sports Medicine, University of Virginia School of Medicine, Charlottesville, Virginia; Team Orthopaedic Surgeon, Jacksonville State University, Jacksonville, Alabama; Staff Orthopaedist, Alabama Sports Medicine and Orthopaedic Clinic, Birmingham, Alabama

Edward J. Corbacio, P.T.
Staff Physical Therapist, Center for Sports Physical Therapy, Wyomissing, Pennsylvania

Marsha A. Eifert-Mangine, M.Ed., P.T., A.T.C.
Staff Physical Therapist, Cincinnati Sportsmedicine and Orthopaedic Center, Cincinnati, Ohio

Andrew R. Einhorn, P.T., A.T.C.
Assistant Director of Physical Therapy, Southern California Center for Sports Medicine, Long Beach, California

Robert P. Engle, P.T., A.T.C.
Adjunct Professor, Department of Physical Therapy, University of Delaware, Newark, Delaware; Clinical Professor, Department of Physical Therapy, Temple University School of Medicine, Philadelphia, Pennsylvania; Director, Knee Rehabilitation Institute, Berwyn, Pennsylvania; Director, Center for Sports Physical Therapy, Wyomissing and Berwyn, Pennsylvania

Daniel P. Giesen, A.T.C.
Director of Athletic Training, Center for Sports Physical Therapy, Wyomissing, Pennsylvania

Debra M. Gill, P.T.A.
Staff Physical Therapy Assistant, Center for Sports Physical Therapy, Wyomissing, Pennsylvania

Lance E. Lauchle, P.T.
Staff Physical Therapist, Center for Sports Physical Therapy, Wyomissing, Pennsylvania

Robert E. Mangine, M.Ed., P.T., A.T.C.
Administrative Director of Sports Medicine, Cincinnati Sportsmedicine and Orthopaedic Center, Cincinnati, Ohio

Kevin A. Mansmann, M.D.
Orthopedic Surgeon, Paoli Memorial Hospital, Paoli, Pennsylvania; Medical Director, Eastern Pennsylvania Rugby Union, Philadelphia, Pennsylvania; Physician, United States Ski Team, Salt Lake City, Utah

Thomas D. Meade, M.D.
Director, Allentown Sports Medicine, Allentown, Pennsylvania

Russell M. Paine, P.T.
Clinical Instructor, Department of Physical Therapy, Louisiana State University Medical Center, Shreveport, Louisiana; Director, Rehabilitation Services of Lake Charles, Lake Charles, Louisiana

Lesley K. Rogan, M.Ed., P.T., A.T.C.
Clinical Assistant Professor, Department of Physical Therapy, Thomas Jefferson University School of Allied Health Sciences; Director of Physical Therapy, University of Pennsylvania Sports Medicine Center, Philadelphia, Pennsylvania

Alexander A. Sapega, M.D.
Assistant Professor, Department of Orthopedic Surgery, University of Pennsylvania School of Medicine, Philadelphia, Pennsylvania

Michael Sawyer, P.T.
Director of Physical Therapy, Southern California Center for Sports Medicine, Long Beach, California

Byron P. Wildermuth, P.T.
Director, Physical Therapy, Orthopedic Arthroscopic Sports Injury Specialists, San Diego, California

Kevin Wilk, P.T.
Clinical Director, Healthsouth Sports Medicine and Rehabilitation Center; Director of Rehabilitation Research, American Sports Medicine Institute, Birmingham, Alabama

Preface

When I decided to undertake the project of writing and editing *Knee Ligament Rehabilitation,* I knew the main challenge would be keeping pace with the rapid changes and varied approaches occurring as the book was in progress. To meet this challenge, I called upon a group of writers whose expertise and experience I highly respect. Their efforts provide important varied insights and styles.

This book provides rehabilitation strategies and techniques that will be useful to practicing physical therapists, athletic trainers, orthopaedic surgeons, and students. The book presents an overview of clinical rehabilitation for selected knee ligament and associated problems beginning with an introduction to anatomy, biomechanics of ligaments, and examination in the first three chapters. Chapter 4 is entirely devoted to instrumented examination, an exciting and relatively new area.

I felt it was important to discuss current concepts and new techniques in meniscus surgery in Chapter 5 before presenting meniscal injury rehabilitation in Chapter 6. Chapters 7 and 8 provide information on medial collateral ligament and posterolateral capsular injury and rehabilitation. Nonoperative treatment is primarily discussed in both chapters.

Anterior cruciate ligament anatomy, biomechanics, diagnosis, surgery, and rehabilitation have become better understood and these fields have changed very rapidly. Chapters 9 through 12 are devoted to the most commonly used approaches and rehabilitation: nonoperative treatment, semitendinosus/gracilis autograft, bone-patellar tendon-bone autograft and allograft, and synthetic substitutes. Posterior cruciate ligament treatment, including nonoperative treatment, an overview of surgical reconstruction, and postoperative rehabilitation, is discussed in Chapters 13 through 15.

Patellofemoral joint problems are associated with operative and nonoperative treatment of knee ligament injuries. Chapter 16 presents considerations for the patella based on an understanding of anatomy, biomechanics, examination, and specific treatment principles. Complications of the rehabilitation process are further discussed in Chapters 17 and 18. Although these chapters contain some overlapping information, I felt that since both sets of authors have done such an excellent job in past writings and presentations it was important to include them.

Bracing, the last chapter topic, has also changed dramatically to keep pace with the trends toward less invasive surgery and earlier, more aggressive rehabilitation. However, the effects of the knee brace and the rationale for its use are still controversial. I felt a separate discussion of this issue would be useful and should be included.

Management of knee ligament injuries is a dynamic, expanding area and aspects of the rehabilitation process are still poorly or incompletely understood. Although considerable progress has been made in understanding the diagnosis, treatment, and rehabilitation of ligament problems, further investigation and clinical research are necessary, and a great deal of progress and change lies ahead. The authors who contributed their time and energy to this project are devoted to making the changes necessary to advance patient care.

Robert P. Engle, P.T., A.T.C.

Acknowledgments

My career has been filled with many special professional relationships and experiences. I would like to thank the following people for their interest, guidance, and strong support: Gary Canner, M.D., Wyomissing, Pennsylvania; Thomas Meade, M.D., Allentown, Pennsylvania; Alex Sapega, M.D., Philadelphia, Pennsylvania; Robert Mangine, P.T., A.T.C., Cincinnati, Ohio; Frank Noyes, M.D., Cincinnati, Ohio; Andrew Einhorn, P.T., A.T.C., Long Beach, California; Byron Wildermuth, P.T., San Diego, California; Fred Allman, M.D., Atlanta, Georgia; Pam Chlad, A.T.C., Collegeville, Pennsylvania; Stanley Grabias, M.D., Reading, Pennsylvania; Don Frey, P.T., A.T.C., Philadelphia, Pennsylvania; and Gregg Johnson, P.T., San Anselmo, California.

Special thanks also go to Kimberly Moore, my loving and supportive sister-in-law, for her editorial work and continuing help with research and education, and to my staff, both past and present, especially Jeff Faust, John Scott, John Moyer, Daniel Giesen, Debbie Gill, Joe Witt, Jason Bowman, Kay Rochowitz, and Michelle Bement. Finally, I would like to acknowledge my parents' guidance and concern, which have strongly influenced my work.

Contents

1

Anatomy of the Knee

DEBRA M. GILL
EDWARD J. CORBACIO
LANCE E. LAUCHLE

INTRODUCTION

Knee injuries are among the most common problems confronting patients, physical therapists, and physicians today. Since the bony structure provides little stability, the soft tissues are required to withstand high forces, often resulting in tissue overload and injury. To properly diagnose and treat an injury, a thorough knowledge of the anatomic structures and biomechanical function of the knee joint is critical.

In this chapter we discuss the anatomy and biomechanics that will ultimately be beneficial in evaluation and treatment of the knee. Thus, we discuss osseous and soft tissue components, along with musculotendinous stabilizers.

OSSEOUS COMPONENTS

The knee joint consists of three bones: the distal femur, the proximal tibia, and the patella. The distal femur flares, forming two weight-bearing condyles separated posteriorly by an intercondylar notch (Fig. 1-1). These condyles blend anteriorly to form a concave trochlear groove providing an articulating surface for the patella. In both the frontal and sagittal planes, the femoral condyles are convex.[1,2]

Although they differ in shape and angulation, the medial condyle is longer in the anterioposterior axis and more symmetric than the lateral condyle.[2,3] The lateral femoral condyle is aligned with the shaft of the femur and thicker in the transverse plane. The height

of the wall of the lateral condyle is greater along the trochlear groove, which helps prevent lateral subluxation of the patella. Hyaline cartilage covers both the condyles and the trochlear groove to aid in movement and weight bearing.

The proximal tibia is divided into two tibial plateaus that are separated from the medial and lateral intercondylar eminences. When flexion occurs, the medial and lateral eminences project into the intercondylar notch of the femur, causing the tibia to rotate along its long axis. Located at the proximal end of the anterior border of the tibia is the tibial tuberosity. This is the insertion site of the patellar tendon. Gerdy's tubercle is located on the proximal tibia (lateral and superior) halfway between the fibular head and tibial tuberosity. The iliotibial band inserts into Gerdy's tubercle.

The lateral tibial plateau differs from the medial plateau in two ways. First, the posterolateral corner extends over the tibial shaft, which allows a facet to articulate with the head of the fibula. Second, the lateral plateau is concave in the frontal plane and convex in the sagittal plane. This geometric difference indicates different motions between the articulating surfaces of the medial and lateral compartments during tibial rotation on the femur.

The articulating surfaces of the tibia and femur are asymmetric in structure. Incongruency between the femoral and tibial condyles produces the motion, which is a combination of rolling, sliding, and spinning of one bony component on another. In a weight-bearing position, the tibia is fixed. Flexion and extension

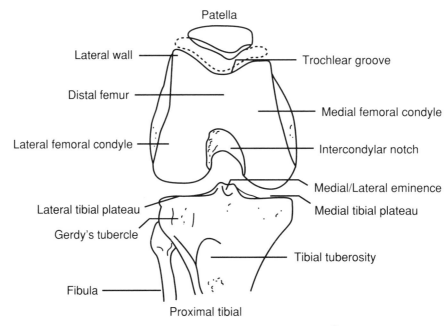

Fig. 1-1. Osseous components of the knee. (Modified from Insall,[63] with permission.)

occur as a result of the femoral condyles rolling, spinning, and sliding on the tibial plateaus.

In the first stage of flexion (0 to 25 degrees), the primary motion is rolling and spinning.[4] Additional flexion occurs by sliding of the femoral condyles on the tibia.[5] As the femoral condyles slide in an anterior direction they also simultaneously roll posteriorly. This ensures contact between the articulating surfaces of the tibia and femur during flexion. The opposite occurs during extension from flexion. The femoral condyles roll anteriorly and simultaneously slide in a posterior direction. The femoral condyles roll and spin on the tibia during the last few degrees of extension.

The screw-home mechanism is a combination of knee extension and external rotation of the tibia. In the normal knee the medial femoral condyle is approximately 1.7 cm longer than the lateral femoral condyle; this creates a spiral motion of the tibia about the femur during flexion and extension.[6] External rotation occurs simultaneously when the tibia glides on the femur from the fully flexed to the fully extended position; it descends and then ascends on the curves of the medial femoral condyle.[6] As a result, screw-home mechanism provides more stability to the knee in any position than would a simple hinge configuration of the tibiofemoral joint.

THE MENISCI

The menisci are circular fibrocartilage disks that rest between the condyles of the tibia and the femur (Fig. 1-2). Both menisci serve to deepen the fossa of the tibia, making the joint surfaces congruous and stabilizing the femur. Shock absorption and lubrication of the surface are other chief functions of the menisci.

The medial meniscus is semicircular and approximately 3.5 cm long. It is considerably wider at its posterior horn than at its anterior horn.[7,8] Anteriorly, the medial meniscus is attached to the tibial plateau in the anterior intercondylar fossa. The anterior horn of the meniscus is attached to the transverse ligament, which merges with the anterior horn of the lateral meniscus. Posteriorly, the medial meniscus is attached to the posterior intercondylar fossa of the tibia. The medial meniscus also attaches at its periphery to the medial capsular structures throughout its length.

The lateral meniscus, on the other hand, is more circular and covers a larger portion of the tibial surface than the medial meniscus. Posteriorly, the lateral meniscus is separated from the joint by the popliteus tendon, which attaches to it. The posterior border also often contains the meniscal femoral ligament of Humphry and Wrisberg.[9] These two ligaments extend from

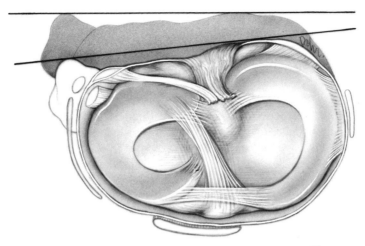

Fig. 1-2. Medial and lateral menisci viewed superiorly. (From Feagin,[64] with permission.)

the medial femoral condyle and attach to the posterior horn of the lateral meniscus.

Vascularization of the medial and lateral menisci is from both the medial and lateral geniculate arteries. Branches of these vessels give rise to a perimeniscal capillary plexus within the capsular tissues and the synovium of the knee point. This plexus is an arborizing network of vessels that supplies the peripheral border of the meniscus throughout its attachment to the joint capsule (Fig. 1-3).[10] Anatomic studies have shown that vascular penetration can be 10 to 25 percent of the width of the lateral meniscus and 10 to 30 percent of the width of the medial meniscus.[11]

Biomechanically, the menisci protract with movement toward extension and retract during flexion of the tibia and femur. During their protraction and re-

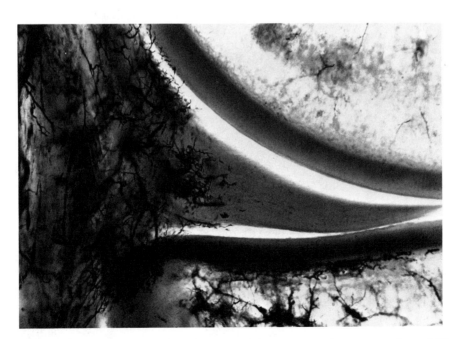

Fig. 1-3. Microvascular zone of the peripheral aspect of the meniscus. (From Arnoczky and Warren,[11] with permission.)

traction movements, the menisci carry varying loads across the joint. Ahmed and Burke[12] demonstrated that 50 percent of the compressive load is transmitted through the menisci in extension and 85 percent at 90 degrees of flexion. These compressive forces from the femur are dispersed in a radial manner across the menisci. These radial forces stretch the meniscal collagen fiber units along their circumferential orientation, thus providing the significant load-bearing support. Rotational weight-bearing movements of the knee are stressful and more difficult to resist for the menisci than are more sagittal movements.

THE PATELLOFEMORAL JOINT

The patella is a triangular sesamoid bone. Anteriorly, the surface is slightly convex in all directions and divided into three parts (Fig. 1-4). The wide base is located superiorly. The middle third contains many vascular orifices. Inferiorly, the patella forms a V-shaped apex that is enveloped by the patellar tendon. The medial border of the patella is thicker than the lateral border, but both receive attachments of the synovium, joint capsule, patellofemoral ligaments and quadriceps expansion. The lateral border receives fibrous expansion from the fascia lata.

The posterior or undersurface of the patella is divided into two parts. Its apex represents 25 percent of the patellar height and is nonarticulating. The superior articulating portion of the posterior surface represents 75 percent of the height of the patella and is completely covered by hyaline cartilage.[12] The cartilaginous coverage reaches 4 to 5 mm of thickness in the midportion of the patella.[13] Hyaline cartilage helps decrease friction and is necessary for transmitting the quadriceps compressive forces around the distal femoral pulley to the tibia. The articulating surface is oval and divided into medial and lateral facets by a vertical ridge.

The articular surface of the lateral facet is concave in both the transverse and vertical planes but may sit in a relative coronal plane.[13] According to some, there are three transverse segments present on the articular surface of the medial and lateral facets that are delineated in the adult by the presence of two transverse ridges at the junction of each third.[14,15] During flexion, these ridges are thought to isolate three segments of different functional significance as the lower, middle, and upper thirds of the patella are brought into contact with the femur. A subtle but relatively constant ridge separating the middle and lower thirds of the patella has been brought to our attention by Emery and Meachim[8] and Ficat and Hungerford.[16] This ridge is often more present on the lateral facet.

The medial facet displays a smaller or "odd" facet along the medial border of the patella. A small secondary vertical ridge separates the odd facet from the remaining medial facet. Each of the major facets separated by the central ridge conforms with its corresponding femoral condyle. One of the most important functions of the patella is facilitating extension of the

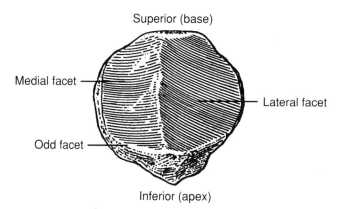

Fig. 1-4. Articular surface of the patella. The various facets and ridges represent the congruence of the patella with the articulating surface of the distal femur. (Modified from Emery and Meachim,[8] with permission.)

knee by increasing the distance of the extensor apparatus from the axis of flexion to extension of the knee. The patella increases the force of the knee extension by as much as 50 percent throughout the entire range of motion.[17]

When the knee moves from full extension into full flexion, the patella glides approximately 7 to 8 cm downward, where it contacts the intercondylar notch.[18,19] It is at this point that the odd facet engages the articulating facet on the medial femoral intercondylar area.[20]

Active knee flexion, in weight bearing, from about 60 to 120 degrees rotates the patella laterally, which engages the lateral facet.[21] When the knee actively moves from full flexion to active extension, the patella glides upward along the central groove until full extension occurs with the quadriceps contracted. At this point the patella is either positioned laterally and incongruently in contact with the lateral aspect of the femoral surface or centered in the patellar groove.[22] In a non-weight-bearing position, the patella rotates in the opposite direction of the femur.[4]

Contact Surface Changes

From full knee extension of the first contact is made by the articular cartilage of the patella contacting the femur between 10 and 20 degrees of flexion. The length of the patellar tendon is the controlling factor. The lateral femur is molded by pressure from the patella, whereas under usual circumstances, the medial ridge does not come in contact with the patella. At 20 degrees the smooth zone of contact extends from the near the secondary ridge between the medial and odd facets to the lateral border of the patella. Even though the medial and lateral facets are considered to be separate facets, there is no corresponding separate zone of contact for each facet. The contact zone moves proximally on the patella as movement proceeds from extension to flexion. By 90 degrees of flexion, the contact zone has reached its proximal patellar border. Throughout this movement the lateral border is in contact, while the medial margin is defined by a cartilaginous ridge between the odd and medial facets. In the first 90 degrees of flexion, most of the patellar articular cartilage, with the exception of the odd facet, is brought into load-bearing contact with the femoral surface. This contact band steadily increases in area as it moves up the patella.[13]

There is a drastic change in the contact pattern by 135 degrees. The medial facet is completely out of contact, lying freely in the intercondylar notch. The entire odd facet is in contact with the lateral border of the medial condyle. A large portion of the lateral femoral condyle is covered by the lateral patellar facet, while the medial condyle is not covered. When the knee is in full extension, the contact area on the femur corresponds to the tibial contact area of the femur. When moving from 90 to 135 degrees, the zone of contact passes over the ridge separating the medial and odd facets.[13] The congruence between the patellar and trochlear facets characterizes the entire patellofemoral contact up to 90 degrees of flexion.

Patellar Stabilizers

The patella is stabilized medially and laterally by the medial and lateral retinaculam respectively (Fig. 1-5). The retinaculam are extensions of the insertion of the medial and lateral vastus muscles. The retinaculum attaches to the medial and lateral borders of the patella and joins with the joint capsule.

The patellofemoral ligaments coincide with the retinaculum to provide passive stabilization to the patella in the mediolateral direction. Patellofemoral structures of the lateral aspect of the knee are considered to be stronger than the opposing medial structures. This is possibly due to reinforcement by the iliotibial tract expansion. Because the lateral femoral condyle is slightly elevated, it reduces the need for a strong capsular restraint on the medial side and provides static stability to the patella.

Patellar Tendon

The patellar tendon extends distally from the inferior aspect of the patella inserting into the tibial tuberosity. Inferiorly, the patellar tendon limits the proximal ascent of the patella from the tibia. According to Ficat and Hungerford,[16] the patellar tendon is 3 cm broad at its insertion into the apex of the patella and 2.5 cm wide at its insertion into the tibial tubercle. It has a length of 5 to 6 cm and is 7 mm thick.

In various degrees of knee flexion, it is the patellar tendon that governs normal posture of the patella at

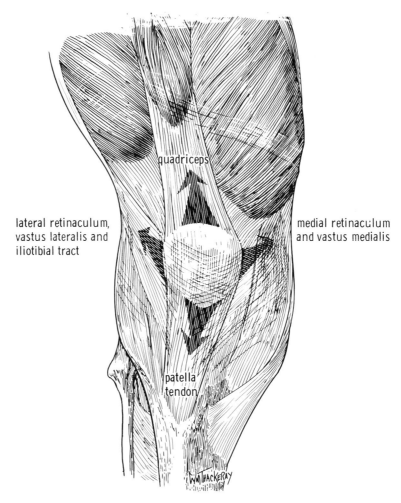

Fig. 1-5. Patellar stabilizers. The medial and lateral reticula are static stabilizers of the knee. The direction of pull from the quadriceps musculature is in line with the femur, and the pull of the patellar tendon is in line with the long axis of the tibia. (From Insall,[63] with permission.)

the end of the femur. At 45 degrees of knee flexion, radiographs illustrate the articular surface of the patella opposing the anterior portion of the femur.[1,23] If the patella is seated lower relative to the femur, it represents patellar baja. Any posture higher than this normal relationship represents patella alta.

Infrapatellar Fat Pads

Located deep to the patellar tendon and anterior to the femoral condyles is the large infrapatellar fat pad. Synovium lines the back of the fat pad, making it highly vascular. As the knee flexes, the fat pad fills the anterior portion of the intercondylar notch. With extension, the

fat pad occupies the patellar groove and covers the trochlear surface of the femur. During knee flexion and extension the fat pad sweeps across the condyles. This disperses a lubricating layer of synovial fluid over the joint surface of the femur prior to contact with the tibia.[24]

Q-Angle

Due to the length difference between the medial and lateral femoral condyles, most knee joints assume a slight valgus angulation in the standing position. The patella acts as a guide for the quadriceps tendon in centralizing different input vectors from the four quadriceps muscles and transmitting these forces through the patellar tendon. The direction of pull of the quadriceps musculature is in line with the femur, and pull of the patellar tendon is in line with the long axis of the tibia. The angle formed between the line of pull of the quadriceps muscles and patellar tendon is known as the quadriceps or Q-angle.

The normal Q-angle is considered to be 10 degrees with the quadriceps isometrically contracted and 0 degrees with the knee flexed at 90 degrees.[25] Quadriceps alteration and an abnormal Q-angle produce a lateral vector tending to displace the patella laterally. This displacement is balanced passively by the medial patellofemoral ligaments and dynamically by the orientation of the distal fibers of the vastus medialis. A breakdown of this equilibrium can result in lateral tracking and instability of the patella.

Plica

During the embryonic stage of life the synovial cavity of the human knee joint forms by fusion of three separate cavities.[1,16] This fusion may be incomplete, leaving a crescent-shaped fold of synovium that attaches laterally in the region of the vastus lateralis tendon insertion into the patella, superiorly at the deep surface of the quadriceps tendon, and medially from the medial femoral condyle to the medial infrapatellar fat pad. This is commonly known as the synovial plica.

Articularis Genu

Another important component of the extensor mechanism is the articularis genu. It is relatively small. Functionally, it retracts the suprapatellar pouch and maintains it in proper position during knee flexion and extension. The function of the extensor mechanism becomes disrupted if there is a suprapatellar and/or medial plica that becomes thickened, scarred, or contracted. This prevents the articularis genu from properly retracting this portion of the synovium in the suprapatellar pouch.[19]

Vastus Medialis Oblique

The angles of insertion of the quadriceps muscles are crucial for stabilizing the patella. The vastus medialis oblique (VMO) normally has a 65 degree orientation of its fibers on the quadriceps tendon and medial border of the patella.[1] A lesser angulation would fail to stabilize the patella during a powerful contraction of the other quadriceps components. A normally developed vastus lateralis appears to be the largest of the four muscles. This causes an increased lateral pull on the patella as it moves into full extension. In many cases of patellar instability, overdevelopment of the vastus lateralis is evident. As the knee flexes, a pull on the patella by the dominant vastus lateralis is visible. This is especially troublesome with insufficient restraints from a low lateral femoral condyle and poor development of the VMO.[23]

CAPSULE

The capsule of the knee surrounds the femoral condyles and tibial plateaus and is the largest synovial joint in the human body (Fig. 1-6). The capsule and ligamentous structures provide static stability to the knee. Insertions of the musculotendinous structures blend with the capsule, providing further dynamic support. The capsule is cylindrical with an anterior window for the patella and is indented posteriorly, forming a partition dividing the joint into medial and lateral compartments. A capsular membrane attaches to the tibia, winding itself around the attachment of the anterior cruciate ligament and in front of the posterior cruciate ligament. Because of this arrangement, the cruciate ligaments are considered extrasynovial but intra-articular. All the articulating surfaces of the knee are enclosed in the capsule inserting into the areas of vascularized bone.

The femoral attachments are proximal to the medial and lateral condyles, excluding the popliteal surface and portions of the intercondylar notch. The anterior portions of the capsule insert around the border of the patella and progress upward 2 to 3 cm to form the suprapatellar pouch or bursa.[2] The bursa helps reduce friction between the femur and quadriceps femoris tendon.

Along the edges of the articulating surface of the plateaus is the tibial capsular attachment. Exceptions are the tibial spines and a portion of the anterior intercondylar region. Posteriorly, the subpopliteal and gastrocnemius bursae are formed from two capsular recesses. The subpopliteal bursa is located between the popliteus tendon and lateral tibial condyle. The gastrocnemius bursa is located deep to the medial

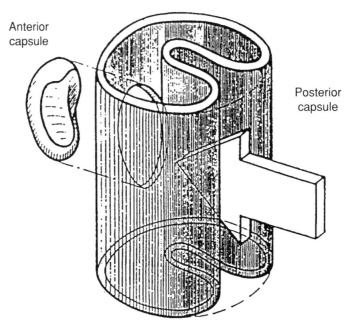

Fig. 1-6. Capsule of the knee. The capsule is cylindrical, with an anterior window for the patella. Posteriorly, the capsule is indented, forming a partition dividing the joint into medial and lateral compartments. The upper and lower ends of the capsule attach to the femur and tibia, respectively. (From Kapandji,[9] with permission.)

head of the gastrocnemius tendon, separating the tendon from the femur. The main function of the capsule and bursae is to move synovial fluid from recess to recess during flexion and extension to lubricate the articulating surfaces, as well as provide joint stability.

CAPSULAR AND COLLATERAL LIGAMENTS

Medial and lateral collateral ligaments are the major ligaments supporting the medial and lateral compartments, respectively. Supporting the capsular structures of the lateral side of the knee is the lateral or fibular collateral ligament. This ligament is a cordlike structure attaching proximally near the lateral epicondyle of the femur. It then slopes posterior and downward to the back of the fibular head. At that distal attachment site, it is attached to and surrounded by the biceps femoris muscle insertion.[1] There is no attachment of the lateral menisci to the lateral collateral ligament. The popliteus tendon separates the lateral meniscus and lateral collateral ligament. As the knee moves from flexion to extension the lateral collateral ligament becomes taut.

The reverse occurs when the knee goes from extension to flexion (Fig. 1-7). The lateral collateral ligament prevents varus stress or lateral joint opening. When the knee is in a flexed position, the anterior portion of the lateral collateral ligament is mostly supporting the knee from a varus stress. When the knee is in an extended position, the posterior part of the lateral collateral ligament provides increased support from varus stress.

The major ligamentous support on the medial side of the knee is the medial or tibial collateral ligament (MCL).[27] There are two distinct divisions of the MCL.[10,28] The first of the divisions is the superficial portion, which extends from a fan-shaped origin just below its adductor tubercle on the medial femoral condyle. It courses inferiorly and anteriorly to insert approximately 3 to 4 cm below the tibial plateau, leading to the pes anserinus.[27,29] Warren and Marshall[5] found that the superficial MCL was separated from the capsule except for the posterior part of the capsule. The superficial fibers of the MCL are vertically oriented, with a few oblique fibers joining the semimembranosus tendon to the posterior medial capsule. Hughston and Eilers[30] named the thickening of the posteromedial corner the posterior oblique ligament.

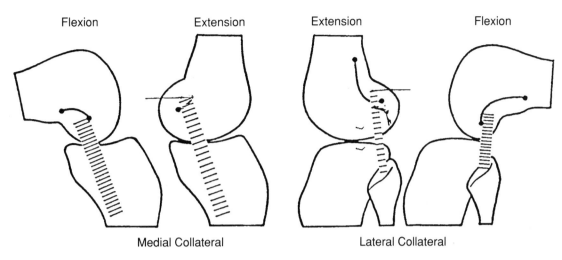

Fig. 1-7. Collateral ligament biomechanics. The collateral ligaments are taut in extension and relaxed in flexion. (From Kapandji,[9] with permission.)

The second division is the deep portion of the MCL, also referred to as the medial capsular ligament. Fibers of the medial capsular ligament are vertically oriented and run from the medial tibial plateau to the margin of the medial femoral condyle.[1,2,27] The periphery of the medial third of the medial meniscus is strongly attached to the deep portion of the medial capsular ligament.[1,27,29]

The suprameniscal and inframeniscal portions of this ligament are also known as the meniscofemoral and meniscotibial ligaments, respectively.[27] The MCL and medial capsule ligament are anatomically separate structures that can rupture at different levels of loading.[27] Like its lateral counterpart the MCL is also taut in extension and relaxed in flexion. When the tibia moves into internal rotation, the fibers of the collateral ligaments become vertical and relax.[19] With tibial external rotation, the collateral fibers become more oblique and taut.[19] Tibial compression with the femur also resists external rotation of the tibia.[19]

Posteriorly, the capsule is strengthened by two ligaments: the posterior oblique popliteal ligament and the arcuate popliteal ligament.[4,31] A portion of the superficial MCL contains a band of fibers which run obliquely to join with a portion of the semimembranosus to reinforce the posteromedial corner of the capsule. The posterior oblique ligament is an expansion of the semimembranosus tendon, that extends from the medial side of the capsule to attach with the medial gastrocnemius muscle and the remaining capsule above the medial femoral condyle.[30] Posteriorly, the oblique popliteal ligaments provide reinforcement to the lateral capsule while it limits anterior medial rotation of the tibia. The ligaments of Wrisberg and Humphry complete the posterior aspect of the knee. These ligaments are frequently absent. When present, they extend from the medial femoral condyle and attach to the posterior horn of the lateral meniscus. They are responsible for reinforcing the capsule during rotational stresses.

Reinforcement of the posterolateral aspect of the knee is provided by the popliteal tendon, the lateral head of the gastrocnemius, the arcuate complex, and the fabellofibular ligament. The arcuate complex is a Y-shaped band of deep capsular fibers that attach distally to the fibular head, fanning proximally over the posterior capsule and a portion of the popliteal tendon. They then join the fibers of the oblique popliteal ligament where it inserts into the femur.[1,2,20]

The fabellofibular ligament is known to be absent in 15 to 20 percent of the population.[20] If the fabella is large, the fabellofibular ligament may be large and the arcuate complex small or absent. The fabellofibular ligament originates on the styloid process of the fibular head and courses vertically with a portion of the arcuate complex to attach to the undersurface of the gastrocnemius muscle and insert into the lateral femoral condyle.

The MCL and medial capsular ligaments are strong stabilizers of the medial side of the knee. They protect against excessive valgus stresses and external rotation stress of the tibia, particularly when the knee is flexed.[27,28] The MCL is composed of two distinct parts. The superficial portion extends from a fan-shaped origin just below the adductor tubercle on the medial femoral condyle inferiorly and anteriorly to insert approximately 3 to 4 cm below the tibial plateau, deep to the pes anserinus. The deep portion of the ligament, also referred to as the medial capsular ligament, extends from the margin of the medial femoral condyle to insert on the middle one-third of the medial meniscus.[1,2,27] These fibers blend with the capsule and have a strong attachment peripherally to the medial meniscus. The MCL and the medial capsular ligaments are anatomically separate structures and can rupture with different levels of stress.

CRUCIATE LIGAMENTS

The anterior and posterior cruciate ligaments (ACL and PCL) stabilize the femur relative to the tibia and are named for their tibial origins, which cross in the sagittal plane.[32,33,34] The ACL is covered in synovial membrane, making it extrasynovial but intra-articular.[32] Distally it attaches anterior to the medial intercondylar eminence of the tibia and travels posteriorly and laterally to the supracondylar notch at the medial surface of the lateral femoral condyle. It has a broad, oblong attachment in a semicircular shape. Odenstein and Gillquist[35] reported an ACL length of 25 to 35 mm, a width of 7 to 12 mm, and a thickness of 4 to 7 mm. Girgis et al.[36] found the average length to be 32.8 mm and the average width to be 11.2 mm (in the middle one-third of the ligament). Kennedy et al.[37] found a length ranging from 37 to 41 mm.

Blood supply to the ACL and PCL arises from the ligamentous branches of the middle genicular artery as well as from some terminal branches of the inferior genicular arteries.[10,38,39] But the blood supply to the cruciates is mainly from the synovial fold covering them. This synovial membrane is richly supplied with vessels, predominantly from the ligamentous branches of the middle genicular artery.[40]

Fibers from branches of the tibial nerve supply the cruciate ligaments. Posteriorly, these fibers penetrate the joint capsule, coursing along with the synovial and periligamentous vessels. There have been smaller vessels observed throughout the substance of the ligament. The majority of these fibers are associated with others observed to lie along the fascicles of the ligament, which could serve some type of proprioceptive or sensory function.[40]

There are at least two major bundles of the ACL, the anteromedial and posterolateral bundles.[2,41,42] These bundles are named for the anatomic location and orientation of the fibers on the tibia and femur. Tibial attachment of the anteromedial bundle is on the anteromedial aspect of the tibia. Likewise, the posterolateral bundle attachment is on the posterolateral aspect of the tibia. This anatomic attachment site of the anteromedial bundle is the isometric attachment site in surgery for substitution of the ACL.[39] The anteromedial bundle is taut in flexion because the ligament is more horizontal in its orientation, whereas the posterolateral bundle is taut in extension (Fig. 1-8).[2,43] However, the ACL is actually a continuum of fibers, a different portion of which is taut throughout the range of motion.[44] This is of great clinical importance because in any position of the knee, a portion of the ACL remains taut.[36] The primary function of the ACL is to limit anterior tibial translation on the femur throughout the range of motion of the knee.[25,45–47]

The PCL is considered the strongest ligamentous structure in the knee joint.[48] It attaches over a broad area on the tibia located on the midposterior portion of the tibial plateau, posterior to the ACL tibial attachment.[9,27] Coursing anteriorly and medially, the broad femoral attachment is on the lateral surface of the medial femoral condyle along the articular margin.[49] This ligament can also be divided into two bundles: a posteromedial band that is taut in extension and an anterolateral band that is more taut in flexion (Fig. 1-9).[9] The primary function of the PCL is to resist hyperextension of the knee and posterior displacement of the tibia relative to the femur.[16,50]

The ACL and PCL work together to stabilize the knee in anterior, posterior, and rotational planes. Both cruciate fibers are always taut during knee motion due to different fiber length.[48] As the knee is flexing from full extension, the ACL becomes more horizontal in relation to the tibial plateaus and relaxes. At 90 degrees

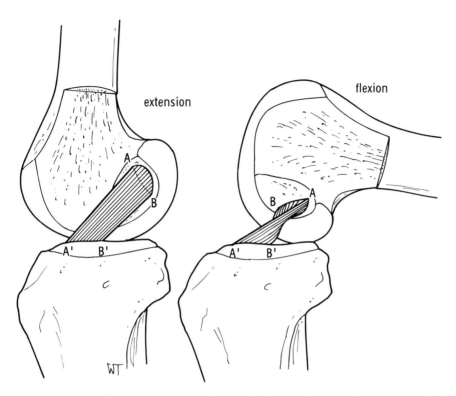

Fig. 1-8. ACL biomechanics. The posterolateral band (B–B′) of the ACL is taut in extension. In flexion, the anteromedial band (A–A′) is taut and the posterolateral band (B–B′) is relaxed. (From Girgis et al.,[36] with permission.)

the ACL is completely horizontal and resting between the two tibial tubercles. Conversely, the PCL is vertical to the tibial plateau when the knee is flexed at 90 degrees. Both cruciates are stretched in hyperextension.[28]

The cruciate ligaments play a very important role in the passive mechanism of rolling and sliding of the femoral condyles on the tibial plateaus during knee motion. During flexion, the ACL is responsible for the sliding movement of the femoral condyle anteriorly, which occurs while the condyle rolls posteriorly.[28] During extension, the PCL is responsible for the sliding movement of the femoral condyle posteriorly, which occurs while the condyle rolls anteriorly.[28] The cruciate ligaments also play a roll in rotational stability of the knee. Internal rotation of the tibia on the femur causes the articular surfaces to approximate as the cruciates intertwine and tighten. The opposite occurs with external rotation, in which they relax.

MUSCULOTENDINOUS STABILIZERS

Musculotendinous units and their interaction with the other stabilizing structures of the knee help provide the balance of the intrinsic and extrinsic forces that Noyes[21] says is necessary for functional knee stability. Analyzing the strategic location and action of the muscles exerting influence at the knee is essential. Using these structures intelligently during the rehabilitation process is critical for obtaining successful results.

Quadriceps

All four heads of the quadriceps attach to the patella. Hughston[1] describes their chief function as deceleration. They are also important for guiding or "tracking" the patella, positioning and stabilizing it in the femoral groove.

Medially, the medial retinaculum arises from the

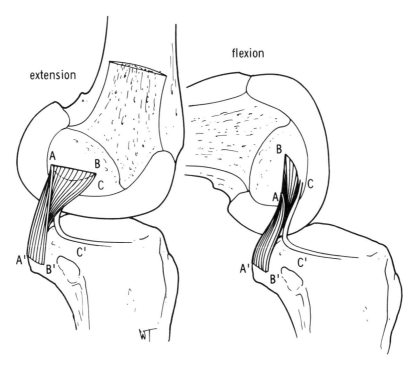

Fig. 1-9. PCL biomechanics. In flexion the bulk of the PCL is taut (A–A'). In extension it is relaxed (A–A'). (From Girgis et al.,[36] with permission.)

medial patellar border and travels to the VMO medial ends. Inferior fibers of the medial retinaculum run deep to the pes anserinus and have an insertion to the MCL on the tibia.[8]

On the lateral side, the lateral retinaculum forms a bridge between the lateral margin of the patella and the distal iliotibial band. The patellofemoral and patellotibial bands relate the lateral border of the patella to both the femur and tibia. The lateral femoral condyle is the site of the patellofemoral band attachment, while the patellotibial band inserts on Gerdy's tubercle.[8]

Two fibrous expansions from the vastus lateralis have an important anatomic course. The vastus lateralis receives a fibrous expansion from the distal iliotibial band. Similarly, a slip from the vastus lateralis travels along the lateral patellar border to the proximal patellar tendon.[8]

Eccentrically, the quadriceps functions antagonistically to the hamstrings and gravity, controlling knee flexion while absorbing compressive forces and decelerating the weighted extremity. Synergistic stabilization of the menisci with the posterior static and dynamic restraints occurs through the meniscopatellar ligaments.[27] Also, the quadriceps tenses both anteromedial and anterolateral joint capsules via the medial and lateral retinacula. MCL strain is decreased by medial quadriceps activity.[27]

The quadriceps have no direct anatomic relationship to the cruciate ligaments. By virtue of their size, orientation, and position, they restrain poterior tibial displacement in synergy with the PCL and the ACL from 90 to 75 degrees of knee extension.[51–53] Conversely, from 75 to 0 degrees of knee extension, the quadriceps translates the tibia anteriorly, making it an antagonist to the ACL.[14,27,37,51,53,54] Greatest strain to the ACL from quadriceps contraction is from 45 to 0 degrees of knee extension.[37]

Control of tibial rotation through the quadriceps mechanism has been discussed.[55] The vastus lateralis is responsible for tibial internal rotation with knee extension. Extension and external tibial rotation are primarily the responsibility of the VMO. Medial patellar tracking is another important VMO function.

Semimembranosus

The semimembranosus attaches by four tendons to the medial tibial condyle, medial capsule, posterior and medial capsule, and medial meniscus.[27,36,56] Besides bolstering the areas of the insertion, the semimembranous internally rotates the tibia along with the semimembranosus gracilis, sartorius, and popliteus and retracts the medial meniscus (Fig. 1-10).

The function of the semimembranosus in resisting external rotation of the tibia has been discussed.[19] At 90 degrees of flexion it exerts great influence as a tibial internal rotator, whereas in extension with its parallel relationship to the medial complex ligaments, it aids in resisting valgus stress.[33]

When considering the semimembranosus in rehabilitation techniques, one should account for its internal tibial rotatory function along with its role in flexion. Its attachment to the medial and posteromedial aspects of the knee qualifies it as a key protector of this origin. Semimembranosus action during rehabilitation of medial meniscus and posteromedial

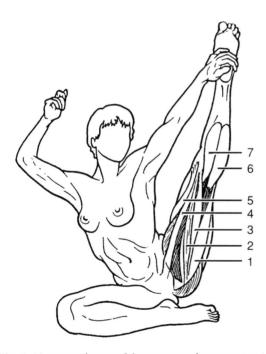

Fig. 1-10. Musculature of the posterior lower extremity (1) Biceps femoris; (2) semitendinosus; (3) semimembranosus; (4) gracilis; (5) sartorius; (6 and 7) gastrocnemius. (From Kapandji,[9] with permission.)

capsular surgeries must be approached cautiously to prevent generation of excessive forces across those structures during healing.

Pes Anserinus

More medially, the pes anserinus (semitendinosus, gracilis, and sartorius) attaches anteriorly to the distal tibial insertion of the MCL. It aids both knee flexion and tibial internal rotation. As knee flexion increases the pes anserinus along with the semimembranosus provides added mechanical advantage to internal rotation. This internal rotational force resists tibial external forces in knee flexion. By virtue of its orientation parallel and superficial to the MCL in relative knee extension, the pes anserinus also aids in valgus stability (Fig. 1-10).[19,20] Dynamic transfer procedures of the pes anserinus were used to increase its internal tibial rotation function.[17,57]

Iliotibial Tract

The lateral function of the iliotibial tract (ITT) is also of great interest. It has been advocated by many surgeons as an ACL substitute with extra-articular and intra-articular procedures because of its strategic location and dynamic contribution through the tensor fascia lata and gluteus maximus.[57,58]

Terry et al.[59] recently outlined in detail the ITT as a functional counterpart of the iliopatellar band. They describe an aponeurotic superficial, medial, deep, and capsulo-osseus layer. Among its identified attachments are the lateral intermuscular septum, lateral femoral condyle, lateral capsular ligament, proximal tibia at Gerdy's tubercle, and fibula. It receives an insertion from the short head of the biceps along its capsulointerosseus layer.

In the final 30 degrees of knee extension, ITT orientation makes it an active knee extensor. With flexion greater than 30 degrees, the ITT takes the role of flexor or decelerator of knee extension.[33] Kapandji[9] calls the tensor fascia lata an internal rotator of the tibia through the ITT insertion. Beyond 30 degrees of flexion, the ITT can exert an external rotating action on the upper tibia along with the long and short head of the biceps.

The ITT is an important static lateral ligament of the knee, but its role in anterolatertal knee instability in surgical procedures is still controversial.[57]

Biceps Femoris

Laterally, the biceps femoris has two thick heads that form a common tendon inserting on the fibular head. Marshall et al.[33] show a rather intimate and complex anatomic relationship to the lateral compartment of the knee. Before reaching the lateral collateral ligament on its way to the fibular connection, the biceps femoris divides into three layers: a superficial, medial, and deep layer.[33]

The superficial layer has three expansions that surround or attach to the lateral collateral ligament, namely, the anterior, medial, and posterior extensions. The deep layer of the biceps femoris tendon arises from a tibial component attaching to Gerdy's tubercle and a fibular component attaching to the fibular head and posterolateral capsule. Biceps tendon fusion with the anterior tibiofibular ligament often occurs, and a fibrous slip is also sent to the ITT, which influences its function with activation.[33]

The multiple attachments have an important functional role in dynamic action on the capsuloligamentous structures. Marshall et al.[33] identified the superficial layer of the common tendon as the major force creating external tibial rotation. The biceps pull on the tibia retracts the joint capsule and pulls the ITT posteriorly, keeping it taut throughout flexion (Fig. 1-10).

Popliteus

Significant functional importance was assigned to the popliteus by Müller[49] and Southmayd and Quigley.[34] It arises from a long vertical attachment and inserts at several key sites at the posterolateral corner of the knee. These include posterior aspects of the lateral femoral condyle, posterior horn of the lateral meniscus, arcuate ligament, and fibular head (Fig. 1-10).

Basmajian[60] identified the popliteus as primarily an internal rotator of the tibia with some activity in the initial phases of flexion to unlock the fully extended knee. As flexion progresses, however, popliteus activity greatly decreases.

Warren et al.[61] concluded from their anatomic research that the popliteus has a dual muscle and ligament function. As a muscle they also say it is an internal tibial rotator.

With the tibia fixed, the popliteus exerts a posterior and lateral pull on the femur.[33] Popliteus stabilization

of the lateral compartment through tendinous reinforcement of the lateral meniscus and posterolateral capsule is a strong functional component of knee stability. Synergistic tibiofemoral stabilization of the PCL has also been indicated.[49,60]

Gastrocnemius

Both heads of the gastocnemius (medial and lateral) take their origin from the posterior femur and joint capsule and run distally below the knee.[62] There they eventually join with the soleus to form the Achilles tendon. Although their primary function is plantar flexion of the ankle, they provide a vital role in dynamic support to the knee. Anterior tibial translation with gastrocnemius activation plays a synergistic role with the quadriceps in controlling posterior subluxation of the PCL-deficient knee (Fig. 1-10).

During midstance of gait, the gastrocnemius maintains knee flexion tension while the knee extends. This prevents hyperextension of the knee. At the end of the contact phase, the gastrocnemius along with the posterior tibialis and soleus decelerates internal rotation of the femur. The gastrocnemius also acts as a knee flexor and external rotator, thus lifting the heel to initiate an upward motion and forward acceleration to the trunk.

SUMMARY

Understanding the anatomy and biomechanics of the knee is essential for proper diagnosis and treatment of the patient with knee dysfunction. The intent of this chapter is to help the clinician accurately evaluate and treat the patient through an understanding of the knee's anatomic structure and function. Having a sound understanding of anatomy will be a valuable foundation for management of injured patients.

REFERENCES

1. Hughston JC: Subluxation of the patella. J Bone Joint Surg 50A:1003, 1968
2. Kennedy JC, Fowler PJ: Medial and anterior instability of the knees: an anatomic and clinical study using stress machines. J Bone Joint Surg 53A:1257, 1971

3. Milch H: Injuries to the cruciate ligaments. Arch Surg 30:805, 1935

4. Montgomery JB, Steadman JR: Rehabilitation of the injured knee. Clin Sports Med 4:333, 1985

5. Warren LF, Marshall JL: The supporting structures and layers on the medial side of the knee. J Bone Joint Surg 61A:56, 1979

6. Nordin M, Frankel VH: Basic Mechanics of the Musculoskeletal System. p. 120. Lea & Febiger, Philadelphia, 1989

7. Ellison AE: Distal iliotibial-band transfer for anterolateral rotatory instability of the knee (ALRI). J Bone Joint Surg 61A:330, 1979

8. Emery IH, Meachim G: Surface morphology and topography of patellofemoral cartilage fibrillation in Liverpool necropsies. J Anat 116:103, 1973

9. Kapandji IA: The Physiology of the Joints. Vol. 2. Churchill Livingstone, Edinburgh, 1970 (from the French, Phisiologie Articulaire, Librane Malone, Paris)

10. Arnoczky SP: Anatomy of the anterior cruciate ligament. Clin Orthop 172:19, 1983

11. Arnoczky SP, Warren RF: Microvasculature of the human meniscus. Am J Sports Med 10:90, 1982

12. Ahmed AM, Burke DL: In-vitro measurements of static pressure distribution in synovial joints. Part I. Tibial surface of the knee. J Biomech Eng 105:216, 1983

13. DiStefano VJ: Functional anatomy and biomechanics of the knee. Athl Train 13:112, 1978

14. Canner GC, Engle RP: The active posterolateral drawer test. (Submitted for publication.)

15. Steindler A: Kinesiology of the Human Body. Charles C Thomas, Springfield, IL, 1955

16. Ficat P, Hungerford DS: Disorders of the Patellofemoral Joint. Williams & Wilkins, Baltimore, 1977 (reprint 1:14; 2:33, 1982)

17. Slocum DB, Larson RL: Pes anserinus transplantation. J Bone Joint Surg 50:226, 1968

18. Fowler, PJ: Functional anatomy of the knee. p. 11. In Hunter LY, Funk FJ (eds): Rehabilitation of the Injured Knee. CV Mosby, St. Louis, 1984

19. Hughston JC, Walsh MW, Puddu G: Patellar Subluxation and Dislocation. Ch. 4. WB Saunders, Philadelphia, 1984

20. Mangine RE: Physical Therapy of the Knee: Anatomy and Biomechanics. Churchill Livingstone, New York, 1988

21. Noyes FR, Butler DL, Paulos LE, Grood ES: Intra-articular cruciate reconstruction. Part I: Perspectives on graft strength, vascularization and immediate motion after replacement. Clin Orthop 172:71, 1983

22. Crock HV: The blood supply of the lower limb bones in man. E & S Livingstone, Edinburgh, 1967

23. Gallie WE, LeMesurier AB: The repair of injuries to the posterior cruciate ligament of the knee joint. Am Surg 85:592, 1927

24. Jackson WO, Drez D, Jr: The Anterior Cruciate Deficient Knee. pp. 17, 55. CV Mosby, St. Louis, 1987

25. Kessler RM, Hertling D: Management of Common Muscuoskeletal Disorders. pp. 402, 440. Harper & Row, Philadelphia, 1983

26. Hey Groves EW: The cruciate ligaments of the knee-joint: their function, rupture, and the operative treatment of the same. Br J Surg 7:505, 1920

27. Daniel D, Lawler J, Malcom L et al: The quadriceps-anterior cruciate interaction. Orthop Trans 6:199, 1982

28. Hunter L, Funk FJ: Rehabilitation of Injured Knees. CV Mosby, St. Louis, 1984

29. Kennedy JC, Hawkins RJ, Willis RB, Danylchuk KD: Tension studies of human knee ligaments. J Bone Joint Surg 58A:350, 1976

30. Hughston JC, Eilers AF: The role of posterior oblique ligaments in repairs of acute medial (collateral) ligament tears of the knee. J Bone Joint Surg 55:923, 1973

31. Seebacher JR, Inglis AE, Warren RF: The structure of posterolateral aspect of the knee. J Bone Joint Surg 64A:536, 1982

32. Fowler PJ: The classification and early diagnosis of knee joint instability. Clin Orthop 147:15, 1980

33. Marshall JL, Girgis FG, Zelko RR: The biceps femoris tendon and its functional significance. J Bone Joint Surg 54:1444, 1972

34. Southmayd W, Quigley TB: The forgotten popliteus muscle. Clin Orthop Rel Res 130:218, 1978

35. Odenstein M, Gillquist J: Functional anatomy of the anterior cruciate ligament and a rationale for reconstruction. J Bone Joint Surg 67A:257, 1985

36. Girgis FG, Marshall JL, Monajem ARS: The cruciate ligaments of the knee joint—anatomical, functional, and experimental analysis. Clin Orthop 106:216, 1975

37. Kennedy JC, Weinberg HW, Wilson AJ: The anatomy and function of the anterior cruciate ligament as determined by clinical and morphological studies. J Bone Joint Surg 56A:223, 1974

38. Marshall JL, Arnoczky SP, Rubin RM, Wickiewicz TL: Microvasculature of the cruciate ligaments. Phys Sports Med 7:87, 1979

39. Sapega A, Moyer R, Schneck C: Testing for isometry during reconstruction of the anterior cruciate ligaments. J Bone Joint Surg 72A:259, 1990

40. Nicholas JA, Hirshman EB: The Lower Extremity and Spine in Sports Medicine. CV Mosby, St. Louis, 1986

41. Andrews JR, Saunders R: A "mini-reconstruction" technique in treating anterolateral rotatory instability (ARLI). Clin Orthop Rel Res 172:93, 1983

42. Johnson LL: Lateral capsular ligament complex: anatomical and surgical considerations. Am J Sports Med 7:156, 1979

43. Hughston JC, Andrews JR, Cross MJ, Meschi A: Classification of knee ligament instabilities. Part II. The lateral compartment. J Bone Joint Surg 58:173, 1976

44. Welsh PR: Knee joint structure and function. Clin Orthop 147:7, 1980

45. Blackburn TA, Craig E: Knee anatomy: a brief review. Phys Ther 60:8, 1981

46. Fowler PJ: Meniscal lesions: the role of arthroscopy in the management of adolescent knee problems. In Kennedy JC (ed): The Injured Adolescent Knee. Williams & Wilkins, Baltimore, 1979

47. Freeman MA: Adult Articular Cartilage. Pitman Medical, London, 1973

48. Insall JN: Anatomy of the Knee. p. 1. In Insall JN (ed): Surgery of the Knee. Churchill Livingstone, New York, 1984

49. Müller W: The Knee: Form, Function, and Ligamentous Reconstruction. p. 22. Springer-Verlag, New York, 1982

50. Finerman G: American Academy of Orthopaedic Surgeons Symposium on Sports Medicine of the Knee; Denver, CO, April 1982. CV Mosby, St. Louis, 1985

51. Arms SW, Pope MH, Johnson RJ, et al: The biomechanics of ACL rehabilitation and reconstructions. Am J Sports Med 12:8, 1984

52. Cailliet R: Knee Pain and Disability. p. 1. FA Davis, Philadelphia, 1987

53. Norkin CC, Levagie PK: Joint Structure and Function. pp. 295, 297, 299. FA Davis, Philadelphia, 1983

54. Sikorski JM, Peters J, Watt I: The importance of femoral rotation in chondromalacia patellae as shown by serial radiography. J Bone Joint Surg 61B:4, 1979

55. McGinty JB: Arthroscopic surgery in sports injuries. Orthop Clin North Am 11:787, 1980

56. Brantigan O, Voshell AF: The mechanics of the ligaments and menisci of the knee joint. J Bone Joint Surg 23:44, 1941

57. Slocum DB, Larson RL: Rotatory instability of the knee. J Bone Joint Surg 50:211, 1968

58. DePalma AF: Diseases of the Knee. JB Lippincott, Philadelphia, 1954

59. Terry GC, Hughston JC, Norwood LA: The anatomy of the iliopatellar band and iliotibial tract. Am J Sports Med 14:39, 1986

60. Basmajian JV, Lovejoy JF: Function of the popliteus muscle in man. J Bone Joint Surg 53B:557, 1971

61. Warren R, Arnoczky SP, Wickiewicz TL: Anatomy of the knee. p. 657. In Nicholas JA, Hersham EB (eds): The Lower Extremity and Spine in Sports Medicine. CV Mosby, St. Louis, 1986

62. Spence A, Mason E: Human Anatomy and Physiology. p. 175. Benjamin-Cummings, Menlo Park, CA, 1979

63. Insall JN: Disorders of the patella. p. 191. In Insall JN (ed): Surgery of the Knee. Churchill Livingstone, New York, 1984

64. Feagin JA Jr: Introduction: Principles of diagnosis and treatment. p. 3. In Feagin JA Jr (ed): The Crucial Ligaments. Churchill Livingstone, New York, 1988

2

Biomechanics and Biomaterials of the Knee

GARY C. CANNER

INTRODUCTION

The design of the human knee joint is such that the features of flexibility and stability are closely interwoven. In the past 20 years, our knowledge of the anatomic characteristics of the knee, knee biomechanics, and knee biomaterials has been advanced greatly. To comprehend the pathomechanics of injuries of the knee, one must have a basic understanding of knee biomechanical and biomaterial properties.

The units of measurement and a definition of the terms used in biomechanical and biomaterial properties are discussed first. An understanding of these principles is a prerequisite to understanding the biomechanics of the various components of the knee joint as well as the biomaterial properties of the osseous structures, the meniscal and articular structures, the ligamentous structures in the knee, and the patellofemoral joint.

Before discussing the static and dynamic relationships of the components of the knee joint, the units of measurement must be defined. The SI (International System) is utilized, with the basic units of the system being length (meter), mass (kilogram), time (second), and temperature (degrees centigrade). The force on a body or object is a function of the mass of the object and the acceleration of the object. In describing force, both the amount and the direction of action are described. For this reason, one describes force as a vector (directional) quantity.

There are several types of forces that are seen in action in the biomechanical functioning of the knee

joint. *Tensile* forces tend to stretch or lengthen the body, while *compressive* forces tend to shorten or compress the body. *Shear* forces generally slide one side of the body over the other, and *torsional* forces usually twist a body. Finally, *bending* forces tend to deform the object in such a way that one side of the object is placed in compression and the other side is placed in tension. A force with a tendency to bend or twist an object or tissue is known as a *moment*.

The effects of forces that are applied to the knee joint can be described by the use of the terms stress and strain. *Stress* is defined as the force acting on the body, divided by the cross-sectional area of the body. *Strain* is the elongation of the body, which is a result of the force applied, and is measured as a percentage of the original total length of the body. In evaluating tissues, a graph can be plotted that depicts the effects of force versus the change in length of the tissue. This is called a *stress-strain curve* and is depicted in Figure 2-1.

The configuration of the curve in a stress-strain graph can be used to determine several properties of that tissue or object. With reference to Figure 2-1, the slope of the initial straight portion defines the *elasticity* of the tissue or object. The greater the slope, the less lengthening occurs for a given amount of stress or force, and thus the less elastic the tissue. The slope of this portion of the curve is different for each material found in the knee. As long as the load that is applied remains in the elastic region of the curve, the tissue will return to its initial length with removal of the load. Once the load exceeds this linear portion (i.e., is

17

greater than F1 in Fig. 2-1), the linear relationship between the stress and strain is no longer present. When this greater load is removed, the tissue will recover from its deformation, but it will not return to its initial length. This area of the curve is known as the *plastic* region. Finally, if sufficient load is applied to the tissue, strain will continue until the tissue fails; this is known as the *strain to failure* (E2 on the curve in Fig. 2-1). A tissue is described as ductile if it has a long portion in the plastic region of the curve. A brittle material will fail either in the elastic region or after a small amount of plastic strain.

In discussing the stress-strain characteristics of a tissue, the influence of time must be considered. If the shape of the stress-strain curve changes for a given tissue with a change in the velocity of application of the stress, then the tissue can be described as viscoelastic. Typically, the slope of the elastic portion of the curve will increase as the rate of loading of the tissue increases. Viscoelasticity is characteristic of virtually all living tissues. The characteristics of viscoelasticity are depicted in Figure 2-2.[1] Two other effects of time on the typical stress-strain curve are described as *creep* and *relaxation*. If a tissue is under constant load, then the percent strain may increase even though there is no increase in the amount of stress applied. This effect is known as creep. Conversely, relaxation is the decrease in stress on a tissue for a given percent strain, or lengthening, if that stretching of the tissue is done over time.

Utilizing these terms and concepts, we can analyze the relationship of the various components of the knee

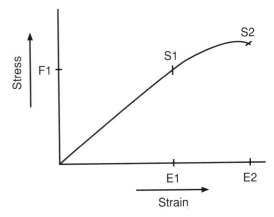

Fig. 2-1. Stress-strain curve. The region of the curve to S_1 is the elastic portion. S_1 to S_2 is the plastic portion. E_2 represents the strain to failure.

joint and understand the mechanics of their interaction. In addition, we can understand the material properties of the tissues and how they change with various stresses, as well as the effects of time and aging. Figure 2-3 summarizes the factors that affect the response of a structure to a load.[1]

THE FEMOROTIBIAL JOINT

To understand the biomechanics of the femorotibial joint, an understanding of the anatomy of the osseous, meniscal and ligamentous structures must be mastered. While much discussion in recent years has centered on the meniscal and ligamentous structures, a

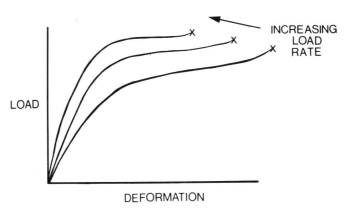

Fig. 2-2. Typical biomaterial properties of a viscoelastic substance. As the rate of application of the stress is increased, the stiffness (increased slope) of the curve increases. (From Dumbleton and Black,[1] with permission.)

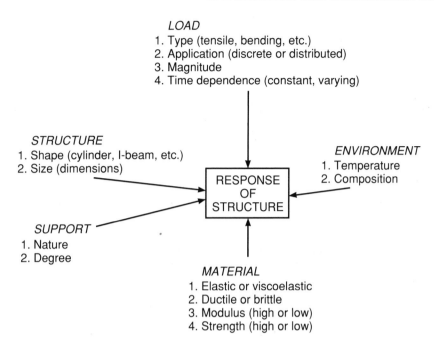

Fig. 2-3. Factors that affect the response of a structure to a load. (From Dumbleton and Black,[1] with permission.)

thorough understanding of the osseous and articular structures is also important. Remember that a great deal of variation in the osseous structures occurs between one person and another, as well as between males and females. For this reason, care must be taken in making generalizations concerning the biomechanical properties of the femorotibial joint.

The femoral condyles are asymmetric, with the medial condyle larger than the lateral condyle. The articular surface of the medial femoral condyle is larger than that of the lateral femoral condyle. Finally, the vertical or long axis of the condyle is less than the anterioposterior axis. The resulting cam effect of the condyles produces a variable tension on the ligamentous structures and compression of the meniscal and articular cartilage structures, depending on the position of flexion or extension of the knee.

There is even greater disparity between the medial and lateral tibial plateaus. The medial tibial plateau is concave and is thus designed for stability. The shorter lateral tibial plateau is slightly convex and is therefore designed for flexibility. Both plateaus are posteriorly inclined with respect to the shaft of the tibia. Conformity between the tibial plateaus and the femoral condyles is significantly improved by the menisci.

When beginning flexion from the locked, completely extended knee position, there is an external rotation of the femur on the tibia, at which time the knee is unlocked. Conversely, since the articular surface of the medial femoral condyle is larger than that of the lateral femoral condyle, when returning to terminal extension, the lateral compartment reaches a position of full extension first. Therefore, final or terminal extension is marked by internal rotation of the femur on the tibia, otherwise known as the screw-home mechanism.

Kinematics is the study of the motion between two objects, in this case the femur and the tibia. As would be true in normal gait, the tibia will be held constant as a point of reference. In discussing the rotation of the femur with respect to the fixed tibia, a center of rotation must be established. In the normal knee there is actually a different center of rotation for each flexion angle of the knee. Frankel and Burstein[2] utilized a four-bar linkage model to determine the instantaneous center of rotation.

A second important factor in determining instantaneous biomechanics of the femur in rotation around the tibia at any position of flexion of the knee is the joint contact point. As demonstrated in Figure 2-4, during the early part of the stance phase of gait, the joint contact point is on the posterior aspect of the tibial plateau. As the knee moves into flexion in midstance, the joint contact point moves anteriorly on the tibial plateau (Fig. 2-5). The positions of these two points (the center of rotation and the joint contact point) are determined by the osseous structures, the meniscal structures, and the cruciate and collateral ligaments.

Utilizing the instant center of rotation and the joint contact point, as well as the direction of the femoral rotation on the tibia, a determination of the direction of the relative surface velocity of the femur on the tibial surface can be made. This velocity is perpendicular to a line drawn from the instant center of rotation to the point of joint contact and is in the opposite direction from the direction of rotation of the femur. If this vector is parallel to the tibial articular surface, then sliding will occur between the femur and tibia (Fig. 2-6). If this vector is not parallel to the surface of the tibia, then either separation of the joint surfaces (Fig. 2-7)

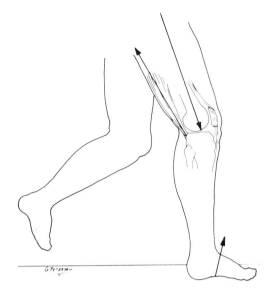

Fig. 2-5. In midstance, with the ground/foot reaction time directed anteriorly, the joint reaction point is anterior on the tibial plateau. (From Burstein,[3] with permission.)

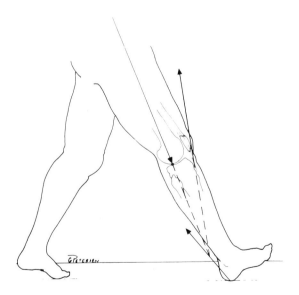

Fig. 2-4. In the early stance phase of gait with the knee near full extension, the joint contact point is posterior on the tibia, due to the posteriorly directed ground/foot reaction force. (From Burstein,[3] with permission.)

or joint compression will occur. This will result in abnormal joint mechanics.

The dynamic factors involved in the maintenance of knee joint equilibrium are three forces—the functional load, the muscle forces controlling this load, and the joint reactive force. Depending on the center of rotation and the joint contact point, the muscle forces can be considerable. The joint reactive, or contact, forces can be two to five times body weight.[3] To counteract a condition of joint separation or distraction resulting from abnormalities of the center of rotation or joint contact, increased compressive loading through voluntary muscle action must occur. Prolonged joint compression in this way can theoretically be deleterious to joint cartilage.

With these principles in mind, it is easy to understand how intra-articular pathology can occur as a result of ligamentous disruption. As a result of anterior cruciate ligament (ACL) deficiency, a decreased resistance to posterior femoral sliding at the joint contact point on the tibia occurs with knee extension. Thus, an increased incidence of meniscal tears is seen in the ACL-deficient knee. In a similar manner, a knee that lacks a functioning posterior cruciate ligament will rely heavily on the extensor mechanism and patella to re-

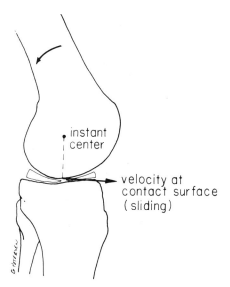

Fig. 2-6. A vector drawn perpendicular to the line between the instant center of rotation and the joint contact point, and originating from the contact point, depicts the velocity of the femur at the contact surface. If this vector is parallel to the tibial joint surface, the femur slides on the tibia. (From Burstein,[3] with permission.)

sist anterior femoral sliding as the knee goes into flexion, frequently resulting in early patellofemoral arthrosis.

ARTICULAR CARTILAGE AND MENISCI

The material qualities of articular cartilage vary with the joint in which they are are contained, as well as their location in that joint. In the femorotibial joint, the articular cartilage resists compressive stresses well, but not shear stress. For this reason, if an increase in the amount of compressive sliding (i.e., shear stress) occurs there will be deleterious effects on this type of cartilage. The articular cartilage will absorb water and therefore be less able to distribute joint forces in the knee. Once this happens, stress localization occurs and stress fractures of the subchondral bone with collapse will soon follow.

The menisci, or semilunar cartilages, have several functions in the knee. They act both to absorb stress and to distribute the stress evenly to the articular cartilage. They also control motion and act as a static sta-

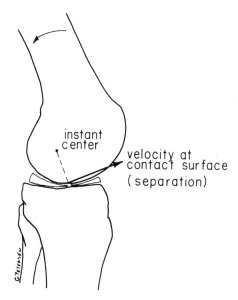

Fig. 2-7. If the velocity of the femur at the contact surface is not parallel to the tibial surface, then separation or compression occurs. (From Burstein,[3] with permission.)

bilizer in the knee. Moreover, they provide nutrition to the articular cartilage.

The meniscal fibers have been described as resembling the hoop shape of a barrel. The hoop concept of meniscal biomechanics states that as load is applied in a compressive form to the meniscus, the tension in the individual bands, or hoops, of the meniscus increases.[4] Only with shear or buckling stress to the meniscus does failure occur. In the same way, radial tears in the meniscus will cause weakening of all the fibers when they are placed in compression between the femur and tibia.

In considering meniscectomy versus meniscal repair, the theoretical importance of the meniscus in preventing degenerative changes must be remembered. Following meniscectomy, distribution of stresses to the joint surfaces is not as widespread and the surface area of contact becomes smaller. The stress per unit area will therefore increase. Some variation exists in stress localization following medial and lateral meniscectomy, depending on the varus or valgus alignment of the knee that has undergone surgery. Following meniscal repair, active extension without sufficient hamstring dynamic protection and ACL static protection will result in stress to the meniscal repair site. For this reason, it is not surprising that meniscal repair success rates diminish in the ACL-deficient knee. Finally, the use of mismatched meniscal allografts or repair with deformed meniscal tissue can also result in stress localization and subsequent degenerative changes.

LIGAMENTS

The analysis of the biomechanical and biomaterial properties of knee ligaments has been a great source of interest in the orthopedic literature in the past 20 years. Ligaments, like other tissues in the knee, are viscoelastic substances. In addition, certain changes occur with aging, such as increased brittleness and decreased maximum load to failure. A ligament is a complex, relatively static collagenous structure whose formation and maturation coincides with that of the femur, tibia, and menisci. Therefore, its function is intimately tied to these structures. One cannot biomechanically analyze a ligament independently, ignoring the bone, menisci, other ligaments, and the dynamic stabilizers. Müller[5] described a four-bar linkage concept, with the ACL and the posterior cruciate ligament (PCL) representing two of the bars, to predict the geometry of the femoral condyles using the tibial plateaus as a base of reference.

To analyze the kinematics of ligaments, one must analyze joint motion three-dimensionally. Grood and Suntay[5] describe 6 degrees of freedom of motion for the knee joint. There are three axes of motion: anteroposterior, mediolateral, and proximodistal. For each axis, there is a rotation and a translation (Table 2-1). On the anteroposterior axis, there are the rotations of abduction and adduction and a translation in the anteroposterior direction. On the mediolateral axis, there are the rotations of flexion and extension with concomitant mediolateral translation. Finally, along the axial or proximodistal axis, there is internal and external rotation, and a translation that can be described as penetration or distraction.

In describing the rotations that can occur, a center of rotation along each axis must be obtained. The determination of the instant center of rotation for flexion and extension on the mediolateral axis has been described. With regard to the longitudinal axis of the knee, lateral compartment rotation is normally increased compared with that of the medial compart-

Table 2-1. Six Degrees of Freedom of Motion, along Three Axes

Axis	Translation	Rotation
Axial	Distraction-impaction	Internal-external
Mediolateral	Mediolateral	Flexion-extension
Anteroposterior	Anteroposterior	Varus-valgus

ment. For this reason, the center of the axis of rotation is normally found in the medial compartment of the knee. This can be altered, however, with injury to the ligamentous structures of the knee. Last, the center of abduction-adduction rotation is usually found in the intercondylar notch region of the knee. However, this center of rotation can move medially or laterally as a result of damage to the ligamentous structures or compression fractures of the femoral condyles or tibial plateaus.

There are several mechanisms by which ligaments control knee motion. The ligaments act in tension to control knee motion in response to stretching. In addition, with certain rotational activities, they can act in compression to prevent excess knee motion. Furthermore, there is most likely a neurologic feedback mechanism, mediated through neural organelles in the ligamentous structures, that activates dynamic stabilizers to prevent excess knee motion.

Remember that ligaments are in fact made up of multiple fiber units. Each unit will work to prevent excess translation in rotation at a given position of knee function. The term *isometricity* has been used to describe two points, one on the femur and one on the tibia, that are equidistant throughout the range of motion of the knee. In reality, different fiber units of the ligamentous structure will maintain a static length, not displaying strain characteristics at various ranges of motion of the knee.

For each rotation and translation, there are primary and secondary ligamentous stabilizers of the knee. The ACL restrains external rotation of the tibia and anterior translation of the tibia or posterior translation of the femur. It comes under a great amount of tensile stress as the knee actively returns to full extension with a posteriorly directed sliding of the femur. The PCL restrains rotation on all three axes, as well as posterior translation of the tibia or anterior translation of the femur on the tibia. The medial and lateral collateral ligamentous structures are primary stabilizers of abduction and adduction rotations. Depending on the flexion angle of the knee, different portions of these two ligaments are taut at any one time.

Several principles of ligament pathology are important to comprehend. Failure of ligaments is a process that occurs serially. It is not clear when neural disruption occurs. Once the ligament experiences neural disruption and significant length change, it loses most of its control over knee motion. Since ligaments act in concert, they typically fail together, with varying levels of loss of integrity.

In discussing surgical reconstruction for ligamentous injury, several principles must be kept in mind. While approximate values for maximum load to failure for the autograft and allograft tissues have been established,[7] if composite grafts are utilized, the overall strength of the graft may only be that of its weakest link. The load to failure value for the attachment sites must also be considered. After grafts have been implanted, they are strong at first, but weaken quickly with resorption and replacement before gradually regaining strength. Rehabilitation principles must take the biomaterial properties of the graft and the host knee into consideration.

THE PATELLOFEMORAL JOINT

Multiple biomechanical variables of the lower extremity must also be taken into account when discussing the patellofemoral joint. The Q-angle, or the relationship of the quadriceps to the patella and its tibial tubercle attachment, has been acknowledged as being extremely important. In addition, factors such as femoral neck anteversion, the varus-valgus alignment of the knee, and tibial torsion also have been suggested to be possible anatomic variations that can contribute to patellofemoral pathology.

The articular cartilage of the patella is much more resistant to shear stress than it is to compressive stresses. There is a change in the area of patellar articular surface contact with respect to the change in the position of the knee. As the knee goes from extension to flexion, the area of contact on the patella moves from distal to proximal. In addition, from 0 degrees to 90 degrees of knee flexion, the total area of contact of the patella increases. The total force increases at a greater rate, however, and thus the force

per unit area increases as knee flexion increases.[8] Active knee extension by quadriceps contraction causes anterior tibial translation at positions of knee flexion from 0 degrees to 70 degrees and posterior tibial translation at positions of knee flexion from 70 degrees to 130 degrees. These concepts must be carefully considered when designing rehabilitation programs utilizing the quadriceps in postinjury or postsurgery situations.

SUMMARY

The biomechanical and biomaterial properties of the various tissue components of the knee have been reviewed. The concept of the functional interrelationship of these components is emphasized in both the normal, nonpathologic state, as well as in several frequently seen combinations of injured tissues following trauma to the knee. A thorough knowledge of these biomechanical and biomaterial properties is essential to allow the orthopaedic surgeon and the physical therapist to proceed with the appropriate treatment of these injuries.

REFERENCES

1. Dumbleton JH, Black J: Principles of mechanics. p. 359. In Black J, Dumbleton JH (eds): Clinical Biomechanics. Churchill Livingstone, New York, 1981
2. Frankel VH, Burstein AH: Orthopedic Biomechanics. Lea & Febiger, Philadelphia, 1970
3. Burstein AH: Biomechanics of the knee. p. 21. In Insall JN (ed): Surgery of the Knee. Churchill Livingstone, New York, 1984
4. Bullough PG, Munvera C, Murphy J et al: The strength of the menisci of the knee as it relates to their fine structure. J Bone Joint 52B:564, 1970
5. Müller W: The Knee. Form, Function, and Ligament Reconstruction. Springer-Verlag, Berlin, 1983
6. Grood ES, Suntay WJ: A joint coordinate system for the clinical description of three-dimensional motion. Application to the knee. J Biomech Eng 105:136, 1983
7. Noyes FR, Butler DC, Grood ES et al: Biomechanical analysis of human ligament grafts used in knee ligament repairs and reconstructions. J Bone Joint Surg 66A:344, 1984
8. Ficat RP, Hungerford DS: Disorders of the patellofemoral joint. Williams & Wilkins, Baltimore, 1977

3
Examination of the Knee

ROBERT P. ENGLE

INTRODUCTION

Examination of the knee with suspected capsuloligamentous injury must be a complete and meticulous process. Each and every structure must be carefully stressed for possible involvement. Only after this kind of evaluation can a course of treatment be properly planned and implemented.

The clinical examination process consists of a subjective and an objective portion. Subjective evaluation, beginning with the patient history, reviews the pathomechanics of injury (onset, nature, location, and behavior of symptoms), past injuries, treatment, and future patient demands.

Objective testing assesses the patient's range of motion, neuromuscular function, patellofemoral joint, and the stabilizing ligaments and capsule.

SUBJECTIVE EVALUATION

Subjective examination begins with the patient's history, noting the onset of the initial symptoms. The examiner must ascertain whether the injury was caused by an acute episode or whether it actually began with a previous injury. Often patients fail to report the exact details of the initial injury unless the examiner specifically questions them about it.

Any additional medical problems should also be noted at this time. Moreover, future functional demands of the patient's sport(s) and/or work need to be determined to set accurate and realistic goals for rehabilitation. Effective rehabilitation is easier to achieve when the patient's specific sport and position are taken into consideration. For example, a weekend golfer would be approached differently from a professional football player, whereas a quarterback's treatment would vary from that of a lineman.

The therapist should then try to recreate the pathomechanics of the injury by determining what position the knee was in when the injury occurred. Was a blow delivered to the lower extremity? If so, what was the direction and magnitude of the force(s)? These questions can lead the therapist to the traumatized structures, which frequently include menisci, articular cartilage, and patellofemoral as well as tibiofemoral restraints. A pop or snap at the time of injury can be distinctly perceived and related to the therapist during the history. Patellar subluxations and (more rarely) dislocations can accompany an anterior cruciate ligament (ACL) tear.

The location of the symptoms should always be discussed with the patient. Pain is not always a reliable indicator of the specific source of dysfunction. Instabilities are often painless but cause other problems, such as giving out, locking, or recurrent effusion. When pain or other complaints are present, note their behavior. What reproduces or aggravates these symptoms? What injuries have occurred in the past? What was the patient told regarding the problem? What was the treatment course and outcome?

Chronic cases of ACL insufficiency have recurrent episodes of giving out, meniscal tears, and articular cartilage destruction. Past surgeries should give the clinician some insight into these specific patient problems and provide direction for management.

If patients are referred to physical therapy postoperatively, it is imperative to discuss the operative findings with the surgeon, including the examination under anesthesia (EUA). Medial and lateral complex,

ACL and posterior cruciate ligament (PCL), and patellar restraints are all more accurately diagnosed with the patient asleep. Without anesthesia, guarding can mask a positive tibiofemoral subluxation test. Arthroscopic examination can assess injuries to the condylar surfaces of the femur and tibia as well as the undersurface of the patella. Meniscal tears can be diagnosed and treated by either excision or repair. Without the surgical details, it is impossible to plan a safe, effective treatment program.

After completing the subjective evaluation, the examiner should have a clear picture of how the knee was injured, the location and behavior of symptoms, past treatment, any medical problems, and the patients' sport and position, as well as the results of arthroscopy and EUA (if applicable).

PHYSICAL EXAMINATION

Effusion

Physical examination can begin in a number of ways. Effusion is the first sign of knee injury and can be evaluated with the knee in full extension or the position of most comfort. Bloody fluid in the joint capsule or hemarthrosis from acute injury can indicate a tear of the cruciate ligaments, patellar dislocation, or osteochondral lesions. Synovitis, meniscal tearing, and articular cartilage degeneration may also lead to effusion.

It is important to establish the presence of an effusion because of its diagnostic significance. Effusion will set up reflex neuromuscular inhibition mechanisms of the quadriceps, also compromising the dynamic component to knee stability. Range of motion can be limited as the result of effusion, and gait patterns will in turn be altered. Limited patellofemoral joint mobility and maltracking can also be created.

The patellofemoral joint can be assessed while maintaining the knee in full extension position. Medial and lateral stabilities are evaluated by passive mobility tests (Fig. 3-1). Lateral patellar subluxation can accompany valgus and external rotation mechanisms of injury with tearing of the medial retinaculum as well as the medial collateral ligament (MCL).

Palpation of the peripatellar structures includes the patellar tendon, medial and lateral fat pads, patellar facets, quadriceps tendon, medial and lateral retinac-

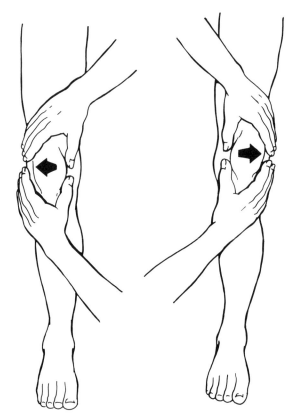

Fig. 3-1. Lateral subluxation with patellar stability testing.

ulum, synovial plica, and vastus medialis oblique insertion. Patellar grinding and other tests to elicit crepitus can be performed, and Q-angle measurements can be taken. Evaluation of the patella with dynamic movement can be made, with range of motion and/or neuromuscular testing later. However, a simple quadriceps isometric test with the knee in extension can demonstrate quadriceps atrophy and patellar tracking problems in full extension.

Range of Motion

Normal range of motion values for the knee vary widely; therefore, a side-to-side comparison should be made. Range of motion can be classified as limited or full, and the degree of limitation is noted by goniometric measurements.

End-feel can give important qualitative information. Simple differentiation is made between painful and painless end-feels, with overstress at the ends of flexion and extension. Abnormalities come from a number of sources and include pain with joint surface contact, meniscal tears, misplaced ligament grafts, scarring of capsular structures, patellofemoral contracture, and other causes.

Another significant distinction is made between elastic and inelastic end-feels. As soft tissue healing proceeds, elasticity will change and motion will be easier to gain. A painful or symptomatic arc with both active and passive motion testing can indicate lesions that represent tendinous, meniscal, or capsular impingement and mechanical instabilities or patellar maltracking. Good, smooth functional range of motion without symptoms is essential to good knee function.

STABILITY EXAMINATION

Reproduction of knee instabilities through a variety of tests follows. Each test stresses a specific aspect of the capsuloligamentous system and helps in diagnosing ligament tears.

The first of these tests is the Lachman examination. With the knee comfortably supported at 20 to 35 degrees of flexion, the examiner simply draws the tibia anteriorly in relation to the femur (Fig. 3-2). Positive findings indicate a tear of the ACL. As important as the

magnitude of the translation present is the end-feel, which is different when compared bilaterally. Torg et al.[1], describe a soft, mushy end point when the ACL has been torn.

From the same position of 20 to 35 degrees of knee flexion, the femur can be stabilized and the tibia externally rotated while assessing passive limits (Fig. 3-3). Increased external rotation on the affected side implicates posterolateral capsule injury. This test is usually painless and is vital in detecting acute posterolateral injury. It can also be performed at 75 or 90 degrees of flexion.[2-4]

Valgus and varus stress tests open the medial and lateral joint lines, respectively (Fig. 3-4). Both tests are done in slight flexion (20 to 30 degrees of flexion). Examiner force is placed on the opposite side of the compartment to be opened. Valgus stress primarily tests the MCL, whereas varus stress tests the lateral collateral ligament. Relative contributions of the secondary restraints depend on the knee position during examination. The posterior aspects of both the medial and lateral capsules increase with testing in relative extension.[5]

Testing the PCL can begin with a simple posterior tibial sag test. The knee is positioned in approximately 75 to 90 degrees of flexion, with the patient in a supine position. If the PCL is torn, the effect of gravity will sag the tibia back into its posteriorly subluxed position.

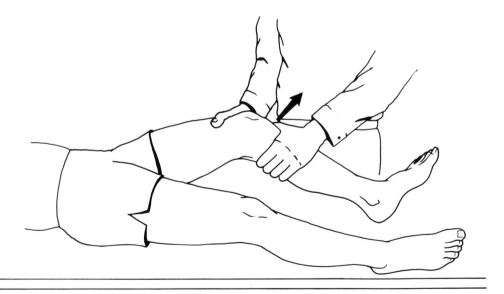

Fig. 3-2. Lachman test for ACL injury.

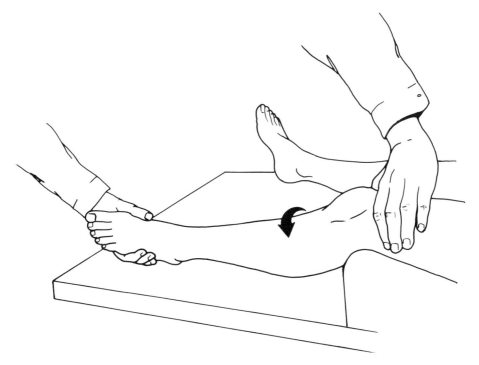

Fig. 3-3. External rotation test for posterolateral instability.

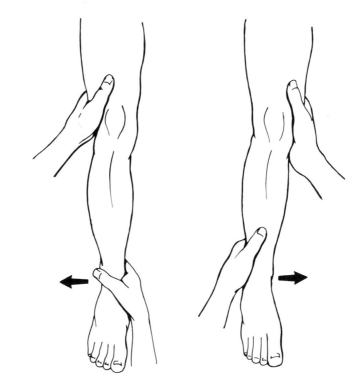

Fig. 3-4. Valgus and varus stress tests for medial complex instability.

From this position, the examiner can secure the patient's foot with the tibia neutral on the surface of the table and provide an anterioposterior translatory force. These anterior and posterior drawer tests assess the ACL and PCL, respectively (Figs. 3-5 and 3-6). Many ACL tears are missed by anterior drawer testing. The posterior horns of the meniscus and hamstring guarding can block the anterior tibial translation in an anterior drawer test, even though the ACL is torn. This problem is negated when using the Lachman test.

Hughston and Norwood[6] the posterolateral drawer, in which the knee is flexed 75 to 90 degrees and the tibia is externally rotated. The examiner then displaces the lateral tibia posteriorly (Fig. 3-7).[6] Subluxation is present with posterolateral capsule injuries. Several other tests have been developed to diagnose posterolateral instability, including the extension/recurvatum,[6] the reverse pivot shift,[7] and the active posterolateral drawer tests.[8]

In the extension/recurvatum test, the patient lies in a relaxed supine position (Fig. 3-8). The examiner lifts both heels off the floor by holding the great toes. Upon lifting of the extremity, the tibia externally rotates and appears to hyperextend relative to the femur. Positive findings reproduce components of increased motion, indicating posterolateral capsule laxity.

In the active posterolateral drawer test, the patient's knee is positioned at a comfortable point in the range of motion, with tibial external rotation similar to that of the passive rotation test, but with the patient sitting (Fig. 3-9). Isolated lateral hamstring contraction in this position will further sublux the lateral tibia posteriorly. Subluxation is elicted by this test in posterolateral instabilities.[8]

Anterolateral instabilities occur when the ACL has been disrupted and laxity of the lateral complex develops.[5] Sudden subluxation can occur to the lateral tibial condyle (relative to the lateral femoral condyle) from approximately 30 degrees of flexion to full extension. Reproduction of this can be attempted through a variety of clinical tests.

Galway and MacIntosh[9] described the pivot shift test (Fig. 3-10). The examiner takes the knee from full extension to flexion while applying valgus and internal rotation stresses. At 30 degrees the tibia reduces from a subluxed position to a normal orientation with the distal femur.

The jerk test described by Hughston and Norwood[10] involves taking the knee from flexion to extension. Valgus and internal rotation stresses are again applied, and at approximately 30 degrees the lateral tibia is subluxed anteriorly throughout the remainder of ex-

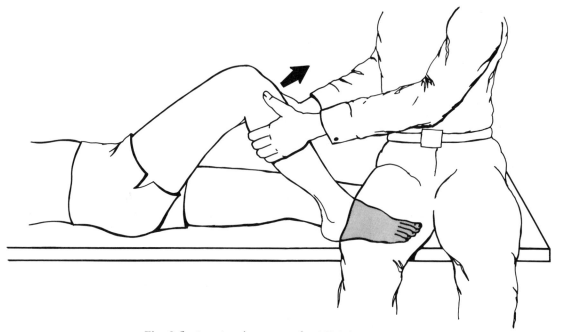

Fig. 3-5. Anterior drawer test for ACL injury.

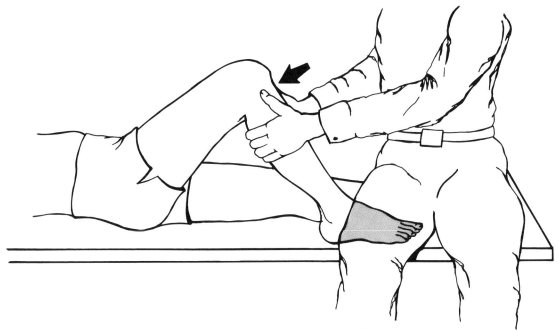

Fig. 3-6. Posterior tibial sag and drawer test for PCL injury.

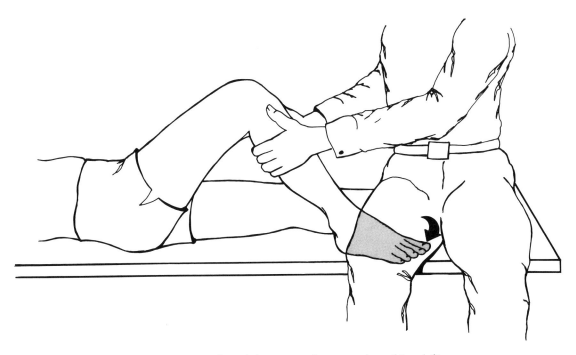

Fig. 3-7. Posterolateral drawer test for posterolateral instability.

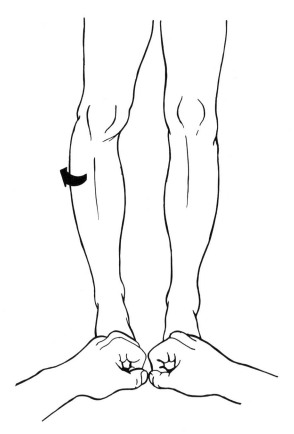

Fig. 3-8. Extension/recurvatum test for posterolateral instability.

tension. Bach et al.[11] and Paulos et al.[12] discuss positive pivot shift test findings with tibial external rotation as well.

Slocum et al.[13] described a gentle anterolateral instability test with the patient sidelying. The examiner flexes and extends the knee passively, while manually attempting to sublux the lateral tibia anteriorly over the final 30 degrees of extension (relative to the lateral femur).

Noyes et al.[14] used the flexion-rotation-drawer test to reproduce the same instability (Fig. 3-11).[14] While flexing the knee from full extension, the examiner provides anterior drawer and internal rotation forces that cause reduction of the anterolateral subluxation from approximately 30 degrees into further flexion. Reproduction of the test creates femoral subluxation on the tibia, while the other tests subluxate the tibia relative to the femur.

Posterolateral instabilities can also elicit sudden shifts in lateral compartmental mechanics. Jakob et al. described the reverse pivot shift, in which the lateral tibia subluxes posteriorly (relative to the lateral femur) from approximately 30 degrees flexion into further flexion (Fig. 3-12). Reduction occurs between 30 degrees of flexion and full extension. Differentation between a positive pivot shift versus a positive reverse pivot shift takes a great deal of examiner experience but is crucial for patient diagnosis and management.

The knee stability examination, a principal com-

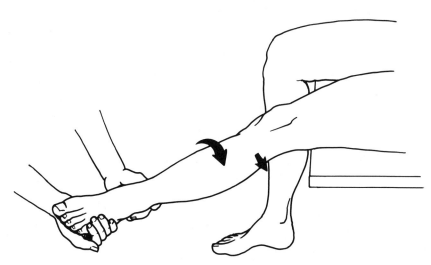

Fig. 3-9. Active posterolateral test for posterolateral instability.

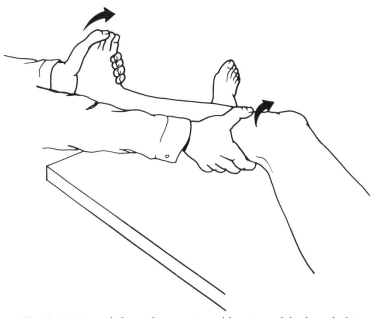

Fig. 3-10. Pivot shift test for anterior subluxation of the lateral tibia.

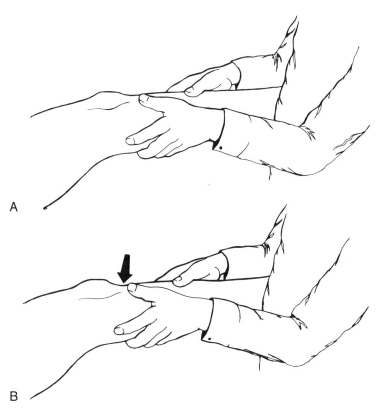

Fig. 3-11. Flexion-rotation-drawer test. **(A)** Lateral subluxation of the tibia relative to the femur. **(B)** Reduction of subluxation in flexion.

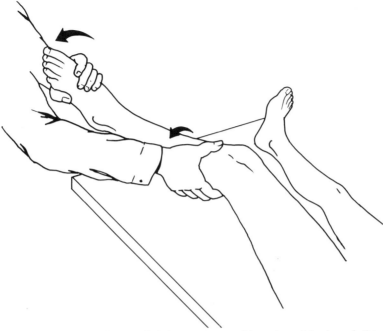

Fig. 3-12. Reversed pivot shift for posterior subluxation of the lateral tibia.

ponent of diagnosis, needs to be well understood in ligament trauma. Conservative and operative treatment are based on the specific structures affected and the degree of injury.

Hughston et al.[15] graded instabilities according to the amount of displacement present (relative to the unaffected side). In grade I injuries, 0 to 5 mm of increased laxity are present. Grade II represents 5 to 10 mm of laxity (greater than the unaffected side). Ten to 15 mm constitutes a grade III or severe instability, while grade IV represents laxity above 15 mm.

INSTRUMENTED STABILITY EXAMINATION

Quantification of the knee stability tests by instrumented methods has provided a certain degree of objectivity to testing procedures. Knee stability can be monitored by these techniques. A great deal of research is necessary, however, to understand more clearly the various devices and the data they generate.

MENISCUS

Meniscus tests are generally difficult to perform, and many tears are diagnosed by history or other methods. Classically, the McMurrays and Apley tests are commonly used to diagnose injuries to the meniscus. Joint line palpation, especially at the meniscus/capsular interfaces, is effective in implicating a tear.

NEUROMUSCULAR EXAMINATION

Neuromuscular function across the joint and throughout the affected extremity is of great importance. Traditional manual muscle testing procedures have been effectively utilized for many years. The introduction of isotonic and isokinetic mechanized devices has allowed for more objectivity with testing. This equipment still does not allow for functional extremity testing (e.g., testing of the hip with the knee and lower leg muscles similar to gait and other normal movement patterns). Conceptually, integrating muscle function with joint mechanics is a crucial concept for the abnormal knee.

Neuromuscular reflex inhibition mechanisms can be present if the patient has a simple synovitis or effusion. In these situations, strengthening exercises may create greater synovial reaction and, in turn, increased reflex inhibition and weakness. Moreover, it must be recognized that the quadriceps control stability and tracking of the patella, as well as translating the tibia anteriorly from 75 degrees to full extension and posteriorly from 75 to 90 degrees with isolated leg extension testing.[16] Changes in neuromuscular function can be directly related to mechanical abnormalities. Inability of these dynamic restraints to effectively control subluxations can also be judged by examination.

Manual techniques give the examiner direct feedback with testing. Joint movements and specific muscles can be isolated or tested with other synergistic lower extremity components. An extensive presentation of procedures is beyond the scope of this chapter. Quadriceps and hamstring function, however, are of prime concern to knee clinicians and will be discussed.

Quadriceps testing can begin with the patient supine or sitting and knee flexed to 90 degrees or greater. Maintaining the tibia in neutral, the patient is resisted in a linear knee extension pattern with concentric and eccentric loading, progressing from gentle submaximal to maximal resistance as testing proceeds. The medial and lateral patellar borders are palpated for subluxation, crepitus, or isolated weakness secondary to inhibitory mechanisms. In addition, in cases of anterior or posterior instabilities, the proximal tibia can be palpated for subluxation or control of subluxation.

The next step is to hold the tibia in internal or external rotation, with leg extension movements to alter forces across both the patellofemoral joint and capsuloligamentous system. External rotation can test vastus medialis restraint of lateral patellar mobility, while internal rotation tests the lateral quadriceps.[17] External and internal rotation with both concentric and eccentric loading dramatically changes forces across the ACL.[18]

ACL forces with quadriceps activation are inherently high over the final 30 degrees of extension but are relatively decreased with external tibial rotation.[19] Internal rotation significantly increases ACL strain over the same range of motion. Eccentric, concentric, and isometric loading all effect the ACL differently.[20]

After testing the knee in an isolated leg extension fashion, the examiner can move to more complex motor functions. For this, I favor the systems of Voss et al.[21] and Johnson and Saliba[22] with modifications (as necessary) to decrease knee forces induced through rotational movements. The possibilities with these procedures are extensive, and a complete review is inappropriate. Combining various components of lower extremity patterns with the quadriceps in spiral-diagonal fashion correlates well with functional movements and provides direction for treatment.

Hamstring activation presents similar important biomechanical aspects. Over the full range of knee motion, hamstring contraction decreases ACL stress and translates the tibia posteriorly.[18] External rotation is created by the biceps femoris, while the semimembranosus and pes anserinus are internal rotators as well as knee flexors. These concepts can be used to reduce excessive anterior translation of both the medial and lateral compartmental instabilities.

For knee flexion testing, position the patient prone, sitting or supine. Evaluate through the full range of motion with isometric, concentric, and eccentric loading. Tibial positioning should be neutral, internal, and externally rotated as indicated. More advanced techniques elicit spiraling from internal to external tibial rotation (and vice versa with knee flexion-extension) to recreate three-dimensional biomechanics.

As with the quadriceps, hamstring testing in diagonal and spiral patterns can be evaluated. Remember that most symptomatic knee instabilities occur at specific positions and with components of flexion-extension and rotation. Look for these neuromuscular insufficiencies in the patterns of knee instabilities previously identified during the examination process.

Testing the entire lower kinetic chain for strength, endurance, stabilization, etc., is vital and must be evaluated. Often a patient's functional activities demand a much higher level of hip and pelvic strength and stabilization than the patient has after injury. Dancers, for example, need tremendous pelvic and lower leg strength, stability, and endurance to function normally.

Evaluation of the neuromuscular system should be concerned with recruitment, including smooth, coordinated efforts. Ability to overcome resistance is important; however, stabilization of specific positions of instability and endurance is equally critical. Beck and Wildermuth[23] have discussed the importance of lower extremity flexibility, proprioception, and other neuromuscular parameters. Testing methods must be introspective and adaptable to be more inclusive and reflective of normal human locomotion.

PALPATION

Palpation of each structure around both the patellofemoral and tibiofemoral articulations is necessary. The patellofemoral structures have already been presented.

Starting anteriorly at the tibiofemoral joint, palpation can begin over the medial and lateral femorotibial condyles and joint lines. The pes anserinus tendon and bursa are palpable on the anteromedial tibia. Medially and laterally the collateral ligaments can be examined. They can be assessed along with the corresponding stability tests (i.e., valgus and varus).

Posteriorly, tenderness can be present at the semimembranosus, popliteus, and biceps femoris bony attachments. The sciatic nerve and femoral artery can be probed centrally over the posterior aspect.

It is important to palpate all the structures mentioned, regardless of patient complaints. Very often patients are unaware of painful structures until the examiner begins this phase of the examination.

FUNCTIONAL TESTS

A significant aspect of the evaluation process is assessing the patient's knee for symptoms by taking the patient through various activities. Depending on the patient's activities, these may vary in importance. Some of the possibilities include squatting, kneeling, sitting, jumping, running, twisting, cutting, and pivoting. Symptoms elicited through these and other tests should be evaluated. Neuromuscular insufficiencies including proprioception can be identified. Decisions can be made regarding appropriate further treatment techniques and the safe progression back to activities from this point.

ASSESSMENT AND PLAN

Once the examination has been completed, the findings can then be summarized. The assessment should take into consideration all aspects and structures of the patient's case. For example, focusing on a chronic ACL insufficiency can lead the examiner away from a particularly symptomatic patellofemoral joint and deficient quadriceps mechanism.

After a detailed clinical assessment is made, the short- and long-term goals of treatment can be established. To reach these goals, treatment approaches should be developed and re-assessed. The frequency and duration of treatment will determine the amount of time required to reach these goals and can be used to motivate the patient. A prognosis can be made based on the rehabilitation program's probability of solving the patient's clinical problems on a long-term basis. The goals, treatment approaches, frequency and duration of treatment, and prognosis are all important aspects of patient documentation.

SUMMARY

Evaluation of the knee is the most important aspect of treatment. The patient's history, including chief complaint, mechanism of injury, behavior of symptoms, and other factors, provides the foundation for diagnosis. This, combined with various aspects of the physical examination, identifies abnormalities in joint function that can be addressed through the treatment process.

REFERENCES

1. Torg JS, Conrad W, Kalen V: Clinical diagnosis of anterior cruciate ligament instability in the athlete. Am J Sports Med 4:84, 1976
2. Gollehon DL, Torzilli PA, Warren RF: The role of the posterolateral and cruciate ligaments in the stability of the human knee. J Bone Joint Surg 69:233, 1987
3. Grood ES, Stowers SF, Noyes FR: Limits of movement in the human knee. J Bone Joint Surg 70:88, 1988
4. Noyes FR: Diagnosis and classification of knee ligament injuries. Paper presented at 1989 Advances on the Knee and Shoulder, Cincinnati, OH, 1989

5. Butler DL, Noyes FR, Grood ES et al: Ligamentous restraints in the human knee: anterior-posterior stability. Orthop Trans 2:161, 1978

6. Hughston JC, Norwood LA: The posterolateral drawer test and external rotation recurvatum test for posterolateral rotatory instability of the knee. Clin Orthop 147:82, 1980

7. Jakob RP, Hassler H, Staeubli H: Observations on rotatory instability of the lateral compartment of the knee. Acta Orthop Scand (suppl. 191) 152:1, 1981

8. Canner GC, Engle RP: The diagnosis of posterolateral laxity in the acutely injured knee. (Unpublished study.)

9. Galway HR, MacIntosh D: The lateral pivot shift: a symptom and sign of anterior cruciate ligament insufficiency. Clin Orthop 147:45, 1980

10. Hughston JC, Norwood LA: Classification of knee ligament instabilities: Part II. The lateral compartment. J Bone Joint Surg 58A:173, 1980

11. Bach BR, Warren RF, Wickiewicz TL: The pivot shift phenomenon: results and descriptions of a modified clinical test for anterior cruciate ligament insufficiency. Am J Sports Med 16:571, 1988

12. Paulos LE, Rosenberg TD, Parker RD: The medial ligaments: pathomechanics and surgical repair with emphasis on the external-rotation pivot-shift test. Tech Orthop 2(2):37, 1987

13. Slocum DB, James SL, Larson RL et al: Clinical test for anterolateral rotatory instability of the knee. Clin Orthop 118:63, 1976

14. Noyes FR, Grood ES, Butler DL et al: Clinical laxity tests and functional stability of the knee: biomechanical concepts. Clin Orthop 146:84, 1980

15. Hughston JC, Andrews JR, Cross MJ, Noschi A: Classification of knee ligament instabilities: Part I. The medial compartment and cruciate ligaments. J Bone Joint Surg 58A:159, 1976

16. Daniels DO, Lawler J, Malcom L: The quadriceps-anterior cruciate interaction. Orthop Trans 6:199, 1982

17. Müller W: The Knee: Form, Function and Ligament Reconstruction. p. 2. Springer-Verlag, New York, 1983

18. Arms SW, Pope MH, Johnson RJ et al: The biomechanics of anterior cruciate ligament rehabilitation and reconstruction. Am J Sports Med 12:8, 1984

19. Paulos L, Noyes FR, Grood DL: Knee rehabilitation after anterior cruciate ligament reconstruction repair. Am J Sports Med 9:140, 1981

20. Renstrom P, Arms Stanwyck TS, Johnson RJ, Pope MH: Strain within the anterior cruciate ligament during hamstring and quadriceps activity. Am J Sports Med 14:83, 1986

21. Voss DE, Ionta MK, Myers BJ: Proprioceptive neuromuscular facilitation. p. 2. Harper & Row, New York, 1986

22. Johnson G, Saliba V: Proprioceptive Neuromuscular Facilitation. Course Notes. Sept. 1987. Baltimore, MD.

23. Beck JL, Wildermuth BP: The female athlete's knee. Clin Sports Med 4:345, 1985

4

Instrumented Examination of the Knee

RUSSELL M. PAINE

INTRODUCTION

The science of medicine requires that the clinician have as much objective information as possible to render decisions regarding treatment of patients to reach the ultimate goal—improvement of care to the patient. The pursuit of this goal has led to the development of devices that attempt to quantify in millimeters the various diagnostic knee examination tests. These results have been previously quantified by a grading system. This grading system has an element of subjective examiner opinion.

Although there have been various claims by manufacturers of these devices to be able to quantify these various diagnostic tests in the knee, reproducible and reliable results have not always been obtainable. To date, the predominant test using instrumented testing that has been reported in the literature is the Lachman test performed between 25 and 30 degrees of knee flexion. Claims by manufacturers of more intricate testing devices able to measure tests other than the Lachman test have yet to be proved reliable. It may well be that some of these devices are ahead of our ability to interpret the data that is recorded during testing. Although we may not be able to interpret the recorded information, the data recorded must be reproducible, reliable, and correlate with suspected pathology.

The purpose of this chapter is to provide an overview of instrumented testing and provide specific clinical techniques that may be useful in obtaining reproducible and accurate results during an instrumented testing examination. The less inherent margin for error a device has, the greater its reliability will be. As is true with any instrument that has been proved to be reliable, its reliability is totally dependent on the expertise of the examiner.

HISTORY

Instrumented testing of the knee began in 1971 when Kennedy and Fowler[1] measured knee laxity with a clinical stress machine and serial radiographs. Kennedy's testing device required the patient to sit in a machine while anterior displacement loads were applied at 90 degrees of flexion. The recorded radiographs were compared, and side-to-side displacements were measured. Torzilli et al.[2] and Jacobsen[3] observed that while Kennedy did measure anterior and varus-valgus laxity, he did not take into consideration tibial rotation. They modified the technique to correct for rotation. The next major study was in 1978 when Markolf et al.[4] used a modified dental chair with potentiometers that measured anteroposterior (AP) translation and constantly measured the amount of applied tibial force. However, it was not until 1983 that Daniel et al.[5] introduced a commercially available device. Since 1983 several devices have been introduced into the marketplace. Oliver and Raab[6] introduced the Genucom device, which was designed to measure all 6 degrees of freedom of the knee. The CA-4000 (formerly KSS) is another device similar to the Genucom. This device was designed to measure 4 degrees of freedom of the knee and was introduced in 1986.[7] The KLT (knee laxity tester) is a device similar to the KT-1000 and was introduced in 1985.[8]

Reliability and reproducibility are major concerns when using any instrumented testing device. There has been a lack of documentation regarding the accuracy of many of the devices, which has led to confusion when interpreting the results obtained during testing with certain devices. A literature review is provided here for each of the devices in hopes of validating results obtained when testing. A detailed description of each device and testing techniques is also provided (Appendix 4-1).

BIOMECHANICS OF THE KNEE

For successful utilization of knee-testing devices, the individual performing the testing must have a working knowledge of the arthrokinematics of the knee. With the aid of bioengineers, the language of knee motion has become more specific. Using engineering terms, motion of the knee can be described as three rotations and three translations about three different axes. The interaction of these movements make up the 6 degrees of freedom in the knee. Combination of these rotations and translations provide coupled motions that are often described as "rolling and gliding" of the femur on the tibia.

The knee is a modified hinge joint, with flexion and extension rotation being its primary motion. Flexion and extension occur about the y axis (mediolateral). The translations that occur along the y axis are mediolateral. Rotations about the x axis (AP) are abduction-adduction. Translations about the x axis are AP. Rotations along the z axis (proximodistal) are internal-external and translations are penetration-distraction. The diagram in Figure 4-1 describes these rotations and translations.

An example of coupled motion that occurs during knee arthrometer testing may be described when performing an anterior drawer test. As the tibia is pulled

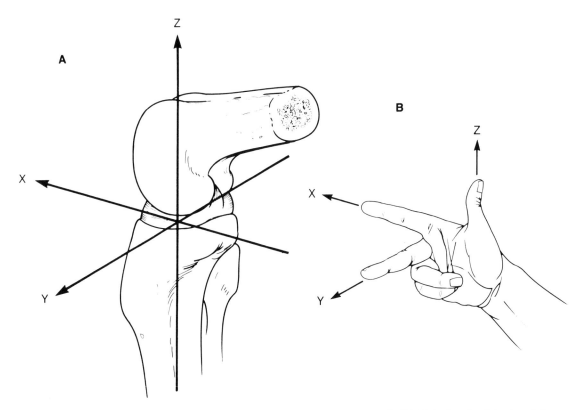

Fig. 4-1. **(A)** The knee with a conventional three-axis system superimposed. **(B)** This sketch of the hand shows a simple way to use the right-hand rule. The index finger is pointed along the x axis, the long finger along the y axis, and the thumb along the z axis. (From Jackson and Drez,[27] with permission.)

anterior, it translates anteriorly and rotates internally. It is the belief of some that constraining this normally occurring motion during an examination would lead to erroneous readings.[9–11] When performing an anterior drawer test, constraining internal rotation of the tibia on the femur may decrease anterior readings. To impose or increase internal rotation of the tibia on the femur would increase anterior translation. This is why it is of utmost importance to apply loads in line with the particular axis that is being tested (Fig. 4-2).

Testing position has definite effects on laxity measurements. Anterior tibial displacement has been reported to be less at 90 degrees of flexion than at 30 degrees. When the anterior cruciate ligament (ACL) has been injured, there is a greater increase in pathologic laxity at 30 degrees than at 90 degrees.[4,12,13] Thus, to maximally demonstrate pathologic laxity for ACL tears, the test position is between 25 and 30 degrees.

Active testing is a new area of interest. Because of the orientation of the patellar tendon's pull on the tibia, there will be an anterior displacement of the tibia with quadriceps contraction when the knee is positioned between 25 and 30 degrees[14] (Fig. 4-3). This active anterior translation is increased in the ACL-deficient knee. As the knee is flexed to approximately 70 degrees, there is a point in the normal knee where the resultant vector of the patellar tendon causes nei-

ther anterior nor posterior displacement of the tibia. Active quadriceps contraction in this position results in no translation of the tibia. Daniel et al.[15] have defined this position as the neutral quadriceps active position. As knee flexion approaches 90 degrees, the vector orientation changes so that there is actually a posterior resultant force acting on the tibia during active quadriceps contraction. In the normal knee this causes a slight posterior displacement of the tibia on the femur (Fig. 4-3). In the posterior cruciate ligament (PCL)-deficient knee, the tibia will be in a posterior sag position at 90 degrees. In the PCL-deficient knee, active quadriceps contraction with the knee positioned at 90 degrees will cause an anterior displacement of the tibia[15] (Fig. 4-4). According to Daniel et al.,[15] an arthrometer reading of anterior displacement at 90 degrees is a positive sign for PCL tears.

Definitions of Biomechanical Terminology

Ultimate tensile strength (breaking point) is the point at which all components of a material fail. For the ACL, the ultimate tensile strength is approximately 1,700 newtons (N).[16]

Plastic deformation occurs when an object does not return to its original resting state when a load is re-

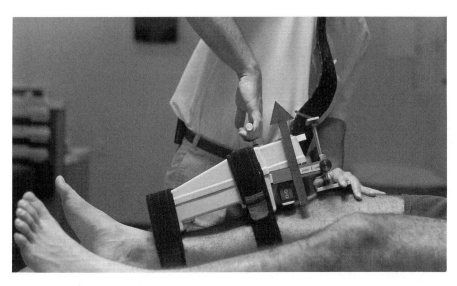

Fig. 4-2. Examiner must apply load perpendicular to axis of rotation (see arrow). Care must also be given not to impose rotation during testing procedure.

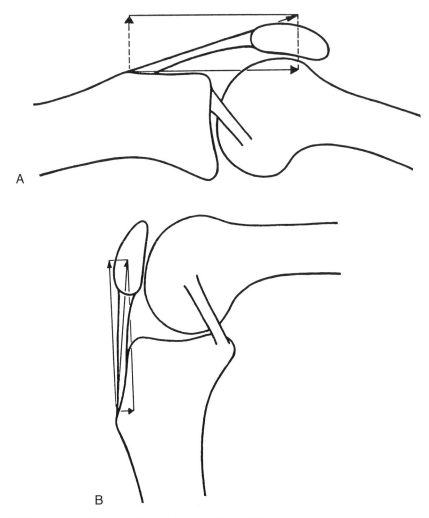

Fig. 4-3. (A) With the normal knee positioned between 25 and 30 degrees, active quadriceps contraction results in anterior tibial translation. This is due to the anterior orientation of the patellar tendon. **(B)** With the normal knee positioned at 90 degrees, the patellar tendon orientation becomes posterior, resulting in posterior translation. (From Daniel,[28] with permission.)

moved. Thus, there has been failure of some of the components of the material.

Elastic deformation is defined as a return to original length of a material after removal of a load.

Elastic hysteresis is the lack of coincidence of curves on a stress-strain curve. The area bounded by the two curves (hysteresis loop) is equal to the energy dissipated within the elastic material. This loop is com-

monly observed when testing with instrumented devices that allow display of a force versus displacement graph (Fig. 4-5).

Stiffness is the amount of force required to deform a ligament a given distance (ratio of the change in force divided by the change in length). The normal stiffness for the ACL is 175 N/mm.[16]

Compliance is the number of millimeters a ligament

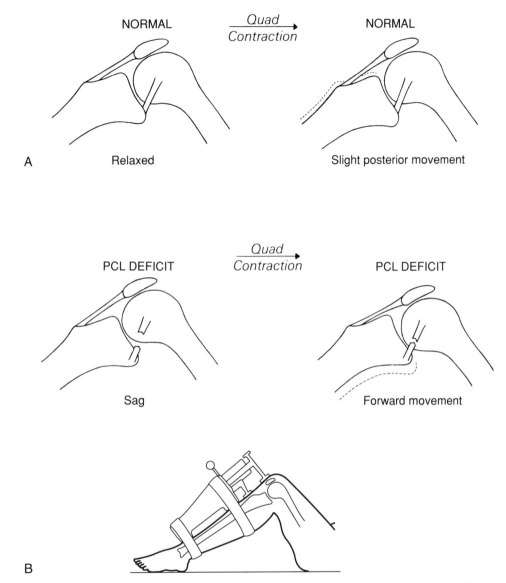

Fig. 4-4. (A) In the normal knee, active quadriceps contraction with the knee positioned at 90 degrees results in 0 to 2 mm of posterior translation. **(B)** In the PCL-deficient knee, a posterior tibial sag is present. Active quadriceps contraction brings the tibia anterior. An instrumented testing device may be used to detect the anterior translation. (From Daniel,[28] with permission.)

deforms when a predetermined force is applied (ratio of the change in length divided by the change in force). For the normal ACL, this is 0.006 mm/N.[16] The compliance figure can be calculated with any of the various devices and is the amount of increase in millimeters of displacement between two displacement loads (e.g., change in length between 15- and 20-lb forces). The compliance figure may well be the most important data retrieved because it tests the actual elasticity of the ligament or graft.

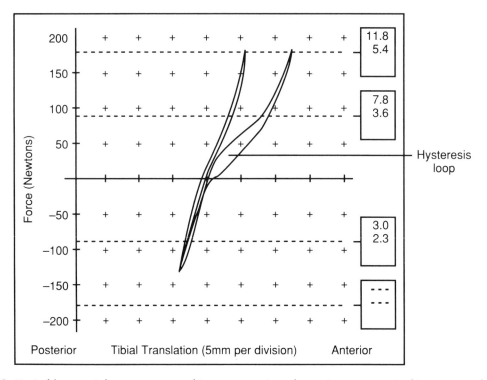

Fig. 4-5. Typical hysteresis loop seen on graphic representation when using computerized instrumented testing devices. Curve shown is taken from force versus displacement graph of CA-4000 device (manufactured by Orthopedic Systems, Inc., Hayward, CA).

CLINICAL USES OF INSTRUMENTED TESTING

As instrumented testing gains greater acceptance through studies documenting reproducibility and reliability, more frequent clinical usage has been observed. Initial skepticism from some clinicians has been overcome as they see the beneficial effects of clinical use of the instrumented testing devices.

One of the primary uses of instrumented testing is that of verification of suspected ACL tears. The data retrieved are not meant to replace the hands of the physician but to act as a finely tuned gauge to document more accurately the severity of suspected pathologic laxity. Decisions regarding treatment options may hinge on accurate assessment by instrumented testing.

It is the general agreement that greater than 3 mm of side-to-side difference is indicative of an ACL tear.[10,17] Daniel (personal communication) has re-

ported on anterior laxity measurements as they relate to "copers" and "noncopers." These data revealed that 89 percent of chronic ACL patients with 8 to 10 mm of side-to-side difference (noncopers) were unable to resume their preinjury activities. The ability to relate numeric values to patient function is an exciting and practical benefit of instrumented testing.

Markolf et al.[4] and Wroble et al.[18] prefer the use of total (anterior plus posterior measurements) AP translation rather than separate anterior and posterior measurements. Wroble et al.[18] believe that reporting total AP translation eliminates the need to identify the neutral position of the knee, thus eliminating this as a possible source of error. Other investigators believe that by adding the posterior and anterior measurements together one may be introducing a source of error rather than reducing a source of error. Thus, as other investigators have reported,[5,8,10,19,20] I prefer to use separate anterior and posterior measurements.

Mangine (personal communication) has suggested

frequent use of instrumented testing during postoperative rehabilitation of the patient with a reconstructed ACL. This program enlists weekly testing to document the compliance and stability of the healing graft.

A more conservative approach may be taken to protect the healing graft if testing reveals a slight increase in side-to-side difference values (greater than 3 mm). This may allow for greater scarring to occur in the posterior capsule to help shield the healing graft.

There is no documentation to support the ability of the graft to tighten after it has undergone plastic deformation. The question remains whether the graft has been strained beyond its yield point and has entered into plastic deformation. Regardless of lack of scientific documentation, it is reasonable to assume a more conservative approach if instrumented testing demonstrates an increase in anterior translation during the postoperative ACL reconstruction rehabilitation period. Conversely, a more aggressive approach may be implemented if the measurements show that the involved knee has lower anterior displacement values than the normal knee.

The CA-4000 testing device offers research applications that are very exciting to knee ligament rehabilitation. This device measures active displacements that occur during various open and closed kinetic chain activities.

TESTING TECHNIQUES TO IMPROVE ACCURACY—KT-1000

The following techniques are specific to the KT-1000 but may also be applied to the other testing devices.

Patient Position

Initial setup of the patient is vital in obtaining accurate and reproducible results. The patient should be supine with the head resting on one pillow. It is helpful to ask patients to rest their hands on their chest. The thigh support should be positioned so that the support rests just above the superior pole of the patella, so as not to reduce measurements by blocking the tibia. The foot rest is then positioned so that support is given just below the lateral malleoli (Fig. 4-6). This position should not constrain rotation and should be equal bilaterally. If excessive external rotation of the tibia on the femur is present, a circumferential thigh strap may be used to decrease rotation. I prefer not to use the thigh strap if possible, so as not to constrain the natural attitude of the knee.

Arthrometer Positioning

Proper position of the arthrometer is of utmost importance for accurate results. The arthrometer is positioned along the crest of the tibia, aligning the V-

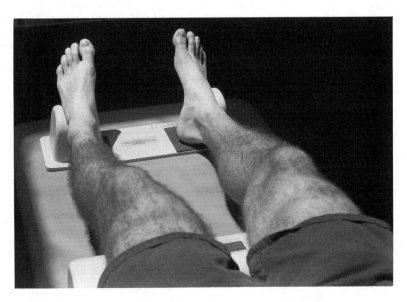

Fig. 4-6. Proper patient positioning showing no constraint to rotation.

shaped undersurface of the arthrometer to the tibial crest. The most proximal portion of the patellar sensor pad is positioned to be even with the inferior pole of the patella. Caution should be used so that the patellar sensor pad is not resting on the patellar tendon. This technique will position the arthrometer properly and is more reproducible and simpler than aligning the instrument by using the joint line arrow located on the side of the arthrometer. The upper strap is tightened firmly. The arthrometer must then be repositioned so it lies in the same plane as the tibial crest. The lower strap is then tightened.

Patient Testing

Most instrumented testing devices enable anterior displacement measurements to be recorded for forces up to 30 lbs. To test for ACL tears, the examiner applies two to three posterior pushes to set the tibia in a starting position. The 20-lb posterior value is then recorded. The tibia is then pulled anteriorly and readings are taken at 15, 20, and 30 lbs of force.

An anterior manual maximum force is then applied to the calf. This anterior force should be applied with the hand positioned just below the head of the fibula (Fig. 4-7). A maximum force is applied by the examiner until there is no further anterior displacement as shown by the device. This test places values that attempt to replicate the Lachman test. I have found the manual maximum test to be the most diagnostic test performed. This test is most useful when testing a large individual who requires more than 30 lbs of force to demonstrate pathologic laxity.

A quadriceps active displacement may also be taken by having the patient lift the heel. I have found the quadriceps active test less accurate for documenting ACL insufficiency.

Markolf[12] and others[9,15,20] have reported that lack of quadriceps relaxation may account for 25 to 50 percent reduction in anterior translation. This is the most common source of lowered anterior translation values. An excellent technique for determining quadriceps relaxation is to palpate the patellar tendon just before testing (Fig. 4-8). If there is stiffness in the ten-

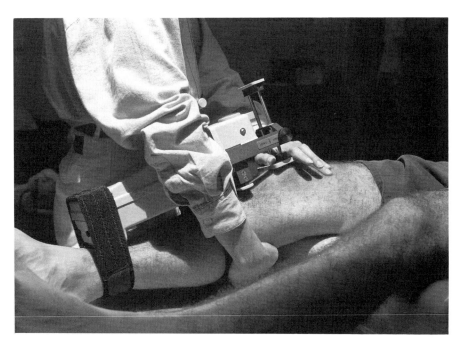

Fig. 4-7. Manual maximum displacement test. Care is taken to load knee below head of fibula. A maximum displacement is applied to the calf until there is no further increase in translation (endpoint is reached). This test is the most diagnostic for ACL tears.

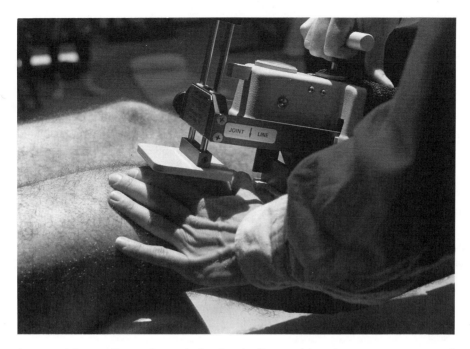

Fig. 4-8. Palpation of the patellar tendon with the thumb allows quick and accurate assessment of quadriceps relaxation. Testing must not proceed if tension is detected in the quadriceps mechanism.

don, the patient should attempt to relax the quadriceps muscle. Techniques for relaxation include oscillating the lower leg, massaging the thigh, and contract-relax proprioceptive neuromuscular facilitation techniques. Testing done with quadriceps tension will result in lowered and inaccurate anterior translation values.

Rotation of the device during testing may cause as much as a 5-mm increase in anterior translation. Care must be taken not to impose rotation during testing. A conscious effort must be made to pull the arthrometer in a plane perpendicular to the shaft of the tibia (Fig. 4-2). Even patellar pressure must also be maintained to obtain accurate results. The examiner should change hand positions when testing right and left knees (right hand pulls on right knee, left hand pulls on left knee).

Visual observation of the displacement needle becomes more accurate by slowing the rate of pull on the force handle. Three reproducible pulls should be made. The latest version of the device, the KT-2000, obviates the need for visual observation of the displacement needle.

In our hands, the manual maximum test is the most

diagnostic of the tests performed. To perform this test properly, it is important not to impose rotation. It is also helpful to apply the anterior load with the hand positioned just below the fibular head.

These techniques may also be applied to the other devices. Patient relaxation must be achieved if accurate results are to be obtained while using any of the devices.

RELIABILITY

As is true with much of the equipment that is introduced into the marketplace today, there is a great need for documentation of the perceived results that manufacturers claim. The following is a review of literature for the various devices.

KT-1000

Daniel et al.[17] have reported that 90 percent of patients with greater than 3 mm of side-to-side difference were shown to have ACL tears. They have also tested cadaveric specimens to verify the reproducibility of the KT-1000.[5] They showed there to be no more than 1 mm difference in measurements between specimens after three repeated tests. Daniel and Stone also tested 10 normal subjects and found that total anterior translation varied by 1 mm or less (personal communication). Involved minus normal differences differed by less than 1 mm. Intertester reliability was addressed in another study by Daniel and Stone in which two examiners tested 34 high school football players (personal communication). All testing was performed on the same day. There was only a 0.9 ± 0.8 mm difference between the two examiners for the right-left difference.

Forster et al.[21] showed that there was substantial inter- and intraexaminer variation in both absolute and side-to-side differences in recorded values when using the KT-1000. The article suggests that two of the four examiners had little experience with testing but were taught according to the manufacturer's instructions. The fact that two examiners were less experienced may have had an effect on data reported. Hanten and Pace[22] reported good correlation between examiners when testing with the KT-1000.

Wroble et al.[18] found no significant difference between trials (within installation) or between installations (within day) for all parameters recorded for the KT-1000. A significant difference was found between days for absolute right and left knee measurements at 89 and 134 N force levels. Most importantly, no significant difference was found between days for the right-to-left differences at both force levels.

Genucom

Reproducibility of the Genucom has been addressed in four known studies. Oliver and Raab[6] tested the Genucom on two cadaver specimens. A series of tests were repeated three times. They reported data of less than 2.2 mm in AP translation at 90 N and 90 degrees of flexion. Highgenboten et al.[23] and Emery et al.[24] also addressed reliability of the Genucom by a test-retest protocol. Neither study quantitated the amount of variability in its tests.

Wroble et al.[25] found no significant differences between tests (AP stress tests at 30 and 90 degrees of flexion and varus-valgus stress tests at 20 degrees of flexion) within a single seating for the group. A significant day-to-day difference was found in individual subjects. Significant differences were also found between the two examiners.

Oliver and Coughlin[19] stated that 95 percent of patients with a demonstrable Lachman test also had a positive Genucom AP test at 30 degrees of flexion. Anderson and Lipscomb[26] found that only 70 percent of clinically detectable acute ACL tears had a positive Genucom 30-degree AP test.

CA-4000

Neuschwander et al.,[7] in comparing the KT-1000 with the CA-4000, reported there to be no significant difference between devices in absolute values for the manual maximum test. There was also no significant difference between devices for the involved and normal values. A significant difference was found between the 20-lb absolute values. These differences were due to dissimilar methods for stabilization of the femur.

Other Devices

Boniface et al.[8] examined 123 normal athletes with no history of knee injury and 30 patients with arthroscopically confirmed ACL injuries using the knee laxity tester. They found that anterior laxity and side-to-side difference correlated with ACL injury; posterior and total AP laxity did not.

Markolf et al.[4] performed a test-retest variability study of two examiners using the UCLA testing device. This study was performed on the normal and ACL-deficient knees of 29 patients. Ninety-three percent of the involved minus normal retest measurements were within 2 mm or less. The mean variation of the involved minus normal values at 20 lbs was 1.2 mm.

Edixhoven et al.[9] tested patients before and after spinal anesthesia. They found no significant differences between anesthetized and unanesthetized states. Drez and Paine (unpublished data) found no significant difference when testing conscious patients versus anesthetized patients. Coaching the patients on relaxation techniques played an important role in results of both these studies.

A need continues to exist for further studies to document the reliability and reproducibility of instrumented testing devices.

FUTURE OF INSTRUMENTED TESTING

As these testing devices gain greater acceptance, and as improvements are made to increase the accuracy of the devices, there will be a greater demand for utilization of objective information obtained from an instrumented knee testing examination. Currently, research efforts that report postoperative results of ACL reconstruction procedures routinely include instrumented knee testing results. As our ability to interpret the various graphs that display rotations and translations improves, there may well be a place for these devices in helping to diagnose rotational instabilities such as posterolateral instability.

SUMMARY

Without question, instrumented testing has been a successful advancement in the care of ligamentous injuries to the knee. Diligent efforts should be used by all clinicians to utilize devices that provide reliable and reproducible results to more objectively quantify measurement of knee laxity.

ACKNOWLEDGMENT

I would like to acknowledge Bradley Chapman, P.T. for his efforts in helping to prepare this chapter.

REFERENCES

1. Kennedy JC, Fowler PJ: Medial and anterior instability of the knee. An anatomical and clinical study using stress machines. J Bone Joint Surg 53A:1257, 1971
2. Torzilli PA, Greenberg RL, Hood RW et al: Measurement of anterior-posterior motion of the knee in injured patients using a biomechanical stress technique. J Bone Joint Surg 66A:1438, 1984
3. Jacobsen K: Stress radiographical measurement of the anteroposterior, medial and lateral stability of the knee joint. Acta Orthop Scand 47:335, 1976
4. Markolf KL, Graff-Radford A, Amstutz HC: In vivo knee stability. A quantitative assessment using an instrumented clinical testing apparatus. J Bone Joint Surg 60A:664, 1978
5. Daniel DM, Malcom LL, Losse G et al: Instrumented measurement of anterior laxity of the knee. J Bone Joint Surg 67A:720, 1985
6. Oliver JH, Raab S: A new device for in vivo knee stability measurement: the Genucom knee analysis system. Company Memorandum #84-1. FAR Orthopaedics, Montreal, 1984
7. Neuschwander D, Drez D, Paine R, Young J: Comparison of anterior laxity measurements in anterior cruciate deficient knees with two instrumented testing devices. Orthopedics 13(3):299, 1990
8. Boniface RJ, Fu FH, Ilkhanipour K: Objective anterior cruciate ligament testing. Orthopedics 9:391, 1986
9. Edixhoven P, Huskes R, de Graaf R et al: Accuracy and reproducibility of instrumented knee-drawer tests. J Orthop Res 5:378, 1987
10. Sherman OH, Markolf KL, Ferkel RD: Measurements of anterior laxity in normal and anterior cruciate absent knees with two instrumented test devices. Clin Orthop 215:156, 1987
11. Sullivan D, Levy IM, Sheskier S et al: Medial restraints to anterior-posterior motion of the knee. J Bone Joint Surg 66A:930, 1984
12. Markolf KL, Kochan A, Amstutz HC: Measurement of knee stiffness and laxity in patients with documented absence of the anterior cruciate ligament. J Bone Joint Surg 66A:242, 1984
13. Nielsen S, Kromann-Andersen C, Rasmussen O, Andersen K: Instability of cadaver knees after transection of capsule and ligaments. Acta Orthop Scand 55:30, 1984
14. Daniel D, Lawler L, Malcom L et al: The quadriceps-ACL interaction. Orthop Trans 6:199, 1982
15. Daniel DM, Stone ML, Barnett P, Sachs R: Use of the quadriceps active test to diagnose posterior cruciate ligament disruption and measure posterior cruciate laxity of the knee. J Bone Joint Surg 70A:386, 1988
16. Noyes FR, Grood ES: The strength of the anterior cruciate ligament in humans and rhesus monkeys. J Bone Joint Surg 58A:1074, 1976
17. Daniel DM, Stone ML, Sachs R, Malcom LL: Instrumented measurement of anterior knee laxity in patients with acute anterior cruciate ligament disruption. Am J Sports Med 13:401, 1985
18. Wroble RR, Van Ginkel LA, Grood ES et al: Repeatability of the KT-1000 arthrometer in a normal population. Am J Sports Med 18:396, 1990
19. Oliver JH, Coughlin LP: Objective knee evaluation using the Genucom knee analysis system. Am J Sports Med 15:571, 1987
20. Shino K, Inoue M, Horibe S et al: Measurement of anterior instability of the knee: a new apparatus for clinical testing. J Bone Joint Surg 69B:608, 1987

21. Forster IW, Warren-Smith CD, Tew M: Is the KT-1000 knee ligament arthrometer reliable? J Bone Joint Surg 71B:843, 1989

22. Hanten WP, Pace MB: Reliability of measuring anterior laxity of the knee joint using a knee ligament arthrometer. Phys Ther 67:357, 1987

23. Highgenboten CL, Jackson A, Meske NB: Measurement of knee laxity using the Genucom knee analysis system. Med Sci Sports Exerc 21:S81, 1989

24. Emery M, Moffroid M, Boerman J et al: Reliability of force/displacement measures in a clinical device designed to measure ligamentous laxity at the knee. J Orthop Sports Phys Ther 10:441, 1989

25. Wroble RR, Grood ES, Noyes FR, Schmitt DJ: Reproducibility of Genucom knee analysis system testing. Am J Sports Med 18:387, 1990

26. Anderson AF, Lipscomb AB: Preoperative instrumented testing of anterior and posterior knee laxity. Am J Sports Med 17:387, 1989

27. Jackson DW, Drez D Jr: The Anterior Cruciate Deficient Knee: New Concepts in Ligament Repair. CV Mosby, St. Louis, 1987

28. Daniel D et al: The Active Drawer Test. Pamphlet presented at the Annual Meeting of the American Academy of Orthopaedic Surgeons, Anaheim, CA, 1983

Appendix 4-1

Knee Testing Devices

KT-1000, KT-2000 (Medmetric Inc., San Diego, CA)

Commercially available since 1983.

Degrees of freedom: 1. Measures anteroposterior laxity.

Forces: 15 (67 N), 20 (89 N), and 30 (134 N) lbs. Detected by audible "beeps"; also able to perform manual maximum test (maximum displacement by examiner's hand).

Estimated side-to-side test time: 5 minutes.

Cost: $3,500.00 (KT-1000); $6,700.00 (KT-2000) (KT-1000 plus x-y plotter).

Advantages:
1. Good reproducibility, extensive research to verify obtained results.
2. Ease of operation.
3. Portable.
4. 5-minute test time.

Disadvantages:
1. Measures only 1 degree of freedom.
2. Unable to effectively perform weight-bearing tests.
3. Not computerized.

GENUCOM KNEE ANALYSIS SYSTEM (Faro Medical, Inc., Montreal, Canada)

Degrees of freedom: 6
  Rotations:
  1. Flexion-extension.
  2. Internal-external.
  3. Mediolateral.
  Translations:
  1. Abduction-adduction.
  2. Compression-distraction.
  3. Anteroposterior.

Forces: 150 N.

Estimated side-to-side test time: 20 minutes.

Cost: Base price of $29,900.00.

Advantages:
1. Proposed measurement of all 6 degrees of freedom.
2. Computerization.
3. Proposed soft tissue compensation.

Disadvantages:
1. Cost.
2. Difficult learning curve.
3. Questionable reliability.
4. Not portable.

CA-4000 (Orthopedic Systems, Inc., Hayward, CA)

Degrees of freedom: 4
 Translations:
 1. Anteroposterior.
 2. Abduction-adduction.
 Rotations:
 1. Internal-external.
 2. Anteroposterior.
Forces:
 1. Calculated 20 (89 N)- and 40 (178 N)-lb forces.
 2. Force applied using force applicator housing strain gauge.
 3. Records up to 200 N.
Estimated side-to-side test time: 15 minutes.
Cost: $13,500.00.
Advantages:
 1. Proposed measurement of 4 degrees of freedom.
 2. Closed kinetic chain measurement.
 3. Greater flexibility with active measurements.
 4. Computerization.
Disadvantages:
 1. Lack of reproducibility and reliability studies.
 2. Slight learning curve.
 3. Semiportable.

KLT (KNEE LAXITY TESTER) (Orthopedic Systems, Inc., Hayward, CA)

Degrees of freedom: 1. Anteroposterior translation.
Forces: 15 lbs (67 N), 20 lbs (89 N).
Estimated test time: 5 minutes.
Cost: $1,500.00.
Advantages:
 1. Ease of operation.
 2. Portable.
 3. Lowered cost.
Disadvantages:
 1. Measures only 1 degree of freedom.
 2. No active measurements possible.
 3. Needs more reproducibility and reliability studies.

5

Meniscus Tears: Diagnosis and Treatment

THOMAS D. MEADE

INTRODUCTION

Although the mammalian meniscus has been present for about 320 million years,[1] it has only been over the past 50 years that traditional perceptions of the meniscus as a functionless vestigial organ[2] have been replaced by its contemporary exalted position as an integral cog in the knee machinery. Menisci have historically been treated like tonsils of the knee joint, being discarded when symptomatic pathology presented. Both clinical and basic science studies[3–7] have documented the appearance of degenerative changes in the knee following meniscectomy, thus prompting a more preservationist attitude toward knee menisci. The intimate relationship between knee ligament injury and meniscal tears, as high as 98 percent in some series,[8] demands a thorough understanding of meniscal biology, biomechanics, and surgical techniques in order to develop and apply appropriate rehabilitative principles.

BIOMECHANICAL FUNCTION

Fairbank's[4] classic article in 1948 on knee joint degenerative changes after meniscectomy was instrumental in providing clinical evidence that menisci indeed participate in load transmission across the knee joint. He documented radiographic arthritic changes 3 months to 14 years following meniscectomies. These included (1) joint space narrowing, (2) flattening of the femoral condyle, and (3) osteophyte formation. This study suggested that meniscectomy is not totally innocuous and may interfere with joint mechanics. It

would take several decades, however, before this and other clinical and animal studies, documenting degenerative-type changes postmeniscectomy, antiquated meniscectomy as a viable surgical procedure.

Joint space narrowing results from the loss of two separate mechanical functions. One is simply the loss of a mechanical spacer. The menisci prevent tibial and femoral articular cartilage contact in the non-weight-bearing situation. Following meniscectomy, this spacer function is lost, allowing articular contact in the unloaded condition. The narrowing resulting from loss of the mechanical spacer alone, however, is small and thought to be no greater than 1 mm.

A second reason for joint space narrowing is a reduction in articular contact area to 40 percent of normal, which significantly increases the strain applied per unit area. Ahmed and Burke[9] have calculated that menisci transmit greater than 50 percent of the total forces across the knee in weight-bearing situations. Grood's[10] excellent analogy of a high-heeled shoe on a soft linoleum floor allows visualization of further joint space narrowing following meniscectomy, due to transmission of weight over a significantly decreased contact area. Large increases in stress per unit area may also induce remodeling changes in the subchondral bone, explaining the femoral condylar flattening described by Fairbanks and others.

Osteophyte formation is commonly seen in the unstable knee because of abnormal periarticular capsular forces resulting from excessive joint translation. The role of the meniscus as a joint stabilizer has been well studied, and it functions to limit joint translation in the face of ligamentous injury. Levy et al.[11] have demonstrated that a meniscectomy performed after an anterior cruciate ligament (ACL) disruption can allow up to 6 mm of additional anteroposterior tibial translation. However, the role of the meniscus as a primary stabilizer of joint motion is less clear. Laboratory studies have shown that in addition to load transmission and stability functions, menisci also participate in joint nutrition, shock absorption, and joint lubrication.[12–14]

Bullough et al.[15] have demonstrated that the major orientation of collagen fibers in the meniscus is circumferential and that this is also the optimal direction in which menisci resist tension. The collagen fibers function very similarly to metal hoops around a wooden barrel in generating hoop tension to prevent peripheral displacement of the meniscus (Fig. 5-1). These hoop forces are transmitted to the tibial plateau through the strong anterior and posterior meniscal attachments. Additional resistance is provided by the intermeniscal ligament and the meniscofemoral ligaments of Wrisberg and Humphry (Fig. 5-2).

Some investigators[16] believe that loss of the ability of a meniscus to generate hoop tension with weight bearing, such as in a complete radial tear or an extensive partial meniscectomy, is tantamount biomechanically to a complete meniscectomy. Others believe that the extra-articular meniscal constraints (collateral ligaments, capsule, popliteus, etc.) play a role in preventing peripheral meniscal displacement.[10]

Partial meniscectomy has been shown to increase the contact stresses on the articular cartilage, but less than that which occurs with a complete meniscectomy, thus affording some stress protection to the joint surfaces. Proportional increases in the peak local contact stress (PLCS) can approach those seen postmeniscectomy if enough meniscal tissue is removed. Meniscal repair, however, has been shown to return PLCS to baseline levels.[17]

MENISCAL INJURY

An appreciation of meniscal blood supply is critical to understanding treatment options and rehabilitation of meniscal injuries. Investigators of embryologic development have shown that the human meniscus is vascularized throughout its substance.[18,19] However, with time, weight bearing, and knee motion, the inner portion gradually becomes avascular. Several investigators have studied the extent of peripheral vascularization in the adult meniscus and have found variations in vascular encroachment from 15 to 33 percent.[20–22] Arnoczky and Warren[20] produced perhaps the most eloquent microvascular investigations, demonstrating 10 to 30 percent peripheral vascularization of the medial meniscus and similar depth of penetration of the lateral meniscus (10 to 25 percent) with an avascular peripheral segment adjacent to the popliteal tendon. Both anterior and posterior horn attachments of each meniscus demonstrated endoligamentous vessels ex-

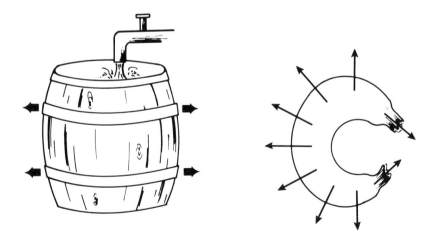

Fig. 5-1. The circumferential collagen fibers of the knee meniscus function in a manner very similar to metal hoops around a wooden barrel. The fibers develop hoop tension in response to femoral condylar loading, which prevents peripheral displacement of the menisci.

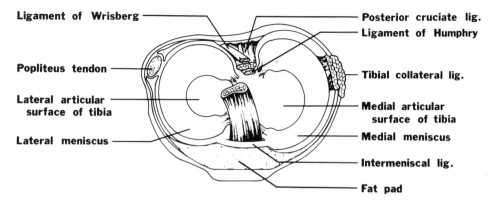

Ligament of Wrisberg

Popliteus tendon

Lateral articular
    surface of tibia

Lateral meniscus

Posterior cruciate lig.

Ligament of Humphry

Tibial collateral lig.

Medial articular
    surface of tibia

Medial meniscus

Intermeniscal lig.

Fat pad

Fig. 5-2. Superior view of the tibial plateau. Hoop stresses generated in the circumferential collagen fibers of the meniscus are transmitted to the tibial plateau through the strong anterior and posterior horn attachments. Additional resistance is provided by the intermeniscal ligament and the meniscofemoral ligaments of Wrisberg and Humphry.

tending into the meniscus and ending in capillary loops. The results of these studies suggest that lesions in the peripheral one-third of the meniscus or in the horn attachment have access to a vascular supply that may be adequate to elicit a healing response (Fig. 5-3). Arnoczky et al.[23] have recently reported on the healing potential of meniscal tears in the avascular portion of the meniscus stimulated with exogenous fibrin clot. Although healing occurs in this situation, it is with histologically different tissue. Biomechanical data are necessary to determine whether this repair tissue is capable of sustaining repetitive clinical loading. Investigators have found successful healing but significantly decreased strength in repaired radial tears in animal models.[24,25] Arnoczky and Warren[26] have also suggested that the "zone of repair" could be extended by creating a vascular access channel across an intact meniscal surface.

MENISCAL REPAIR

King[12] concluded in 1936 that semilunar menisci serve to protect the hyaline articular cartilages and that probably operative excision should be limited to removal of the mobile portion. This advice, plus an additional 50 years of clinical evidence documenting articular demise after meniscectomy, has converted most orthopaedic surgeons from performing open complete meniscectomies to doing partial arthroscopic resec-

tion. In fact, partial arthroscopic meniscectomy is presently one of the most commonly performed surgical procedures. A physician comfortable with arthroscopic techniques finds this procedure to be quick, easy to perform, associated with a very low complication rate, and often completed under local anesthesia. The patient likewise appreciates the outpatient procedure, little pain, and often rapid recovery with early return to activities. So why change?

Although short-term patient satisfaction is high, increasingly, studies are showing that partial meniscectomy may be deleterious to the knee in the long run. DiStefano[27] and Cox et al.[3] in separate studies found that partial meniscectomy leads to less severe degenerative changes than complete meniscectomy; however, the degree of change is directly related to the

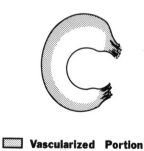

▨ **Vascularized Portion**

Fig. 5-3. The peripheral one-third of the meniscus is the optimal location for meniscal repair owing to adequate vascularization.

amount of meniscus removed. Borne et al.[28] confirmed increased strain on the proximal tibia with both complete and partial meniscectomy. Manzione et al.[29] reported 60 percent unsatisfactory long-term results in children with partial or complete meniscectomy. Additionally, many clinical studies have documented high healing rates, low re-rupture rates, and symptomatic relief following meniscal repair.[30–35]

In ligamentous instability, preservation of the meniscus is even more essential. It is not uncommon in an active sports medicine practice to see the 20- to 35-year-old athlete with an ACL deficiency, who has had a subsequent total or subtotal meniscectomy, present with advanced medial joint arthrosis and pain. It is less common to see identical changes in a similar patient with intact menisci.[36] With accumulating evidence documenting the benefit of retaining meniscal tissue, one might wonder why there exists resistance to change.

First, clinical and basic science studies documenting benefits of meniscal repair surgery are less than 10 years old, a relatively short period on the orthopaedic calendar. Second, meniscal repair requires advanced arthroscopic skills, experienced assistants, and increased operative times and is associated with a higher complication rate. Patients are exposed to increased anesthesia time and prolonged rehabilitation necessitating greater rehabilitation expertise. However, I and others believe the long-term benefits of preserving meniscal tissue are well worth the short-term inconveniences and any slight increase in surgical risk.

Meniscal repair is not a new procedure. Annandale[37] is credited with the first surgical repair of a torn meniscus in 1863. King[12] followed with eloquent studies on meniscal repair in the animal model in 1936. However, it was not until 1976 that the first case of arthroscopically assisted meniscal repair was reported.[38] Many clinical and basic science studies have since documented the healing potential of the meniscus, but noticeably lacking are studies documenting satisfactory biomechanical function of healed menisci. This is analogous to gluing together a split in one's jeans; coapting the tear with paste does not ensure continued cohesion under the stress of daily wear. Recent investigations by Newman et al.[24] have documented both healing and normal mechanical function in repaired canine menisci with peripheral longitudinal tears. Repaired radial tears demonstrated spreading at the in-

jury site, adversely influencing mechanical function. Long-term clinical studies documenting the lack of degenerative Fairbank-type changes following meniscal repair associated with good clinical results will determine the ultimate benefit of repair procedures.

The geometric configuration of a meniscal tear is an important factor in determining suitability for repair (Fig. 5-4). Fortunately, the single longitudinal type of tear is very common in the younger active population, and when it is located in the peripheral vascularized one-third of the meniscus, is the most rewarding to repair. Performing a partial meniscectomy of a tear located in the outer one-third would easily involve removing between 12 and 35 percent of the meniscus, resulting in joint contact forces increasing by 300 to 400 percent.[39]

Several additional factors associated with an increased healing potential have been reported by Henning et al.[40] These include a peripheral location, length less than 300 mm, acute tears (less than 8 weeks), rasp abrasion, and exogenous clot insertion. Radial tears can also be repaired if they can be coapted anatomically and there is vascular access to the periphery. Although radial tears have been shown to heal in both human and animal models, spreading at the repair site may render the meniscus less able to sustain hoop tension, resulting in increased tibial plateau contact stresses. A longer period of protected weight bearing is indicated in radial repairs.

There exist a group of meniscal tears that require no surgical treatment. Often, surgeons will discover a meniscal tear during arthroscopy that is located in an area that was not noted to be symptomatic preoperatively. Lesions that can be left alone include full-thickness meniscal tears less than 5 mm long that are stable to probing, radial tears less than 5 mm long, and partial-thickness tears that are stable to probing and less than 50 percent complete. Performing the diagnostic portion of the arthroscopy under local anesthesia is extremely helpful for the occasional meniscal tear that fits nonoperative criteria but elicits pain with probing. This lesion is then treated with either repair or partial excision. Only recently has healing of meniscal tears treated nonoperatively been documented.[41]

The decision to partially excise the loose meniscal fragment or repair it is becoming less clear-cut. There is little doubt about the healing potential of the pe-

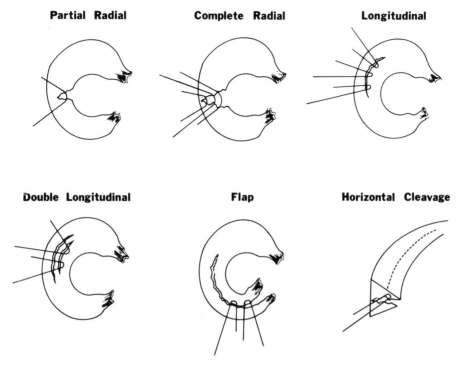

Partial Radial   **Complete Radial**   **Longitudinal**

Double Longitudinal   **Flap**   **Horizontal Cleavage**

Fig. 5-4. Meniscal tears may assume an infinite number of configurations. The six most common tears are depicted. Complex tears involve two or more of the above configurations in a single meniscus.

ripheral meniscus. Many studies have documented healing rates as high as 90 percent in this area.[30–32, 34,35] Newer techniques such as inserting fibrin clot[23] in the avascular tear or placing fascial patches[42] as scaffolding over complex tears are rapidly expanding the limits of meniscal repair. These techniques permit us to believe that the decision to repair meniscal tears is based less on the location of a tear and more on the surgeon's ability to adequately reduce and stabilize the meniscus.

SURGICAL TECHNIQUES

Various surgical techniques to repair menisci have been described since Annandale's first report of meniscal repair in 1885.[37] Until 1976, when the first report[35] of arthroscopically aided meniscal repair appeared, meniscal repair was performed by open direct suturing of the meniscus to the capsule. Often this was associated with severe medial or lateral joint disrup-

tion or knee dislocation. Dehaven[43] presently advocates an open technique to repair meniscal lesions if they are within 2 mm of the meniscosynovial junction. Most arthroscopic repair techniques are variations of either an inside-out or an outside-in type of repair (Fig. 5-5). The inside-out techniques using a posteromedial or posterolateral incision as described by Henning and colleagues[35,42] affords the greatest ability to reduce and hold the meniscus anatomically; additionally, it allows the surgeon to place a maximum number of sutures while protecting the neurovascular structures with a popliteal retractor. Various outside-in techniques utilize a blind approach to the meniscal tear. The surgeon does not visualize the suture placement until the needle has penetrated the meniscus from the outside-in. If malplacement of a suture has occurred, multiple passes through the meniscus are necessary to attain optimal placement. Utilizing the inside-out technique, suture needles are passed through the meniscal tear under direct arthroscopic visualization, avoiding the hit-or-miss approach.

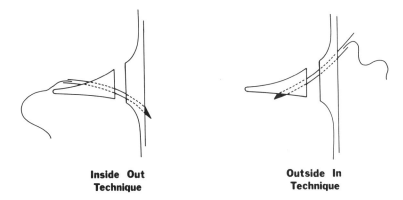

Inside Out Technique

Outside In Technique

Fig. 5-5. Meniscal suture. The two most popular arthroscopically assisted meniscal repair techniques differ in the initial direction of suture passage.

MENISCAL PATHOLOGY

Meniscal lesions necessitating arthroscopic surgery are not limited to traumatic tears. Discoid menisci occasionally occur in childhood or adolescents with pain or locking symptoms, most commonly in the lateral compartment. Surgery often involves partial meniscectomy with contouring of the discoid shape into a more normal semilunar cartilage to render the patient less symptomatic.

Inflammatory disorders of the knee such as rheumatoid arthritis can cause destruction of the articular cartilage and meniscus by the invading pannus. Arthroscopic resection of the pannus and necrotic menisci along with extensive synovectomy are often indicated to help alleviate symptoms in advanced cases. Similarly, joint sepsis can cause extensive cartilage necrosis necessitating partial meniscal debridement and high-volume joint irrigation.

Chondrocalcinosis articularis (pseudogout) is a metabolic disorder with clinical symptoms mimicking gout. Calcium pyrophosphate crystals are laid down in both the hyaline and fibrocartilage and act as irritants to the joint. Clinically, the patient can suffer from repeated episodes of severe joint pain, swelling, tenderness, warmth, and erythema. Although arthroscopy is not a primary mode of treatment for patients with acute exacerbations of pseudogout, as an adjunct to pharmacologic control, the patient can benefit by removal of some crystalline load from the cartilage surface with copious irrigation. This may inhibit or delay degenerative meniscal lesions such as intermeniscal cysts or ossicles associated with chondrocalcinosis.

LASER APPLICATIONS TO MENISCAL SURGERY

The laser (light amplification by simulated emission of radiation) has been added to the arthroscopist's armamentarium for use in meniscal surgery. Of the several hundred types of lasers that exist, the three which have been used in meniscal surgery include the carbon dioxide (CO_2) laser, the argon laser, and the neodymium-yttrium aluminum garnet (Nd-YAG) laser. Their primary use is that of a laser scalpel to remove and contour menisci and excise synovium. Additionally, lasers have been shown to elicit a healing response in articular cartilage. All use of lasers in the knee should be considered experimental at present.

CO_2 lasers are somewhat inconvenient to use since the surgeon must perform arthroscopy in a gas medium. This requires constant switching from a liquid to gas medium, which also results in considerable subcutaneous emphysema. The wattage level employed on meniscal tissue meticulously removes tissue one cell layer at a time and significantly prolongs a simple partial meniscectomy when compared with conventional techniques. One advantage might be an ability to smoothly contour an irregular meniscal tear.

The argon laser utilizes wavelengths best absorbed by pigmented tissue such as blood vessels and melanin. This seems to be a more beneficial tool for the ophthalmologist and dermatologist. The relatively unpigmented menisci and articular cartilage would therefore require significantly higher power densities to vaporize. More research is necessary to convert this laser into an effective arthroscopic tool.

The Nd-YAG laser loses excessive amounts of energy due to light scattering. Newer probes have been developed to allow use of this laser as a contact vaporizer. Its purported advantages include (1) use in a saline medium, (2) small size, (3) variable probe tips, (4) fiberoptic application, and (5) less articular scuffing.[44]

Not withstanding the many advantages lasers may offer in treating intra-articular pathology, there are major concerns about educating surgeons in the use of a new technology whose primary purpose is to remove meniscal tissue, when current research trends indicate the value of preserving menisci through repair techniques. The uneducated health care consumer may mistakenly believe "laser arthroscopy" is a significant scientific advance in treating meniscal tears, when in reality it may prove to be an expensive method to perform a partial meniscectomy.

FUTURE TRENDS

Several exciting basic science developments occurring in laboratories across the country will shape the future of meniscal surgery. Investigators have performed successful meniscal allograft transplants in animal models.[10,11] Tissue evaluation has documented both healing and biomechanical function in these models. Arthroscopically performed meniscal allografts have been performed in humans; however, clinical follow-up is too short to make any valid conclusions. Meniscal transplantation has its widest application in the young patient with a previous meniscectomy who is now demonstrating early degenerative symptoms. Advanced arthrosis would be a relative contraindication to a meniscal transplant, since the major goal is to prevent these late degenerative changes.

Cell mediators, such as angiogenin,[45] a blood vessel-inducing protein, are being used to induce angiogenesis in the avascular portion of the meniscus. This is yet another advance directed at preserving valuable meniscal tissue to obviate the need for complete or partial meniscectomies.

In vitro culturing of meniscal tissue is an important laboratory tool to evaluate the biologic potential of the fibrocartilage matrix and cells. Products of such experimentation will allow for better understanding of the biologic milieu and conditions necessary to optimize meniscal healing.

Finally, collagen-based scaffolds that act as biologic superstructures for meniscal regeneration are being developed in some laboratories.[46] Early results in animals appear promising. If such a model proves successful in humans, the ability to grow fibrochondrocytes into functioning, vascularized menisci would be a quantum leap in our efforts to replace absent or damaged menisci and preserve articular cartilage.

REFERENCES

1. Dye SF, Via MW, Andersen C: An evolutionary perspective of the knee. Orthop Trans 10:70, 1986
2. Sutton JB: Ligaments. Their Nature and Morphology. H. K. Lewis & Co., London, 1897
3. Cox JS, Nye CE, Schaefer WW et al: The degenerative effects of partial and total medial meniscus in dogs knees. Clin Orthop 109:178, 1978
4. Fairbank TJ: Knee joint changes after meniscectomy. J Bone Joint Surg 30B:664, 1948
5. Jackson RJ, Kettelkamp DB, Clark W et al: Factors affecting late results after meniscectomy. J Bone Joint Surg 56A:719, 1974
6. Jackson JP: Degenerative changes in the knee after meniscectomy. J Bone Joint Surg 49B:584, 1967
7. Tapper EM, Hoover NW: Late results after meniscectomy. J Bone Joint Surg 51A:517, 1969
8. Warren RF, Marshall JL: Injuries of the anterior cruciate and medial collateral ligaments of the knee: a retrospective analysis of clinical records—Part I. Clin Orthop 136:191, 1978
9. Ahmed AM, Burke DL: In vivo measurement of static pressure distribution in synovial joints. Part I: Tibial surface of the knee. J Biomech Eng 105:201, 1983
10. Grood ES: Menisci function. Adv Orthop Surg 4:193, 1984
11. Levy M, Torzilli PA, Warren RF: The effect of medial meniscectomy on anterior-posterior motion of the knee. J Bone Joint Surg 64A:883, 1982
12. King D: The function of semilunar cartilages. J Bone Joint Surg 18:1069, 1936
13. Seedham BB: Loadbearing function of the menisci. Physiotherapy 62:223, 1976

14. Cabaud HE, Rodkey LG, Fitzwater JE: Medial meniscus repairs. An experimental and morphologic study. Am J Sports Med 9:129, 1981

15. Bullough PG, Munver AL, Murphy J, Weinstein AM: The strength of the menisci of the knee as it relates to their fine structure. J Bone Joint Surg 52B:564, 1970

16. Shrive NG, O'Conner JJ, Goodfellow JW: Loadbearing in the knee joint. Clin Orthop 131:279, 1978

17. Lanzer WL, Komenda G: Changes in articular cartilage after meniscectomy. Clin Orthop 252:41, 1990

18. Clark CR, Ogden JA: Development of the menisci of the human knee joint. J Bone Joint Surg 65:538, 1983

19. Kaplan EB: The embryology of the menisci of the knee joint. Bull Hosp Joint Dis 16:111, 1955

20. Arnoczky SP, Warren RF: Microvasculature of the human meniscus. Am J Sports Med 10:90, 1982

21. Davies DV, Edwards DAW: The blood supply of the synovial membrane and intra-articular structures. Ann R Coll Surg Eng 2:142, 1948

22. Scapinelli R: Studies on the vasculature of the human knee joint. Acta Anat Basel 70:305, 1968

23. Arnoczky SP, Warren RF, Spivak JM: Meniscal repair using an exogenous fibrin clot. J Bone Joint Surg 70A:1209, 1988

24. Newman AP, Anderson OR, Daniels AV: Mechanics of the healed meniscus in a canine model. Am J Sports Med 17:164, 1989

25. Krause WR, Burdette WA, Loughran TP: Properties of the normal and repaired canine meniscus. Orthop Trans 15:207, 1989

26. Arnoczky SP, Warren RF: The microvasculature of the meniscus and its response to injury. Am J Sports Med 11:131, 1983

27. DiStefano VJ: Function post traumatic sequelae and current concepts of management of knee meniscus injuries. Clin Orthop 151:143, 1980

28. Bourne RD, Finlay JB, Papadopoulos P, Andreae P: The effect of medial meniscectomy on strain distribution in the proximal part of the tibia. J Bone Joint Surg 66A:1431, 1984

29. Manzione M, Pizzutillo PD, Peoples AB, Schweizer PA: Meniscectomy in children: a long-term follow-up study. Am J Sports Med 11:111, 1983

30. Cassidy RE, Shaffer AJ: Repair of peripheral meniscus tears. Am J Sports Med 9:209, 1981

31. Dehaven KE: Peripheral meniscus repair—an alternative to meniscectomy. J Bone Joint Surg 63B:463, 1981

32. Hamberg P, Gillquist J, Lysholm J: Suture of the new and old peripheral meniscus tears. J Bone Joint Surg 65A:193, 1983

33. Price CT, Allen WC: Ligament repair in the knee with preservation of the meniscus. J Bone Joint Surg 60A:61, 1978

34. Rosenberg TO, Scott SM, Coward DB et al: Arthroscopic meniscal repair evaluated with repeat arthroscopy. Arthroscopy 2:14, 1986

35. Scott GA, Jolly BL, Henning CE: Combined posterior incision and arthroscopic intra-articular repair of the meniscus. J Bone Joint Surg 68A:847, 1986

36. Lindenfeld TN: Arthroscopically aided meniscal repair. Orthopedics 10:1293, 1987

37. Annandale T: An operation for displaced semilunar cartilage. Br Med J 1:779, 1885

38. Ikeuchi H: Surgery under arthroscopic control. p. 57. In Proceedings of the Societé Internationale d'Arthroscopie, Copenhagen, Denmark, 1975. Rheumatologie [Basel] (special issue), 1976

39. Seedhom BB, Hargreaves DJ: Transmission of the load in the knee joint with special reference to the role of the menisci: Part II. Experimental results, discussion and conclusions. Eng Med 8:220, 1979

40. Henning CE, Clark JR, Lynch MA et al: Arthroscopic meniscus repair with a posterior incision. American Association of Orthopaedic Surgeons Inst. Course Lect. 37:209, 1988

41. Weiss CB, Lundberg M, Hamberg P et al: Non-operative treatment of meniscal tears. J Bone Joint Surg 71A:811, 1989

42. Henning CE, Lynch MA, Yearout KM et al: Arthroscopic meniscal repair using an exogenous fibrin clot. Clin Orthop 252:64, 1990

43. Dehaven K: Decision-making factors in the treatment of meniscus lesions. Clin Orthop 252:49, 1990

44. Obrien SJ, Miller FV: The contact neodymium-yttrium aluminum garnet laser—a new arthroscopic approach to arthroscopic laser surgery. Clin Orthop 252:95, 1990

45. King TV, Vallee BI, Rosenberg AE: Induction of angiogenesis in the knee meniscus using argiogenin. Orthopaedic Research Society Trans 14:206, 1989

46. Stone KR, Rookey WG, Webber RJ et al: Future directions: collagen-based prosthesis for meniscal regeneration. Clin Orthop 252:129, 1990

6

Rehabilitation Following Meniscal Surgery

JOHN T. CAVANAUGH

INTRODUCTION

Meniscal injuries are common in today's exercise-minded world. The population, in general, has become more athletically active, and people stay active longer. Meniscal lesions can be either traumatic or degenerative in nature. Surgical intervention, in the form of total or partial meniscectomy or meniscal repair, may often be necessary. This chapter discusses the physical therapist's role in postoperative meniscus rehabilitation.

ANATOMY, CLINICAL BIOMECHANICS, AND FUNCTION

The medial meniscus is oval or C-shaped and is larger in diameter than the lateral meniscus. The entire border of the medial meniscus is attached to the tibia by thick coronary ligaments. The semimembranosus attaches to the posterior aspect of the medial meniscus. The lateral meniscus, on the other hand, is more circular or O-shaped and may cover up to 70 to 90 percent of the articular surface. The popliteus tendon inserts at the posterior horn. The capsular attachment to the lateral meniscus is weak, allowing greater mobility. This increased mobility may contribute to the lesser occurrence of tears on the lateral side.[1]

Meniscal tissue is hydrated, soft, and fibrocartilaginous. The concentration of collagen in meniscal fibrocartilage is slightly greater than that in articular cartilage.[2] The vascular supply to the menisci originates from the capsule and synovial attachments where vessels penetrate the periphery to supply the outer one-third, leaving the inner two-thirds avascular.[3]

The menisci are designed to move with the tibia. The menisci move anteriorly and medially during extension; with flexion, the menisci move posteriorly and laterally, with an emphasis on the action of the popliteus and semimembranosus muscles. The amount of rotation allowed by the mobile lateral meniscus may be as much as 15 to 20 degrees.[4]

The menisci function to: (1) distribute weight-bearing loads; (2) increase joint congruency, thus aiding stability; (3) limit abnormal motions; and (4) possibly improve articular nourishment.[5]

As the anterior horns of the menisci go forward, they act as a buffer to hyperextension and dampen the pendulum effect of the leg during the swing-through phase of gait.[6] Cadavers with an intact anterior cruciate ligament (ACL) showed a 14 percent increase in rotatory laxity after medial and lateral meniscectomy.[7] The medial meniscus has been shown to be a significant restraint to anterior tibial displacement, especially in the absence of the ACL.[8]

MECHANISM OF INJURY

Noncontact stresses are the most frequent mechanisms of injury to the menisci.[9] These stresses result from a sudden acceleration or deceleration in combination with a change in direction (e.g., when a soccer or lacrosse player "plants and cuts" to elude an opponent). In jumping sports such as volleyball or basketball, the additional element of vertical force with angular momentum upon landing can contribute to a meniscal tear. This scenario worsens when significant rotation between the tibia and femur is accompanied by hyperextension or hyperflexion stress.

Degenerative meniscal lesions may occur in older, active individuals with minimal stress, such as swinging a golf club or squatting to pick up an object.

Contact injuries also contribute to meniscal lesions. This usually occurs when the involved extremity is fixed and receives a blow, resulting in a valgus, varus, or hyperextended moment with the knee flexed and rotated. Ligamentous lesions are usually associated with this scenario (the "unhappy triad"). The end result of most of these mechanisms is a shear stress, rupturing the meniscus.

The incidence of meniscal injury in patients who suffer acute ACL injury has been estimated by De-Haven[10] to be 65 percent. In acute ACL injury, the lateral meniscus has been reported injured almost as frequently as the medial meniscus.[11] In chronic ACL insufficiency, the incidence of meniscal pathology can approach 98 percent.[12] The medial meniscus injury rate in chronic ACL deficiency has been found to be higher (86.9 percent versus 28.9 percent for the lateral side).[13]

Meniscal lesions may have varied clinical symptoms. Displaced tears, such as bucket handle tears, can produce locking and giving way. Nondisplaced tears can alter meniscus mobility and produce abnormal traction stresses to the capsule and synovium, accounting for the pain associated with such lesions.[9]

SURGICAL INTERVENTION

The surgical approach to meniscus tear is multifaceted and depends specifically on the type of tear, its location within the meniscus, associated ligament injuries, and the age and activity level of the patient.[14]

With the advancement of arthroscopic techniques and finer instrumentation, total meniscectomy is seldom done. Studies of partial and total meniscectomy have shown diminished morbidity when a partial meniscectomy has been performed.[15] In 1948, Fairbank[16] was the first to call attention to degenerative changes in the knee joint postmeniscectomy. More recent studies have shown decreased shock-absorbing capability, higher peak stress, and increased stress concentration following total meniscectomy.[17,18]

Partial meniscectomy attempts to decrease second-ary changes associated with total meniscectomy. By providing more of the biomechanical, load-bearing functions of the meniscus and fine tuning or controlling of the joint, increased protection is provided.[19]

The recognition of the importance of the meniscus has led to more frequent attempts to preserve, rather than remove, a torn meniscus. Meniscal repair is preferred because it offers the chance to restore normal anatomy and function to the knee. Thomas Annandale[20] reported the first meniscal repair in 1883 in Edinburgh, Scotland. Meniscal repair, however, has only been widely performed in the last 20 years. Current concepts are based on experience with open suturing of peripheral tears. More recent developments with arthroscopy permit repair of nonperipheral as well as peripheral lesions. Current technology employs vascular access channels,[21] which potentiate a healing response in the avascular zone of the meniscus, PDS absorbable sutures, and the insertion of a fibrin clot. Based on the work of Arnoczky et al.,[22] insertion of fibrin clots in the avascular zone of a meniscal defect has promoted healing. Clinical success rates for meniscus repairs have approached 90 percent, and healing by arthrographic or arthroscopic criteria has been documented to be approximately 80 percent.[23]

IMPLEMENTING A REHABILITATION PROGRAM

The most important principle in implementing a rehabilitation program is individualization. Too often therapists look for a cookbook approach to therapy. It is vital to recognize that no two meniscectomy or meniscal repair patients are alike. Components of the individualized program are listed in Table 6-1.

Preinjury Status

It is necessary to identify the physical condition of the patient prior to surgery. Is the patient a recreational athlete who regularly competes, or is the patient an occasional athlete who golfs, plays tennis, or skis intermittently? Perhaps the patient is a competitive athlete who, as a member of a team, sustains an injury during the season. The patient may be an elite athlete of international notoriety, or a nonathlete sustaining an injury during an activity of daily living. Media re-

Table 6-1. Components for an Individualized Program Status after Meniscus Surgery

Preinjury status	Nonathlete/recreational athlete/ elite athlete
	Physical condition
Type of surgery	Open versus arthroscopic
	Partial versus total meniscectomy
	Size/site of lesion excised
	Size/site of repair
Associated pathology	Chondromalacia
	Degenerative joint disease
	Ligament insufficiency
Comprehensive evaluation	History
	Observations
	Subjective complaints
	Physical examination
Postoperative goals	Surgeon/therapist/patient
	Short term/long term
	Patient compliance
Treatment plan	Functional progression
	SAID principle
	Rules of rehabilitation

ports of professional athletes returning quickly to sport following arthroscopic surgery often frustrate the recreational athlete, who takes longer to rehabilitate. Here the professional's preinjury state is appreciated.

Type of Surgery

Should surgery be open or arthroscopic? Partial versus total meniscectomy? Meniscal repair? Seldom are two surgeries the same. It is important to know the specifics of how the surgery was performed. This can be achieved by obtaining a copy of the operative note and/ or discussing the operation with the patient's surgeon. The surgical technique (including the type and number of incisions) has a direct effect on the progression of the patient's rehabilitation program. The more soft tissue dissection there is, especially capsular incisions and repairs, the more hemarthrosis and muscle inhibition will occur postoperatively.[24] It has been shown that knee joint effusion can cause quadriceps muscle inhibition.[25] Mechanoreceptors in the joint capsule respond to changes in tension and in turn inhibit the motor nerves supplying the quadriceps muscles. Therefore, a smaller postoperative effusion will lead to decreased quadriceps inhibition, resulting in a faster return of muscle function.

The site of partial meniscectomy is relevant as well.

An excised lesion from an avascular region will result in less hemarthrosis than, for example, a peripheral lesion, thus shortening the postoperative course.

Northmore-Ball et al.[26] compared the results of 219 knees after arthroscopic partial, open partial, and open total meniscectomies. The arthroscopic group spent far less time on crutches and returned to sport activity in one-half the time compared with those in the open groups.

The meniscal repair patient offers a greater challenge to the therapist than the arthroscopic meniscectomy patient. Here communication between the therapist and surgeon is imperative, as the type and location of the repair will influence the postoperative course. Specifics are discussed later in this chapter.

Associated Pathology

From the postoperative note or communication with the surgeon, one can ascertain any associated knee pathology that may alter the individualized program. For example, a patient with ACL insufficiency will need increased proprioceptive training, while a patient with chondromalacia patellae may not be a candidate for certain isotonic or isokinetic exercises. A patient with degenerative arthritis will take longer to rehabilitate depending on the severity of the disease. Gillquist and Oretorp[27] found that the recovery time was approximately twice as long in patients with degenerative changes than in patients who had normal articular surfaces.

Comprehensive Evaluation

An evaluation sets the basis from which progress is measured. It tells us where we are and where we are going. Postoperatively, a comprehensive evaluation is the key in formulating a treatment plan. Here, preinjury state, type of surgery, and associated pathology are taken into consideration with evaluative findings when formulating an assessment.

In taking a history, several questions require answers. When did the injury occur (acute or chronic)? How did it happen (mechanism of injury)? What symptoms were present (locking, swelling, pain)? How was the injury managed (rest, physical therapy, immobilization)? How long ago was the surgery? What has the patient done for the knee since surgery?

Observations should document the patient's weight-bearing status and the use of any assistive device. The presence of an effusion should be noted as well as the amount of atrophy compared with the uninvolved extremity. Anatomic alignment is an important observation as the patient may present with a valgus or varus deformity.

The patient's subjective complaints are of the utmost importance throughout the rehabilitation process. Reports of pain (when, where, and description), lack of mobility, and weakness will alter the postoperative course.

During the physical examination, it is important to document active and passive range of motion within the guidelines of physiologic healing restraints (as in the case of meniscal repair). Girth measurements should be taken at, above, and below the knee joint bilaterally. Manual muscle tests may reveal a proximal or distal weakness. Quadriceps testing is usually not applicable immediately postoperative as swelling and patellofemoral discomfort accompany this test. Neurovascular integrity should be checked with distal pulses and sensation testing. Laxity tests to include Lachmann, anterior and posterior drawer, pivot shift, and varus and valgus testing can rule out associated ligamentous pathology. Meniscal tests are seldom appropriate postoperatively. Palpation of medial and lateral joint lines, as well as medial and lateral aspects of the patella, can help rule out contributory lesions. Assessing patellar mobility and tracking can be valuable when later implementing specific quadricep exercises. Flexibility assessment is important because tight muscles about one joint can alter forces at another joint in the closed kinetic chain. Older patients with degenerative meniscal tears notoriously present with tight hamstrings. This can alter knee joint kinematics and possibly contribute to the mechanism of injury. Gait evaluation (when applicable) can be useful in assessing the patient's biomechanical profile.

With all the data considered, an objective assessment can then be made.

Postoperative Goals

The collected information should be discussed with the patient and the realistic goals of the surgeon, therapist, and patient set. The patient should be brought to understand the magnitude of the surgery and the timetable for recovery. Differences between patient's pathologies can drastically alter goal setting. An intercollegiate basketball player may return to full activity in 2 weeks after resection of a clean flap tear, whereas a middle-aged weekend tennis player, after excision of a bucket handle tear with degenerative joint changes, may take several months to regain the desired level of activity. Goals should be specific to the needs of the individual patient, that is, what the patient wants to be able to do. Typical short-term goals should include decreasing pain and joint effusion, facilitating a normal gait pattern, and restoring normal range of motion. Long-term goals include improved muscle strength, endurance, and flexibility throughout the involved extremity, improved proprioception and conditioning, and the eventual return to the full activity of choice.

It should be emphasized to patients that they play a vital role in the rehabilitation process. Patient compliance to therapy and home exercises are key to a complete recovery.

Treatment Plan

The final component of implementing an individualized rehabilitation program is the formation of a treatment plan. The underlying message of the treatment plan should be a functional orientation to exercise. It is important that the rehabilitation program follow a functional progression. This concept has been defined by Kegerreis[28] as an ordered sequence of activities enabling the acquisition or reacquisition of skills required for the safe, effective performance of athletic endeavors. One must look at the specific components of the activity that the patient wants to return to and prescribe an appropriate exercise or activity to improve those components. For example, a football lineman should emphasize an exercise with maximal effort of short duration. A soccer player, on the other hand, would be best off working on repetitive submaximal contractions over a prolonged time.

In association with a functional progression, the therapist should follow the SAID principle[29] (specific adaptation to imposed demands). The body adapts to specific activities based on the type of stress experienced, and the type of adaption that takes place will be specific to the type of training performed. This concept is demonstrated throughout the rehabilitation process in various closed kinetic chain (body movement performed with one or both feet in a stationary position) exercises, which impose different forces at the knee in multiple planes. Therefore, in following a functional approach to rehabilitation, emphasis should be placed on treatment in a closed kinetic state when appropriate.

To initiate the treatment plan, it is imperative to follow certain rehabilitation rules. These have been described by Gray[30]: (1) create a safe environment for optimal healing; (2) don't hurt the patient; (3) be as aggressive as you can without breaking rule 2. The treatment plan can be made effective by understanding the specific effects of the treatment, the cause of the patient's symptoms, the functional biomechanics of the knee joint, stages of tissue healing, and the patient's specific injury or surgery.

REHABILITATION GUIDELINES FOLLOWING ARTHROSCOPIC MENISCECTOMY

Rehabilitation following arthroscopic meniscectomy can be divided into four phases (Table 6-2): protection, moderate protection, early functional, and late func-

tional. The word guideline is used instead of protocol as it allows for individualization.

Protection Phase

This immediate postoperative phase is characterized by soft tissue bleeding and effusion, pain, and quadriceps inhibition. Prior to discharge from the hospital, the patient's involved extremity is placed in a Jobst cryotemp (Fig. 6-1) in an elevated position for 20 minutes. By utilizing the intermittent compression device, RICE (rest, ice, compression, and elevation) is quickly applied. The patient is then instructed in a series of home therapeutic exercises, which include quadriceps setting, straight leg raises (SLR) in multiple planes, and an active-assisted range of motion exercise. The patient is fitted with crutches and instructed in ambulation training weight bearing as tolerated on all surfaces. The patient is encouraged to follow the RICE principle and to curtail any excessive walking throughout this first phase, which usually lasts 5 to 7 days postoperatively. Nonsteroidal anti-inflammatory drugs (NSAIDs) are prescribed, as they have been shown to decrease pain and effusion throughout the postoperative period following arthroscopic meniscectomy.[31]

Table 6-2. Rehabilitation Guidelines Following Arthroscopic Meniscectomy

Phase	Goals	Treatment
Protection	Decrease pain and effusion Decrease quadriceps inhibition	RICE AAROM[a] Quadriceps setting SLR (multiple planes) WBAT[b] with crutches NSAIDS
Moderate protection	Improve range of motion Decrease pain and effusion Normalize gait Improve muscle strength Improve flexibility	Stationary bike Proximal PRE Hamstring PRE Quadriceps isometrics at multiple angles Gait training Stretching Home program Ice/TENS
Early functional	Restore normal range of motion Improve muscle strength, power, and endurance Improve flexibility Improve proprioception Improve conditioning	Quadriceps isotonics (limited arc) Closed kinetic chain exercises Quadricips/hamstring isokinetics
Late functional	Restore normal muscle strength, power, and endurance Restore normal flexibility Full return to sport activity	Advanced closed chain activities Velocity spectrum training Sport-specific activities Return to sport assessment

[a] AAROM, Active assisted range of motion.
[b] WBAT, Weight bearing as tolerated.

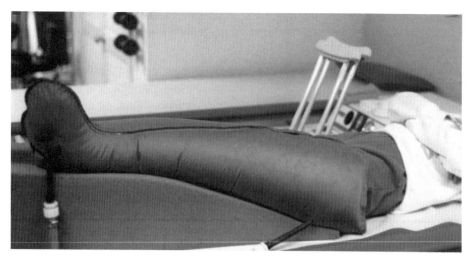

Fig. 6-1. Jobst cryotemp.

Moderate Protection Phase

The moderate protection phase is characterized by decreased pain, mild effusion, range of motion greater than or equal to 90 degrees, and weakness.

At the beginning of this phase, approximately 1 week postoperatively, the patient begins rehabilitation. History, measurements, and tests consistent with an initial evaluation are taken. The patient is allowed to discontinue using crutches upon demonstrating a normal gait pattern. The patient is reminded that "every step is therapy," as normal gait will help facilitate normal range of motion. Using cuff weights, multiple plane SLR are continued in a progressive resisted exercise (PRE) manner. The leg lift in the supine position should be performed with the involved knee in a slightly flexed position to improve the effect of the exercise on the vastus muscle group. Proximal (hip) musculature and hamstring isotonic exercises are added to the program, utilizing various progressive resisted machines (Bodymaster, Nautilus, etc.). In keeping with the concept of total leg strength, calf raises off a step are begun. Submaximal multiple angle quadricep isometrics are performed to improve static muscular strength without causing further joint irritation. Strength gains are angle specific, and physiologic overflow is about 20 degrees in either direction.[32] This exercise is useful in strengthening the vastus medialis oblique, as it has been found to have maximal output in the 60- to 70-degree range of mo-

tion. Electrical stimulation and/or biofeedback are used in conjunction with the isometric exercise for the patient with advanced quadriceps inhibition.

Stationary cycling is initiated to improve range of motion and build muscle strength and endurance. Ergometric cycling has been shown to be an excellent mode of rehabilitation since tibiofemoral compressive forces induced during cycling approach only 1.2 times body weight. This is significantly lower than activities of daily living such as walking (two to four times body weight) or stair climbing (three to seven times body weight).[33] Seat height should be kept high because patellofemoral joint compressive force increases with decreased seat height.[34] When range of motion is limited to less than 100 degrees, a short crank (90 mm) ergometer is employed, decreasing the arc of motion necessary to cycle.[35] This gives the patient a psychological boost because it allows for aerobic exercise (Fig. 6-2).

Flexibility exercises (in the form of hamstring and calf stretching) are started, preferably after cycling since increased tissue temperature promotes a more effective stretch.

Cold application is continued for its analgesic and anti-inflammatory effects. Transcutaneous electrical nerve stimulation (TENS) is used for patients with increased pain.

The patient's home program is expanded to include cuff weight PRE, stationary bike (if available), and stretching. The patient is also provided with a Ther-

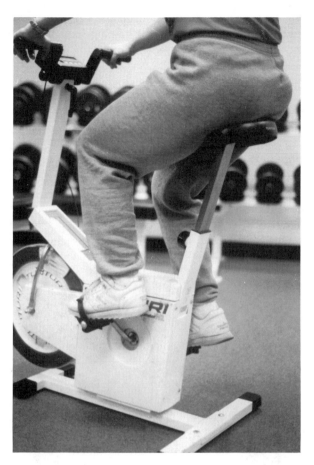

Fig. 6-2. Short-crank ergometer.

aband for standing hip extension, abduction, adduction, and seated knee flexion.

Early Functional Phase

The early functional phase is characterized by an absence of pain, minimal or no effusion, range of motion greater than or equal to 120 degrees, and weakness.

Isotonic knee extension exercise inside a limited arc is begun with low resistance. Initially, a 90- to 30-degree arc is employed since patellofemoral forces are displaced over a wider surface area in this range. The therapist should palpate for crepitus and note any discomfort throughout the range of motion. The arc of motion should then be modified accordingly.

As we function with our feet on the ground, so should we rehabilitate. In this phase, several closed

chain exercises are implemented, keeping in mind the functional progression discussed earlier in this chapter. Contralateral Theraband exercises (Fig. 6-3) provide isometric cocontraction and proprioceptive input throughout the involved extremity. The uninvolved extremity attached to Theraband at the ankle performs hip extension and flexion and/or hip abduction and adduction with the involved extremity in a weight-bearing state with the knee slightly flexed. The resultant forces to the involved knee occur in a sagittal and coronal plane, respectively.

The patient is instructed in a proper squatting technique inside a pain-free and crepitus-free arc. Range of motion is limited to no greater than 90 degrees of knee flexion. The use of sport cord (Fig. 6-4) assists the patient in maintaining proper form, making sure the knees stay behind the feet, decreasing patellofe-

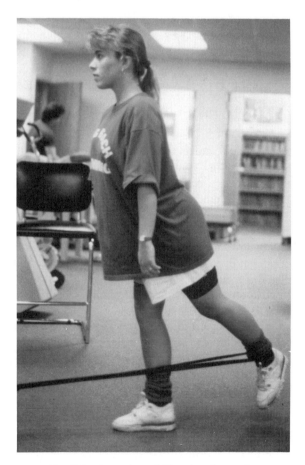

Fig. 6-3. Contralateral Theraband exercise.

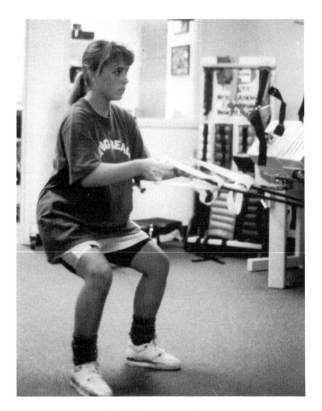

Fig. 6-4. Sport cord squat.

moral forces. Similar technique is reinforced as the leg press machine is utilized bilaterally progressing to unilateral exercise. Lateral step-ups are added to the program with gradual height increments, starting with a phone book and progressing to a normal step.

BAPS (Biomechanical Ankle Platform System; Camp Medical Products, Jackson, MI) is started to facilitate proprioception training to the involved knee joint. From the ground up, changes are seen throughout the closed kinetic chain. For example, as the foot pronates, the tibia internally rotates, causing a valgus force at the knee. Hence, the knee joint acclimates itself to forces in multiple planes, much like those experienced in sport activity. Proprioception is further challenged by increasing the BAPS level (1 to 5) and providing the patient with dumbbells, adding the element of intrinsic loading to the exercise (Fig. 6-5).

Isokinetic exercise is initiated using short arc, submaximal effort, and intermediate speeds (150 to 210 degrees/sec) and progressing to full arc, submaximal effort, and fast speeds. It has been reported that the angular velocity of the knee during gait is 233 degrees/sec.[36] Therefore, specificity of training for functional activities shows the need for training at high speeds.

Late Functional Phase

The late functional phase is characterized by full range of motion, no effusion, and improved muscle strength and flexibility.

Advanced closed chain exercises are added in this stage. The Pro Fitter (Fig. 6-6) continues proprioceptive and balance training. Stairmaster and Versaclimber are utilized to build muscular strength and endurance as well as aerobic conditioning.

Quadriceps and hip musculature stretching are

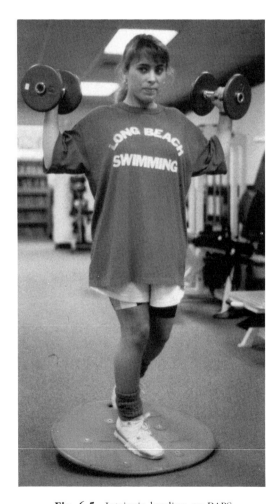

Fig. 6-5. Intrinsic loading on BAPS.

netic speeds.[37] When running forward the patient is encouraged to maintain a controlled sprint rather than a jog. By staying on the ball of the foot, vertical or compressive loading is decreased.

Before allowing the patient to return to sport activity, the therapist needs to do more than achieve normal range of motion and muscle strength. The components of the patient's sport or activity should be incorporated into the rehabilitation program as well. For example, basketball players need to jump and land. Therefore, jumping activities (jump rope, box drill, etc.) should be included in their program. More importantly, they should be taught how to land to protect their knees. Golfers rely on a great deal of tibial rotation throughout the swing; their program, therefore, should include an assessment of their swing and a modification made if necessary. Agility drills in the form of figure eights, carioca, and cutting maneuvers are included

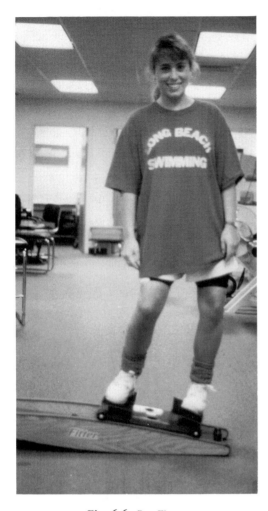

Fig. 6-6. Pro Fitter.

added as increased emphasis is placed on flexibility in this stage.

Isokinetic exercises include the progression to velocity spectrum training (60 to 400 degrees/sec), depending on the needs of the individual patient.

Running is initiated when quadriceps strength approaches 80 percent. At first, an underwater treadmill system (Fig. 6-7) is used since the buoyancy of the water decreases the amount of force incurred at the knee joint. The patient then progresses to retrorunning on a treadmill, as it has been shown that ground reaction force is significantly less during retrorunning versus forward running. Retrorunning has also been found to increase quadriceps strength at slow isoki-

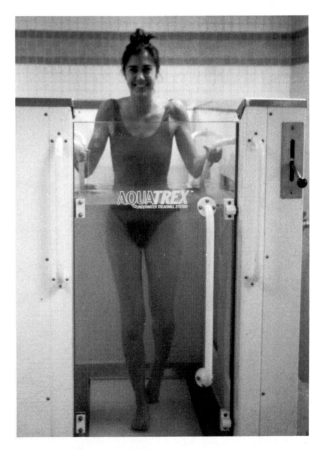

Fig. 6-7. Underwater treadmill system.

here as they replicate components of most team and racquet sports.

Prior to discharge from rehabilitation and the full return to sport activity, a series of tests must be satisfactory:

1. Full range of motion.
2. Flexibility acceptable for the needs of the activity.
3. Total work within 10 percent of the noninvolved extremity as muscle strength is measured isokinetically.
4. Muscular endurance within 10 percent of the noninvolved extremity as measured by the number of leg press repetitions using one-half the patient's body weight.
5. Functional power as measured by standing broad jump.
6. Proprioception measured on BAPS board.
7. Apprehension (lack of) with sport specific activities.

REHABILITATION GUIDELINES FOLLOWING ARTHROSCOPIC MENISCAL REPAIR

Following arthroscopic meniscal repair, a more conservative approach to postoperative management and rehabilitation is taken. Communication with the surgeon is vital. Anatomic site of the repair (vascular [red] or nonvascular [white]) and location of the repair (anterior or posterior) will directly affect the postoperative regimen. For example, the rehabilitation program for a nonvascular (white) posterior repair will be less aggressive than that for a peripheral (red) anterior repair.

Guidelines following meniscal repair will vary in proportion to the number of orthopaedic surgeons performing repairs. Morgan and Casscells[38] recommend immobilization of the knee in full extension for 4 weeks, allowing immediate weight bearing as tolerated. Rosenberg[39] advocates immobilization of the knee for 3 to 4 weeks with non-weight bearing. Bert,[40] on the other hand, recommends knee immobilization in extension, non-weight bearing for 6 weeks, and no sport activity for 6 months.

At the Hospital for Special Surgery, the guideline following meniscal repair includes weight bearing as tolerated and ambulation with crutches for 4 to 6 weeks with the postoperative brace locked at 0-degree extension. During this protection phase, range of motion exercises are limited to 0 to 90 degrees. Multiple-plane straight leg raises in a PRE fashion are employed, as are proximal strengthening exercises. After this protection phase, the patient follows a guideline similar to that discussed earlier in this chapter with the exception that running and sport activity do not begin until 4 months postoperatively.

SUMMARY

Reassessment of the patient at the beginning of each therapy visit is vital. Too rapid a progression in therapy and/or normal functional activities will be demonstrated by increased effusion. This is most likely related to muscular fatigue leaving the articular surfaces unprotected against compressive forces.

To achieve a successful result, a team contribution must be made by the surgeon, the therapist, and the patient. Each plays a vital role since even the finest surgery can lead to failure without proper rehabilitation and patient compliance.

Rehabilitation programs following meniscal surgery should be individualized and based on a functional progression. The therapist, with an understanding of the patient's injury, healing restraints, and knee joint biomechanics, can be progressive, aggressive, and effective in the postoperative program.

ACKNOWLEDGMENTS

I would like to thank Nicholas Sgaglione, Robert Schwartz, Russell Warren, and Thomas Wickiewicz for their help and encouragement in preparing this chapter.

REFERENCES

1. Goldman A, Waugh TR: The menisci of the knee. Orthop Rev 14:67, 1985
2. Arnoczky SP, Adams ME, DeHaven KE et al: Meniscus. p. 427. In Woo SL-Y, Buckwalter JA (eds): Injury and Repair of the Musculoskeletal Soft Tissues. American Academy of Orthopaedic Surgeons, Park Ridge, IL, 1988

3. Arnoczky SP, Warren RF: Microvasculature of the human meniscus. Am J Sports Med 10:90, 1982

4. Müller W: The Knee. Springer-Verlag, New York, 1982

5. Walker P, Erkmann MJ: The role of the meniscus in force transmission across the knee. Clin Orthop 109:184, 1975

6. DiStefano VJ: Function, post-traumatic sequelae and current concepts of knee meniscus injuries: a review. Clin Orthop 151:143, 1980

7. Tapper EM, Hoover NW: Late results after meniscectomy. J Bone Joint Surg 56A:161, 1974

8. Levy IM, Torzilli PA, Warren RF: The effect of medial meniscectomy on anterior-posterior motion of the knee. J Bone Joint Surg 64A:883, 1982

9. DeHaven KE: Injuries to the menisci of the knee. p. 905. In Nicholas JA, Hershmann EB (eds): The Lower Extremity and Spine in Sports Medicine. CV Mosby, St. Louis, 1986

10. DeHaven KE: Diagnosis of acute knee injuries with hemarthrosis. Am J Sports Med 8:9, 1980

11. Cerabona F, Sherman MF, Bonamo JR, Sklar J: Patterns of meniscal injury with acute anterior cruciate ligament tears. Am J Sports Med 16:603, 1988

12. Warren RF, Marshall J: Injuries of the anterior cruciate ligament and medial collateral ligament of the knee. Clin Orthop 136:191, 1978

13. Kornblatt I, Warren RF, Wickiewicz TL: Long term follow-up of anterior cruciate ligament reconstruction using the quadriceps tendon substitution for chronic anterior cruciate ligament insufficiency. Am J Sports Med 16:444, 1988

14. Rosenberg T, Scott S, Paulos L: Arthroscopic surgery: repair of peripheral detachment of the meniscus. Contemp Orthop 10:43, 1985

15. McGinty JB, Guess LF, Marvin RA: Partial or total meniscectomy. J Bone Joint Surg 59A:763, 1977

16. Fairbank TJ: Knee joint changes after meniscectomy. J Bone Joint Surg 30B:664, 1948

17. Ahmed AM, Burke DL: In-vivo measurements of static measure distribution in synovial joints. Part I. Tibial surface of the knee. J Biomech Eng 105:216, 1983

18. Voloshin AS, Wosk J: Shock absorption of meniscectomized and painful knees: a comparative in-vivo study. J Biomed Eng 5:157, 1983

19. Krause WR, Pope MH, Johnson RJ et al: Mechanical changes in the knee after meniscectomy. J Bone Joint Surg 58A:599, 1976

20. Annandale T: An operation for displaced semilunar cartilage. Br Med J 1:779, 1885

21. Arnoczky SP, Warren RF: Microvascular of the meniscus and its response to injury. An experimental study in the dog. Am J Sports Med 11:131, 1983

22. Arnoczky SP, Warren RF, Spivak JM: Meniscal repair using an exogenous fibrin clot. J Bone Joint Surg 70A:1209, 1988

23. O'Brien SJ, Warren RF, Wickiewicz TL et al: Meniscal repair using open techniques. Submitted for publication.

24. Zarins B, Boyce J, Harris BA: Knee rehabilitation following arthroscopic meniscectomy. Clin Orthop Rel Res 198:36, 1985

25. Kennedy JC, Alexander IJ, Hayes KC: Nerve supply of the human knee and its functional importance. Am J Sports Med 10:329, 1982

26. Northmore-Ball MD, Dandy DJ, Jackson RW et al: Arthroscopic open and partial total meniscectomy. J Bone Joint Surg 65B:400, 1983

27. Gillquist J, Oretorp N: Arthroscopic partial meniscectomy. Contemp Orthop 167:29, 1982

28. Kegerreis S: The construction and implementation of a functional progression as a component of athletic rehabilitation. J Orthop Sports Phys Ther July-Aug:14, 1983

29. Wallis EL, Logan GA: Figure improvement and body conditioning through exercise. Prentice-Hall, Englewood Cliffs, NJ, 1964

30. Gray G: Successful strategies for closed chain testing and rehabilitation. Chain Reaction Seminar. May 1989

31. Ogilvie-Harris DJ, Baver M, Correy P: Prostaglandin inhibition and the rate of recovery after arthroscopic meniscectomy. J Bone Joint Surg 67B:567, 1985

32. Knapic JJ, Ramos MU, Wright JE: Non-specific effects of isometric and isokinetic strength training at a particular joint angle (abstract). Med Sci Sports Exerc 12:120, 1980

33. Ericson MO, Nisell R: Tibiofemoral joint forces during ergometer cycling. Am J Sports Med 14:285, 1986

34. Ericson MO, Nisell R: Patellofemoral joint forces during ergometer cycling. Phys Ther 67:1365, 1987

35. Schwartz RE, Asnis PD, Cavanaugh JT et al: Short crank cycle ergometry. J Orthop Sports Phys Ther 13:95, 1991

36. Wyatt MP, Edwards AM: Comparison of quadricep and hamstring torque values during isokinetic exercise. J Orthop Sports Phys Ther 3:48, 1981

37. Threlkeld AJ, Horn TS, Wojtowicz GM: Kinematics, ground reaction force and muscle balance produced by backward running. J Orthop Sports Phys Ther 11:56, 1989

38. Morgan CD, Casscells SW: Arthroscopic meniscal repair. Arthroscopy 2:1, 1986

39. Rosenberg T: Meniscus Repair and Rehabilitation. Presented at Annual University of Utah Arthroscopy Course, Snowbird, Utah, Jan. 1990.

40. Bert J: Meniscus Repair and Rehabilitation. Presented at Annual University of Utah Arthroscopy Course, Snowbird, Utah, Jan. 1990.

7

Medial Collateral Ligament Injuries: Diagnosis, Treatment, and Rehabilitation

KEVIN WILK
WILLIAM G. CLANCY, JR.

INTRODUCTION

Ligamentous injuries to the knee are a very common occurrence in sports and account for 25 to 40 percent of all knee injuries.[1,2] Sprains of the medial collateral ligament (MCL) occur most frequently.[3] Sprains are clinically classified by severity into three grades. Grade I sprains consist of microtrauma to the structure with no increased laxity. Grade II sprains occur as a result of moderate trauma with a slight increase in clinical laxity, and grade III sprains result from severe trauma with complete disruption and significant laxity. With the frequent occurrence of MCL sprains in sports, it is important for the clinician to understand the basic sciences and clinical sciences related to the identification and treatment of MCL injury.

This chapter discusses the anatomy, biomechanics, and healing process following injury of the MCL. In addition, it discusses the mechanism of injury and the evaluation of the medial aspect of the knee. The treatment of MCL sprains is discussed in detail. We explore operative and nonoperative treatment and explain the scientific basis and clinical rationale for both treatment choices.

ANATOMY

The literature has produced at times significant confusion concerning the accurate delineation of what structures comprise the MCL of the knee. Some con-

sider the posterior oblique ligament to be part of the MCL, while others describe it as a separate ligament. The MCL has frequently been described as one structure, whereas Warren and Marshall[4] emphasized the contribution of the midmedial capsule.

The MCL (frequently referred to as the tibial collateral ligament) provides the main ligamentous restraint on the medial side of the knee. The MCL has three portions (Fig. 7-1). The deep portion is a thickening of the medial capsule that originates from the edge of the medial femoral condyle and extends vertically to the periphery of the medial tibial plateau. This portion has a strong attachment to the medial meniscus. The second portion of the MCL is the superficial portion (Fig. 7-2). This portion is delta shaped, with a wide origin just below the adductor tubercle of the medial femoral condyle. This superficial portion extends inferiorly and narrows to insert distally 3 to 4 cm below the tibial plateau beneath the tendons of the pes anseriuns. The MCL and pes anserinus tendon are separated by the pes anserinus bursa. Brantigan and Voshell[5] and subsequently Warren and Marshall[4] have demonstrated that the superficial portion is separate from the deep portion by a bursa, the bursa of Voshell. The third portion of the MCL is the point where these two structures blend together in the posteromedial portion of the knee to form the posterior oblique ligament. Hughston and Eilers[6] have termed the thickness of the posteromedial corner the posterior oblique ligament. The superficial

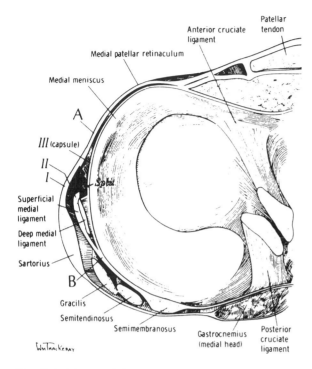

Fig. 7-1. The medial meniscus. (From Warren and Marshall,[23] with permission.)

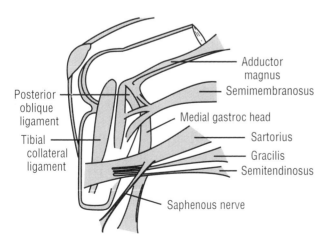

Fig. 7-2. Anatomy of the medial compartment.

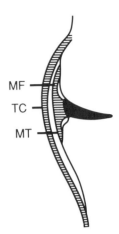

Fig. 7-3. Meniscofemoral (MF) and meniscotibial (MT) portion of the medial capsular ligament. Tibial or medial collateral ligament (TC).

fibers are vertical and contain a band that runs obliquely to join with several slips of the semimembranosus muscle. This serves to reinforce the posteromedial corner of the knee. In addition, proximally the superficial portion of the MCL has been noted to attach to the vastus medialis oblique (VMO) portion of the quadriceps femoris muscle near the ligamentous femoral attachment site. The attachment of the MCL to the VMO would appear to be very important from a neurologic control standpoint, providing feedback from the ligament to the muscle regarding tension.

The deep portion of the MCL has a firm attachment to the medial meniscus. This attachment is most significant in the posteromedial aspect. The capsular attachments to the menisci have been classified as the meniscofemoral and meniscotibial ligaments (Fig. 7-3).

BIOMECHANICS

The biomechanics of the MCL is well documented in the literature.[4,6–12] The MCL is the primary restraint to medial opening (or abduction) of the knee at both 5 and 25 degrees of knee flexion. Grood and associates[7] have demonstrated with selective tissue sectioning that

Table 7-1. Rehabilitation of Grade I, II, and III Isolated MCL (and Lateral Collateral Ligament) Sprains

This program may be accelerated for grade I MCL/LCL sprains or may be extended depending on the severity of the injury. The following schedule serves as a guideline to help return an athlete to a preinjury state.

Note that if there is any increase in pain or swelling or loss of range of motion the progression of the patient may be too rapid.

Phase I—Maximal Protection Phase

Goals:
1. Early protected range of motion (ROM)
2. Prevent quadriceps atrophy
3. Decrease effusion and pain

A. Day 1
1. Ice, compression, elevation
2. Knee hinge brace, nonpainful ROM (brace worn at night)
3. Crutches with weight bearing as tolerated
4. Passive range of motion (PROM)/active assisted range of motion (AAROM) to maintain ROM
5. Electrical muscle stimulus to quadriceps (8 h/d)
6. Isometric quadriceps, quad sets, 60 repeats; 3 × day
   Straight leg raises (SLR), 3 sets of 15; 3 × day

B. Day 2
1. Continue isometrics (quad sets, SLR)
2. Hamstring setting
3. Well leg exercises
4. Whirlpool for ROM (cold for first 3 to 4 days, then warm)
5. High voltage galvanic stimulation (HVGS) to control swelling
6. Continue above

C. Days 3–7
1. Continue above
2. Crutches with weight bearing as tolerated
3. ROM as tolerated
4. Eccentric quadriceps work
5. Bicycle for ROM stimulus
6. Multiangle isometrics with electric stimulus to quadriceps
7. Initiate hip abduction and extension, 3 sets of 15
8. Brace worn at night; brace at day as needed

Phase II—Moderate Protection Phase

Criteria for Progression:
1. No increase in instability
2. No increase in swelling
3. Minimal tenderness
4. PROM 10–100 degrees

Goals:
1. Full painless ROM
2. Restore strength
3. Ambulation without crutches

A. Week 2
1. Continue strengthening program with progressive resistive exercises (PREs)
2. Continue electric muscle stimulus
3. Continue ROM exercises
4. Multiangle isometrics with electric stimulus
5. Discontinue crutches
6. Bicycle for endurance (Fitron interval)
7. Water exercises, running in water forward and backward
8. Full ROM exercises

9. Flexibility exercises, hamstrings, quadriceps, iliotibial band, etc.
10. Proprioception training
11. Initiate active knee extension 90–40 degrees
12. Initiate minisquat program

B. Days 11–14
1. Continue as week 2
2. PREs emphasis quadriceps, medial hamstrings, hip abduction
3. Initiate isokinetics, submaximal → maximal effort, fast contractile velocities
4. Jogging (no cutting)

Phase III—Minimal Protection Phase

Criteria for Progression:
1. No instability
2. No swelling or tenderness
3. Full painless ROM

Goals:
1. Increase strength/power/endurance
2. Improve neuromuscular coordination

A. Week 3
1. Continue strengthening program
   Emphasis
      Fast-speed isokinetics
      Eccentric quadriceps
      Isotonic hip adduction, medial hamstrings
      Knee extensions, minisquats (time bouts)
      Tubing exercises (time bouts)
      Leg press, squats, plyometric jumps, step-ups (time bouts)
2. Isokinetic test
3. Proprioception training
4. Endurance exercises
      Stationary bike 30–40 minutes
      Nordic Trac, swimming, etc.
5. Continue jogging, full-speed straight lines
6. Continue water running—straight lines → figure eights

Phase IV—Return to Activity Phase

Criteria for Progression:
1. No instability
2. No tenderness, swelling
3. Full ROM

Goals:
1. Regaining athletic ability specific to players' sport and position
2. Endurance and strength
3. Emphasis on sport-specific training

Continued

Table 7-1. (*continued*)

Phase IV—Return to Activity Phase

A. Week 4
1. Continue same as week 3 with strengthening exercises
2. Repeat isokinetic test
3. Agility drills
   Figure eights
   Circles
   45-degree cutting over 20 yards
4. Acceleration-deceleration speed drills of 20, 40, and 60 yards
5. 20-, 40-, 60-yard sprints
6. Continue proprioception training
7. Implement drills related to player's sport and position
8. Athlete returns to contact sport with lateral knee brace

Return to Activity Criteria:
1. No instability
2. Full ROM
3. Isokinetic test that fulfills criteria
4. Satisfactory clinical examination

Maintenance Program:
1. Continue strengthening program
2. Continue flexibility exercises
3. Continue proprioception exercises

Table 7-2. Methods of Interpreting Test Data

Nine critical isokinetic test parameters
1. Peak torque to body weight ratio
2. Bilateral mean peak torque comparison
3. Torque curve analysis
4. Bilateral total work comparison
5. Unilateral peak torque ratio
6. Average power to body weight ratio
7. Bilateral peak torque comparison
8. Time ratio to torque development
9. Endurance ratio (first repetition to last repetition)

Quadriceps torque to body weight ratios

	Men (%)	Women (%)
60 degrees	100–115	80–95
180 degrees	60–75	50–65
300 degrees	40–55	30–45
450 degrees	30–40	20–29

Hamstring/quadriceps unilateral ratio[a]

60 degrees	6–69%
180 degrees	70–79%
300 degrees	80–94%
450 degrees	95–100%

[a] Anterior cruciate ligament patients add 10%; posterior cruciate ligament patients subtract 10%.
(Adapted from Wilk,[54] with permission.)

at 25 degrees of knee flexion the MCL affords 78 percent of the restraint to medial opening. The secondary restraints to the abduction loads are the anterior and posterior cruciate ligaments (13 percent) and the medial and posteromedial capsule (7 percent). At 5 degrees of knee flexion, the MCL affords 57 percent of the restraint and the capsular restraint increases from 7 to 25 percent, while the cruciate ligaments afford essentially the same restraint. In addition, Kennedy and Fowler,[8] Markolf et al.[10] and Mains et al.[9] have reported significant increases in valgus laxity after sectioning of the MCL. Thus, these reports document that as knee extension increases, the posterior portion of the MCL, namely, the oblique posterior ligament portion, becomes taut and provides increased stability. Conversely, as the knee flexes to 30 degrees, the posterior portion of the MCL becomes lax and the anterior portion of the MCL provides the majority of the restraint to medial opening.

A portion of the MCL is taut throughout the range of motion of the knee. This is due in part to the semicircular point of origin on the femur. The tautness of the MCL increases as the knee reaches full extension. Warren and Marshall[4] noted that the anterior 5 mm of the MCL remains taut as the knee goes into flexion and that the entire MCL remains taut as the knee goes into extension (Fig. 7-4). This suggested to them that the anterior-most fibers of the MCL are the prime stabilizers. With increasing loads and ultimate failure of the tibial collateral ligament and mid-medial capsule, then the posterior oblique ligament exhibits significant damage.[12] Note that these studies were done on specimens in which both the flexion angle and rotation were fixed.

Müller[11] noted that the MCL prevents external rotation of the tibia. Sectioning studies by Warren et al.[12] documented that after sectioning of the MCL there is an increase in tibial external rotation with the knee in flexion. Others[6] have suggested that the posterior oblique ligament and the posterior portion of the MCL are the primary restraint to external rotation. It has been clinically evident that forced external rotation may produce partial injury to the MCL but probably seldom produces complete disruption without an additional valgus force.

In summary, the anterior-most fibers of the MCL are the primary restraints to a valgus force. The postero-

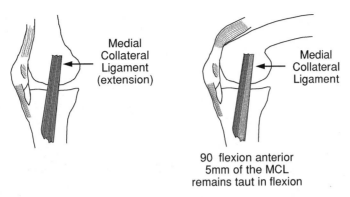

Fig. 7-4. Biomechanics of the medial collateral ligament.

medial fibers of the MCL become a very important restraint to a valgus force only after injury to the anterior-most fibers. Sectioning of the MCL will also produce increased external rotation of the tibia. The anterior and posterior cruciate ligaments act as secondary restraints to valgus opening of the knee when there is complete disruption of the MCL, but they have no effect on resisting excessive external tibial rotation owing to their anatomic insertions.

There are injuries in which a complete disruption of the anterior cruciate or posterior cruciate ligament occurs with only a partial injury to the MCL. These injuries are not a result of pure abduction forces but are a combination of rotation, hyperextension, abduction, and quadriceps deceleration forces.

MECHANISM OF INJURY

The MCL is most often injured as a result of a valgus force or combined valgus and external rotation forces. This injury can be caused by an external force such as a blow to the lateral aspect of the knee or falling to the side with the ipsilateral leg kept firmly fixed. Injury to the MCL is often associated with contact sports such as football in which there are frequent blows to the lateral side of the knee.

Some believe that medial meniscus pathologies can also lead to MCL injury. The deep portion of the MCL attaches to the periphery of the medial meniscus, and this firm attachment can often cause a peripheral tear due to a valgus force. However, unpublished studies by Clancy (personal communication) have docu-

mented by arthroscopy that in isolated MCL injuries there is rarely a true meniscal tear. The tear occurs in the meniscotibial or meniscofemoral portion of the deep capsule. These capsular injuries do not require surgery or immobilization (Clancy, personal communication).

Maturation also has effects on the site of MCl failures. Tipton et al.[13] and Woo et al.[14] have demonstrated changes in the structural properties of the MCL bone complex during maturation in animals. Their findings indicated that the ligamentous attachment site was weak until the epiphyses closed. Thus, the MCL is affected by the proximity of the tibial growth plate. In their studies, the MCL failed by tibial avulsion in the skeletally immature. In contrast, after closure of the epiphysis, only 12 percent of failures were due to tibial avulsion.[14] It would also appear in older individuals (more than 50 years of age) that there is a higher incidence of bone avulsion failure compared with younger persons.[15] Thus, when evaluating the skeletally immature or, in contrast, the older patient the clinician must be sure to clinically evaluate (radiograph) for avulsion fracture. In individuals from epiphysis closure to 50 years of age midsubstance tears of the ligamentous tissue are most prevalent.

CLINICAL EXAMINATION

A careful and thoroughly detailed history is obtained, including a complete description of the mechanism of injury, as well as the occurrence of any previous knee injuries. This is followed with a thorough clinical examination, which is essential to help clarify the degree of injury. Examination of the knee begins with the patient's leg relaxed so the knee can be adequately evaluated. In some cases, an examination with the patient under spinal or general anesthesia may be required to obtain adequate muscle relaxation. Knee examination is performed with the patient supine and the thigh supported by the table, which assists in relaxation of the thigh musculature. The least painful tests are performed first. The Lachman test, performed at 20 degrees of flexion, and the anterior drawer test are the least painful and most important tests to determine anterior cruciate ligament integrity. The knee is then flexed to 90 degrees, and the anterior tibial step is assessed as well as posterior cruciate ligament status (posterior drawer test). Valgus stress testing with the knee in full extension (Fig. 7-5) and then in 30 degrees of flexion (Fig. 7-6) is performed to determine the

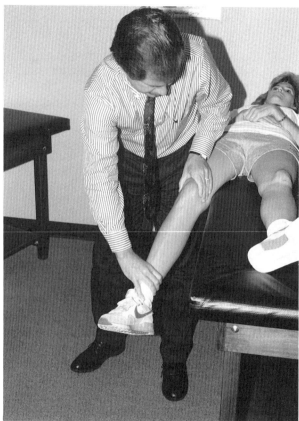

Fig. 7-6. Valgus stress test in flexion.

extent of damage to the MCL and medial capsule. The degree of medial opening is compared with that of the contralateral knee to determine the extent of the injury. The amount of valgus opening is noted and classified to document the degree or severity of the injury.

Mild medial laxity with applied valgus stress with the knee in full extension indicates damage to the MCL, the posterior oblique ligament, and the medial capsular ligament. If there is gross instability (increased medial opening) at full extension, injury to the cruciates should be suspected and specific cruciate tests should be performed at that time (Fig. 7-7). With the knee in 30 degrees of flexion, the posterior capsule and posterior oblique ligament become lax. Medial opening with applied valgus is indicative of damage to the MCL (Fig. 7-8).

In addition, to measure quantitively the amount of medial opening with applied valgus stress, the ex-

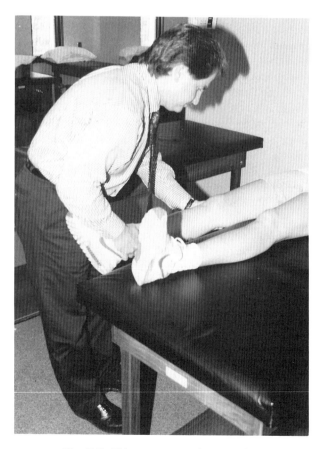

Fig. 7-5. Valgus stress test in extension.

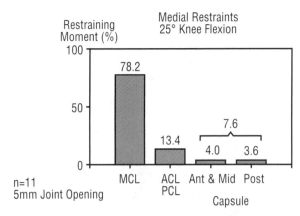

Fig. 7-7. Valgus stress test restraints in flexion. (From Grood et al.,[7] with permission.)

aminer should also assess the quality of the end point or end-feel. With normal knee stability, valgus stress would elicit a firm end point. In complete grade III tears of the MCL, there is no end point until the secondary restraints have been encountered. The quantity and quality of the joint opening should always be compared with that of the contralateral side.

When performing valgus stress testing of the knee, care should be taken to control and prevent axial rotation. This rotatory motion may be misinterpreted as increased medial laxity.[16] Care should be taken to perform single-plane testing to ensure specific ligamentous structural testing.

In addition, careful and meticulous palpation of bony and soft tissue should be part of a comprehensive

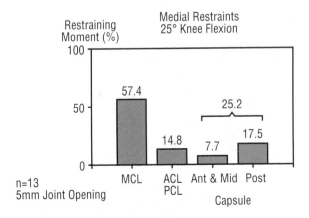

Fig. 7-8. Valgus stress test restraints in extension. (From Grood et al.,[7] with permission.)

clinical examination. The patient can present with point tenderness on the adductor tubercle and/or along the MCL on the joint line (Fig. 7-9). Anterior joint line tenderness may indicate medial meniscus injury, and careful examination must be performed (Fig. 7-10). Active range of motion may elicit pain near the terminal extension point, and pain with knee flexion past 90 and 100 degrees may be present in the acute phase. Mild soft tissue swelling is present and easily palpated on examination. A large hemarthrosis is present when anterior cruciate ligament injury has occurred. When the classic "unhappy triad" of O'Donoghue[25] is present, the hemarthrosis may be minimal due to extravasation of blood through the tear of the medial capsule.

As mentioned earlier, when evaluating for an MCL injury, care must be taken to evaluate the medial meniscus and anterior cruciate ligament for possible injury. Persistent joint line pain on or near the MCL should be carefully evaluated for medial meniscus pathology. The traditional McMurray's test and Apley compression test have been used for evaluation of menisci pathology. However, unfortunately these two tests are not reliable when performed on patients with MCL injury. This is because a rotatory movement is performed by the examiner on the tibia, which loads the injured MCL and produces pain. The use of magnetic resonance imaging (MRI) may be most beneficial. If there exists any question whether there is a first-degree MCL sprain (no laxity present on clinical examination) or a medial menisci tear, an MRI should be obtained.

Unfortunately, the size of the effusion present does not necessarily correlate with the injury. A small effusion may be present with a complete disruption of the MCL as the fluid may extravasate through the capsular deficit.

TREATMENT

Presently, there exist two primary principles in the treatment of MCL injuries. One principle is to protect the injury site from further damage in the early stages of healing by a period of immobilization. The other principle is to promote and accelerate the remodeling of healed tissue by the application of controlled stresses immediately following injury (early or im-

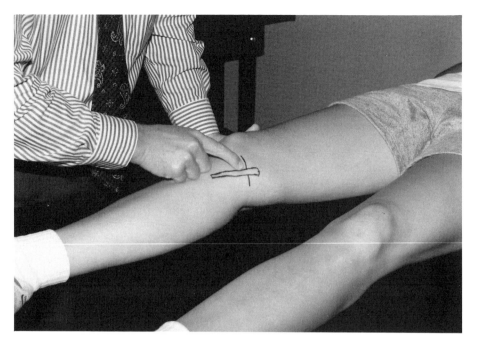

Fig. 7-9. Palpation of medial collateral ligament.

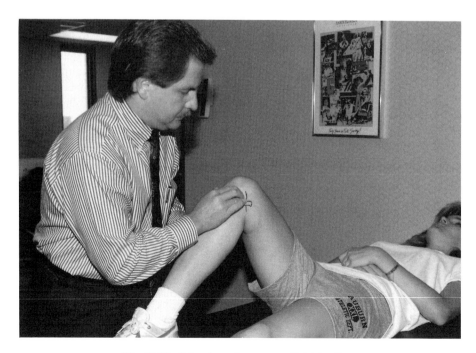

Fig. 7-10. Palpation of anteromedial joint line.

mediate mobilization). In the past, clinicians have utilized the former. Presently, however, most clinicians advocate the latter for treatment of MCL injuries.

Ellasasser et al.[16] reported 98 percent successful return to professional football only 3 to 8 weeks following MCL injury when the treatment consisted of mobilization and early exercise and no surgery. Derscheid and Garrick[17] reported successful return to football 3 weeks after a grade II MCL injury when treatment consisted of nonoperative early motion. Jones et al.[18] reported good results with nonoperative treatment in MCL sprains in high school football players. Frank and coworkers[19-21] reported spontaneous healing of sectioned MCLs in animals without surgery and immobilization. Vailas et al.[22] stated that "the repair process was delayed by immobilization and accelerated by early motion." Goldstein and Barmada[23] found that mobilized MCL sprains were stronger than immobilized MCL sprains in sectioned rabbit knees.

In contrast, several investigators[6,24] have reported excellent results treating MCL sprains with surgery and immobilization. O'Donoghue[25] recommended surgical repair followed subsequent immobilization. Goshall and Hansen[26] recommended primary surgical repair of the injured MCL. Other investigators[6,26-28] have also reported excellent results following primary repair of a completely torn MCL. Indelicato[29,30] reported excellent results treating grade III MCL sprains with 2 weeks of immobilization, followed by several weeks of restricted motion. Similar results were reported by Fetto and Marshall[31] without surgery and immobilization.

Thus, some controversy exists among researchers on two basic principles: (1) whether to surgically repair the grade III MCL injury and (2) whether to allow mobilization or immobilization during the early rehabilitation phases.

Healing Response of the MCL

Woo et al.[44] investigated the question of immobilization. In their study of sectioned canine MCL they investigated three groups: group 1, no repair and immediate activities; group 2, repair and 3 weeks of immobilization; and group 3, repair and 6 weeks of immobilization. They evaluated the MCL for laxity and structural properties at 6, 12, and 48 weeks postoperatively. It was determined that the unrepaired and

immediate motion group had the best results. The valgus-varus laxity and structural properties returned to values comparable to the contralateral side at 12 weeks. However, the mechanical properties of MCL were slower to return and did not become completely normal even at 48 weeks. They concluded that "early mobilization is the treatment of choice of *isolated MCL injuries*." In addition, Woo and associates[32] noted increased bone avulsion failure in the MCL complex after immobilization. This weakening of the periosteal insertion site was also noted by Noyes et al.[33] when investigating the effects of immobilization on the anterior cruciate ligaments-bone unit. These investigators[32,33] and others[34,35] observed subperiosteal resorption of bone, causing a weakening of the ligamentous fibers attaching to the insertion site. Thus, an increase in avulsion failure was noted. Several researchers[8-11,36,37] have supported the hypothesis that the prognosis of MCL healing is poor when combined with injury to other structures of the knee, particularly the anterior cruciate ligament. Therefore, with complete loss of the anterior cruciate ligament the healing response of the MCL is greatly diminished.[11,37] In addition, there is a marked deterioration of joint surfaces and periarticular osteophyte formation.

The healing process of the injured MCL has been described by Jack,[38] Frank,[21] and Laws.[36] The process has been divided into several phases.[42,43] Phase I (acute inflammation and reaction) occurs during the first 72 hours. There is hematoma formation manifested by swelling, redness, warmth, and pain that occurs owing to cellular interaction. Phase II (repair and regeneration) lasts from 48 to 72 hours after the injury until approximately 6 weeks after the injury. It is characterized by subsidence of the inflammation and the onset of healing. Phase III (remodeling and maturation) requires an extended period (12 months or more) to become maximal. During this phase the healing ligament becomes progressively stronger. It has been noted[21,44] that the original tensile strength is not regained, and probably the maximum return is 70 to 75 percent. In complete midsubstance MCL injuries, the unrepaired or immobilize injuries heal by scar formation rather than true ligament regeneration. Motion and stress appear to accelerate some of the processes.[6,22]

The MCL, being a periarticular ligament, probably

heals through the production and remodeling process of scar tissue. Thus, there are many factors that will influence the healing process (age, nutritional status, anemia, diabetes mellitus, uremia). In addition, other factors such as degree of injury, infection, associated injuries, synovial environment, blood supply, mechanical stress, and mediators of inflammation will influence the healing process.

We have discussed the associated anatomy and biomechanics of the MCL. In addition, the mechanism of injury, clinical examination, and the healing process have been described. Now we will discuss the surgical and nonsurgical treatment of MCL sprains.

Treatment of MCL Injuries

There is little debate now regarding whether or not to surgically repair the MCL. The literature suggests that certain conditions must be met before optimal healing of the MCL can occur: (1) the torn ligament fibers must remain in continuity or be confined within a well-vascularized soft tissue bed; (2) controlled, functional stresses help stimulate and direct the healing process; and (3) there must be some protection against harmful stresses during collagen synthesis and the remodeling or maturation phases. Thus, we have come to adopt the following criteria for surgical repair of the medial collateral ligament: (1) failed conservative nonoperative treatment; (2) complete rupture of the MCL with concomitant anterior cruciate ligament instability (in this case, the anterior cruciate ligament should be reconstructed).

The severity of injury determined on physical examination determines the rehabilitation course and duration. The rehabilitation program is the same for minor to severe (grade I to grade III) MCL sprains. However, the duration of treatment in each phase may be extended. The nonoperative rehabilitation of MCL sprains is based on five basic rehabilitation principles:

1. The effects of immobilization must be minimized.
2. Never overstress healing tissue.
3. The patient must fulfill specific criteria to progress from stage to stage.
4. The program must be based on current clinical and scientific research.
5. The program must be adaptable to each patient.

With these basic principles in mind, our rehabilitation program is based on early motion, early weight bearing, early control of pain and effusion, and retardation of muscle atrophy (especially the quadriceps). This program has been successful in 98 percent of the cases, with the average days lost from athletics being 9.2 days for grade I injuries and 17.8 days for grade II injuries.[45]

The program is divided into four phases: maximal protection, moderate protection, minimal protection, and return to activity/maintenance. The complete program is outlined in Table 7-1.

In the first phase, the maximal protection phase, goals are to (1) achieve early protected range of motion, (2) prevent quadricep atrophy, and (3) decrease pain and effusion. The treatment consists of ice, compression, elevation, and a brace that will allow full nonpainful range of motion. In addition, crutches are used for the first few days for protection and weight bearing as tolerated. Immediately following the injury, aggressive supervised physical therapy is initiated aimed at retarding muscle atrophy and restoring full range of motion. Electrical muscular stimulation is used to re-educate the quadriceps muscle and also to retard quadriceps muscular atrophy.[46–48] Range of motion exercises are initiated immediately using passive and active assisted range of motion and then progressing to active range of motion. The purposes of the range of motion exercises are to re-establish normal range of motion and also to allow proper alignment of newly synthesized collagen tissue. This ensures strong elastic scar formation. Other advantages to early motion include retarding capsular contractures, maintaining articular cartilage nutrition, and decreasing disuse effects.[49–53] By the end of the first week, more aggressive strengthening exercises such as minisquats, leg press, and quadriceps eccentrics can be initiated.

The patient who has nearly full range of motion, minimal tenderness, and no change in instability or swelling can progress to phase II, the moderate protection phase. The goals in this phase are to regain the remaining range of motion, achieve unrestricted ambulation without assistive devices, and restore muscular strength, power, and endurance.

The emphasis of this phase is strengthening. More aggressive strengthening exercises are begun (isokinetics, heavy progressive resisted exercise, and also a pool running program). In addition, flexibility and proprioceptive training are emphasized. The progressive resisted exercise program for knee extension must be monitored for patellofemoral joint irritation, crepitation, and/or pain. If this occurs the program must be modified to a range that is pain-free and crepitus-free to prevent further articular cartilage breakdown.

The next phase of the program is the minimal protection phase. In this phase the goals are to increase strength, power, and endurance and to improve neuromuscular coordination. The emphasis is now on functional return and the exercises are geared toward function. A running program is initiated as well as high-speed exercise. Agility drills, balance drills, and endurance bouts are used. In this phase we emphasize functional exercises in the closed kinetic chain.

The final phase, return to activity and maintenance, is initiated once the patient fulfills specific criteria. The patient must present with no pain or tenderness, no instability, an isokinetic test that fulfills a specific criteria (Table 7-2),[54] and a satisfactory clinical examination. An athlete who obtains these parameters can return to sport training and begin a maintenance program. At this time a program is designed to continue the strengthing process of the musculotendinous unit and continue to facilitate the attainment of power, endurance, and neuromuscular control. This is usually accomplished through functional exercises such as close kinetic chain and by continuing to strengthen the quadriceps while guarding against patellofemoral irritation and articular cartilage breakdown.

Surgical Management

In severe (grade III) sprains to the MCL complex, some physicians believe a primary surgical repair should be performed.[11,24] Müller[11] states that spontaneous healing of grade III MCL sprains is rare and therefore recommends surgical repair.·

The primary repair should include reapproximation of torn structures to promote the healing process. The isometric position must be carefully checked by repeatedly flexing and extending the knee; there should be consistent tension throughout the range. If not, tension should be applied or diminished.

At the time of surgery, there should be careful evaluation and visualization of the meniscus and anterior

and posterior cruciate ligaments. If any of these structures are involved, appropriate surgical procedures should be performed.

The rehabilitation program following primary repair of the MCL is more aggressive today than before. Immediate postoperatively we allow as much motion as possible. In addition, full weight bearing is allowed with a brace locked at 0° of extension. Early strengthening is initiated and the program progresses in a manner similar to that of the nonoperative program as previously described (Table 7-1).

REFERENCES

1. Powell J: 636,000 injuries annually in high school football. Athl Train 22:19, 1987
2. DeHaven KE, Litner DM: Athletic injuries: comparison by age, sport, and gender. Am J Sports Med 14:218, 1986
3. Woo SLY, Buckwalter JA: Injury and Repair Of The Musculoskeletal Soft Tissue. American Academy of Orthopaedic Surgeons Symposium, 1988
4. Warren LF, Marshall JL: The supporting structures and layers on the medial side of the knee—an anatomical analysis. J Bone Joint Surg 61A:56, 1979
5. Brantigan OC, Voshell AF: The mechanics of the ligaments and menisci of the knee joint. J Bone Joint Surg 23A:44, 1941
6. Hughston JC, Eilers AF: The role of the posterior oblique ligament and repairs of acute medial (collateral) ligament tears of the knee. J Bone Joint Surg 55A:923, 1973
7. Grood ES, Noyes FR, Butler DL et al: Ligamentous and capsular restraints preventing straight medial and lateral laxity in intact human cadaver knees. J Bone Joint Surg 63A:1257, 1981
8. Kennedy JC, Fowler PJ: Medial and anterior instability of the knee. An anatomical and clinical study using stress machines. J Bone Joint Surg 53A:1257, 1971
9. Mains DB, Andrews JG, Stonecipher T: Medial and anterior posterior ligament stability of the human knee, measured with stress apparatus. Am J Sports Med 5:144, 1977
10. Markolf KL, Mensch JS, Amstutz HC: Stiffness and laxity of the knee—the contribution of supporting structures. J Bone Joint Surg 58A:583, 1976
11. Müller W: The Knee: Form, Function, and Ligament Reconstruction. Springer-Verlag, New York, 1983
12. Warren LF, Marshall JL, Girgis F: The prime static stabilizer of the medial side of the knee. J Bone Joint Surg, 56A:665, 1974

13. Tipton CM, Mathies RD, Martin RK: Influence of age and sex on strength of bone-ligament junctions in knee joints of rats. J Bone Joint Surg 60A:230, 1978

14. Woo SLY, Orlando CA, Gomez MA, et al: Tensile properties of the medial collateral ligament as a function of age. J Orthop Res 4:133, 1986

15. Noyes FR, Grood ES: The strength of the anterior cruciate ligament in humans and rhesus monkeys: age-related and species-related changes. J Bone Joint Surg 58A:1074, 1976

16. Ellasasser JC, Reynolds FC, Omohundro JR: The non-operative treatment of collateral ligament injuries of the knee in professional football players. J Bone Joint Surg 56A:1185, 1974

17. Derscheid GL, Garrick JG: Medial collateral ligament injuries in football; non-operative management of grade I & II sprains. Am J Sports Med 9:981, 1981

18. Jones RE, Henley MB, Francis P: Non-operative management of isolated grade III collateral ligament injury in high school football players. Clin Orthop 213:137, 1986

19. Frank C, Akeson WH, Woo SLY, et al: Physiology and therapeutic value of passive joint motion. Clin Orthop 185:113, 1984

20. Frank CB, Schachar N, Dittrich D: Natural history of healing in the repaired medial collateral ligament. J Orthop Res 1:179, 1983

21. Frank C, Woo SLY, Amiel D, et al: Medial collateral ligament healing—a multidisciplinary assessment in rabbits. Am J Sports Med 11:379, 1983

22. Vailas AC, Tipton CM, Matthes RD et al: Physical activity and its influence on the repair process of medial collateral ligaments. Connect Tissue Res 9:225, 1981

23. Goldstein WM, Barmada R: Early mobilization of rabbit medial collateral ligament repairs: biomechanic and histologic study. Arch Phys Med Rehabil 65:239, 1984

24. Hughston JC, Barrett GR: Acute anteromedial rotary instability. Long-term results of surgical repair. J Bone Joint Surg 65A:145, 1983

25. O'Donoghue DH: Surgical treatment of fresh injuries to the major ligaments of the knee. J Bone Joint Surg 32A:721, 1950

26. Godshall RW, Hansen CA: The classification, treatment and follow-up evaluation of medial collateral ligament injuries of the knee. J Bone Joint Surg 56A:1316, 1974

27. Pickett JC, Altizer TJ: Injuries of the ligaments of the knee. Clin Orthop 76:27, 1971

28. Smillie IS: Injuries of the Knee Joint. Williams & Wilkins, Baltimore, 1946

29. Indelicato PA: Non-operative treatment of complete tears of the medial collateral ligament of the knee. J Bone Joint Surg 65A:323, 1983

30. Indelicato PA: Injury to the medial capsuloligamentous complex, p. 197. In Feagin JA (ed): The Crucial Ligaments, Churchill Livingstone, New York, 1988

31. Fetto JF, Marshall JL: Medial collateral ligament injuries of the knee: a rationale for treatment. Clin Orthop 132:206, 1978

32. Woo SLY, Gomez MA, Sites TJ et al: The biomechanical and morphological changes in the medial collateral ligament of the rabbit after immobilization and remobilization. J Bone Joint Surg 69A:1200, 1987

33. Noyes FR, DeLucas JL. Toruik DJ: Biomechanics of anterior cruciate ligament failure: an analysis of strain-rate, sensitivity and mechanism of failure in primates. J Bone Joint Surg 56A:236, 1974

34. Laros GS, Tipton CM, Cooper RR: Influences of physical activity on ligament insertions in the knees of dogs. J Bone Joint Surg 53A:275, 1971

35. Barfred T: Experimental rupture of the Achilles tendon: comparison of various types of experimental rupture in rats. Acta Orthop Scand 42:528, 1971

36. Laws G, Walton M: Fibroblastic healing of grade III ligament injuries. J Bone Joint Surg 70B:390, 1988

37. Woo SLY, Young EP, Ohland KJ: The effects of transection of the anterior cruciate ligament on healing of the medial collateral ligament. J Bone Joint Surg 72A:382, 1988

38. Jack ER: Experimental rupture of the medial collateral ligament of the knee. J Bone Joint Surg 32B:396, 1950

39. Ogata K, Whiteside LA, Andersen DA: The intra-articular effect of various postoperative managements following knee ligament repair: an experimental study in dogs. Clin Orthop 150:271, 1980

40. Hastings DE: Non-operative treatment of complete tears of the medial collateral ligament of the knee joint. Clin Orthop 147:22, 1980

41. Warren LF, Marshall JL: Injuries of the anterior cruciate and medial collateral ligaments of the knee. A long-term follow-up of 86 cases—part II. Clin Orthop 136:197, 1978

42. Oakes BW: Acute soft tissue injuries. Aust Fam Phys, suppl. 10:3, 1982

43. Van Der Meuler JC: Present state of knowledge on processes of healing in collagen structures. Int J Sports Med 3:4, 1982

44. Woo SLY, Inoue M. McGuik-Burleson E et al: Treatment of the medial collateral ligament injury: II. Structure and function of canine knees in response to differing treatment regimens. Am J Sports Med 15:22, 1987

45. Wilk KE, Corzatt RD: Non-operative Rehabilitation of Grade I & II Sprains on the Medial Collateral Ligament in Athletes. Presented at the Combined Sections Meeting of the American Physical Therapy Association, Washington DC, 1988

46. Lossing I, Grimby G, Jonsson T et al: Effects of electrical muscle stimulation combined with voluntary contractions—after knee ligament surgery. Med Sci Sports Excer 20:93, 1988

47. Delitto A, Rose SJ, McKowca JM: Electrical stimulation vs voluntary exercise in strengthening thigh musculature after anterior cruciate ligament surgery. Phys Ther 68:660, 1988

48. Eriksson E, Haggmark T: Comparison of isometric muscle training and electrical stimulation supplementing isometric muscle training in the recovery after major knee ligament surgery. Am J Sports Med 7:169, 1979

49. Dehne E, Tory R: Treatment of joint injuries by immediate mobilization—based upon the spinal adoption concept. Clin Orthop 77:218, 1971

50. Haggmark T, Eriksson E: Cylinder of mobile cast brace after knee ligament surgery: a clinical analysis and morphologic and enzymatic studies of changes in the quadriceps muscle. Am J Sports Med 7:48, 1979

51. Perkins G: Rest and motion. J Bone Joint Surg 35B:521, 1954

52. Coutts R, Rothe J, Kaita J: The role of continuous passive motion in the rehabilitation of the total knee patient. Clin Orthop 159:126, 1981

53. Salter RB, Hamilton HW, Wedge JH et al: Clinical application of basic research on continuous passive motion for disorders and injuries of synovial joints. J Orthop Res 1:325, 1984

54. Wilk KE: Dynamic muscle strenth testing. p. 123. In Amundsen L (ed): Muscle Strength Testing. Churchill Livingstone, New York, 1990

55. Levy M: Posterior meniscal capsuloligamentous complexes of the knee. p. 207. In Feagin JA Jr (ed): The Crucial Ligaments. Churchill Livingstone, New York, 1988

8

Posterolateral Instability: Diagnosis and Treatment

ROBERT P. ENGLE
GARY C. CANNER

INTRODUCTION

Diagnosis and treatment of both acute and chronic injuries to the posterolateral ligaments of the knee is challenging and difficult even for experienced clinicians. Acute examination often overlooks injury to this corner of the knee.[1,2] Without proper management, increased instability, recurrent meniscal tearing, and joint surface erosion frequently result.[3-10]

LITERATURE REVIEW

Posterolateral instability occurs when the lateral tibial plateau subluxes posteriorly relative to the lateral femoral condyle (Fig. 8-1).[11] There is some controversy as to the lesion responsible for this instability. Jakob et al.[9] studied the effects of ligament sectioning on cadaver knees and concluded that the popliteus or arcuate ligament was primarily affected.

Grood et al.[12] in their research, also performed on cadaver knees, thought that the lateral collateral ligament was an equally important structure restraining posterolateral laxity. Gollehon et al.[1] demonstrated an increase in posterior tibial translation, varus rotation, and external tibial rotation with posterolateral ligament insufficiency. They and others discuss the role of the lateral and posterolateral structures in conjunction with injuries to both the anterior and posterior cruciate ligaments.[2-8,10,11,13-15]

The most commonly reported mechanism of injury was a blow to the anteromedial tibia with varus in relative knee extension.[3-5,7] These mechanisms frequently result in injuries to various other structures, including osteochondral components, patellofemoral restraints, one or both of the cruciate ligaments, and the peroneal nerve. Chronic laxity in the lateral and posterolateral structures can be seen in anterior cruciate ligament- and posterior cruciate ligament-deficient knees.

This chronic increase in laxity, which may initially be relatively mild, is most likely secondary to the large role of the lateral collateral ligament in anterior cruciate ligament deficiency. As these structures become overloaded while attempting to control anterior subluxation, stretching begins and laxity increases. Joint axis of motion then shifts more medially, which causes increasingly rapid stretching to occur to the point of functional knee instability and, ultimately, disability.

In posterior cruciate ligament insufficiency, the posterolateral and lateral structures provide significant secondary restraint to both flexion and extension positions.[12] They undergo a similar stretching over time that leads to progressive laxity, meniscal tears, functional instability, and joint surface erosion. Gollehon et al.[1] stressed the importance of a comprehensive examination of the knee and appreciation for posterolateral compartment injury.

CLINICAL EXAMINATION

Several tests for posterolateral instability have been described in the literature. Hughston and Norwood[8] described the posterolateral drawer and extension/recurvatum tests. In the posterolateral drawer test, the

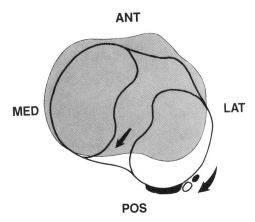

Fig. 8-1. Posterolateral subluxation of the tibial relative to the femur.

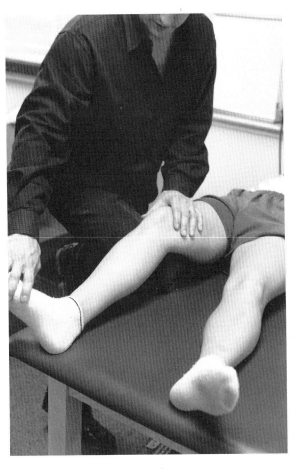

Fig. 8-2. External rotation test.

examiner attempts to sublux the lateral tibial condyle posteriorly relative to the lateral femoral condyle with the knee in 90 degrees of flexion and with the patient supine with both knees resting in full extension. The examiner is positioned facing the patient's feet and holds the great toe of each lower extremity. Each toe is lifted to bring the knee into further extension and into increased recurvatum and external tibial rotation.

Varus stress testing has been described by several investigators as a test for lateral and posterolateral instability. Noyes et al.[15] have documented the relative contributions of both the lateral and posterolateral ligaments with varus stress in both the flexed and extended positions. They contend that when performing a varus stress test, the contribution of the posterolateral structures is greatest the closer the knee gets to full extension. Increased varus has been shown by several others as well.[1,3–5,7–9,11,12,14]

Grood et al.[12] demonstrated that the greatest laxity due to the posterolateral complex could be elicited at 20 to 40 degrees of flexion by simply testing passive external rotation of the tibia (Fig. 8-2). Jakob et al.[9] seemed to agree that the 20 to 40 degrees was equally important when they described the reversed pivot shift in 1981.

In the reversed pivot shift test, the knee is taken from 70 to 80 degrees of flexion to full extension, with a valgus force applied to the knee similar to the pivot shift test of Galway and MacIntosh.[16] If posterolateral instability is present, the lateral tibia will be subluxed relative to the lateral femoral condyle at the starting position.

At approximately 40 degrees of extension, the tibia will reduce from its subluxed to a normal position. With extension back to flexion, the tibia begins from its now reduced position and subluxes. Often this reduction is audible, palpable, and visible, like the pivot shift associated with anterolateral instability. Many times the reversed pivot shift is incorrectly interpreted as a positive pivot shift. Symptoms of functional instability are often reproduced with this test.

Patient guarding can negate the reversed pivot shift secondary to pain and apprehension. In mild cases of posterolateral injury, the test findings are minimal and a great deal of examiner experience and patient cooperation is required.

The external rotation test can usually be performed in the same position as the Lachman examination and is relatively comfortable for the patient in both acute and chronic cases. Further posterolateral subluxation can be elicited if the patient is asked to flex the knee while the examiner holds the tibia in its maximally externally rotated position (Fig. 8-3). Biceps femoris activity pulls the tibia backward against the injured posterolateral structures.

Further laxity can be palpated at the posterior aspect of the lateral tibial condyle. Pain is commonly elicited and can reproduce the patient's symptoms. This pain can be secondary to a number of problems, including tears of the lateral meniscus, posterolateral capsule, popliteus tendon, or biceps femoris complex, as well as damage to the peroneal nerve.

This active posterolateral drawer (APLD) test has been used by us as part of both acute and chronic examinations when possible. We prospectively studied 70 consecutive patients who suffered acute knee ligament injuries.[13] Initial examinations, performed by one examiner (G.C.C.), revealed 6 of these 70 patients as having a positive APLD test acutely.

Of these six patients with positive findings, all had findings of posterolateral injury and instability on arthroscopy and examination under anesthesia. Follow-up over 18 months was negative for posterolateral instability because of the initial recognition and proper management of this problem. Treatment was provided in most cases for concomitant injury to the osteochondral elements, menisci, patellofemoral joint, and cruciate and collateral ligaments.

TREATMENT

Conservative Management

As with most knee ligament instabilities, there exist a variety of both surgical and nonsurgical options. Even the most experienced surgeons acknowledge the difficulty of repairing the posterolateral and lateral ligaments of the knee. Many of these procedures are performed with other cruciate ligament surgeries. Posterolateral repairs have been discussed by several investigators.[3–7,10]

Nonoperative or conservative management depends on a comprehensive rehabilitation program that attempts to provide an adequate counterforce to the resultant pathomechanics. An appreciation of the musculotendinous restraints is necessary, as is a thorough initial and on-going re-examination of the patient.

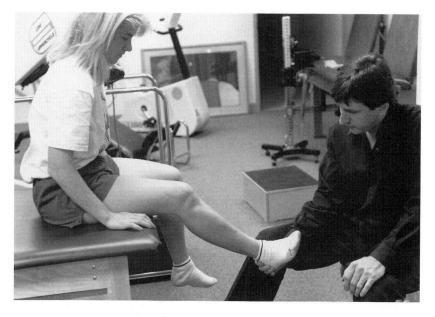

Fig. 8-3. Active posterolateral drawer test.

Acute-Phase Rehabilitation

Acute injuries to the posterolateral structures can be graded according to the degree of laxity, as described by Hughston et al.[11,14] Mild injuries should be treated by a brief period of immobilization, whereas moderate to severe injuries should be placed in an immobilizer or cast brace system for 10 to 21 days.

Initially constraining the joint by avoiding the terminal 20 to 30 degrees of extension slackens the posterior capsule, allowing it to heal without stress. Nonweight bearing or partial weight bearing will further relieve these structures of deforming forces. Full weight bearing should not be allowed for 3 weeks or longer until initial healing has occurred and neuromuscular support to the joint has improved.

A rehabilitative exercise program should begin as soon as possible, with proper precautions and constraints specific to this instability. Electrical muscle stimulation can augment the exercise program. Ice should be used following treatment to minimize pain, swelling, and inflammation.

Chronic-Phase Rehabilitation

Most chronic cases show some pain and dysfunction at the patellofemoral joint. This must be clearly understood prior to beginning rehabilitation and planned into the program.

Since the acute phase has already passed in these patients, immobilization and restricted weight bearing are necessary only for those patients who are experiencing recurrent synovitis, pain, and/or degenerative changes to the joint that are limiting their everyday activities. Neuromuscular techniques are essential to regaining stability.

Musculotendinous Anatomy

Marshall et al.[17] detailed the extensive anatomy of the biceps femoris relative to its lateral and posterolateral attachments. They characterized its function as a tibial external rotator as well as a knee flexor. Through this work one can clearly see the antagonist relationship between the biceps group and the posterolateral capsule with knee flexion exercises that allow the tibia unconstrained external rotation.

Basajian and Lovejoy,[18] Southmayd and Quigley,[19] and Müller[20] each discuss the function of the popliteus in posterolateral stability. It functions primarily as an internal tibial rotator with a component of knee flexor during initial flexion (0 to 15 degrees) and acts as a dynamic restraint to posterolateral instability. Quadriceps activity is also a dynamic stabilizer. In this same (0 to 15 degree) range, however, quadriceps facilitation should be performed in a manner that does not allow for excessive external rotation. This is especially important immediately following injury when ligamentous healing is just beginning.

Therapeutic Exercise Techniques

Restoration of neuromuscular function is important to provide full strength, endurance, and mobility. However, specific techniques must be chosen that do not take the patient into unrestrained posterolateral subluxation. This will only lead to further problems.

Several manually applied proprioceptive neuromuscular facilitation procedures as described by Voss et al.,[21] and others modified by us, have proved to be important. These include techniques that emphasize internal or neutral tibial rotation with synergistic knee extension and flexion. Lower extremity diagonal patterns from Voss et al.[21] are used, avoiding external tibial rotation (Fig. 8-4). To avoid posterolateral stress, the knee can be isometrically stabilized in range of motion outside of terminal extension. Isolated knee flexion and extension techniques can also be applied with manual and various resistive exercise approaches, with appropriate external rotation restraint (Fig. 8-5).

Weight-bearing functional training exercises are valuable, both when applied manually and when performed using equipment. These can include balance boards, leg press, squats, stair climbing, cross-country skiing, walking, and other methods (Fig. 8-6).

Patellofemoral precautions must be taken in rehabilitation with these patients. Abnormal tibial translation and rotations are commonly associated with articular cartilage shear stresses over the patella. Manual procedures other than those already described can be helpful with patellar stabilization and tracking. Procedures described by Beck and Wildermuth[22] can be modified to avoid posterolateral subluxation while protecting the patellofemoral joint.

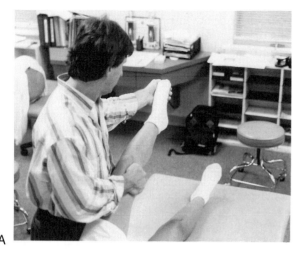

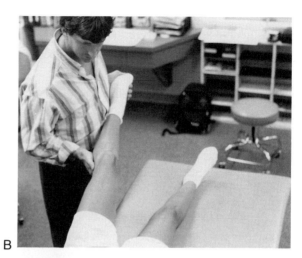

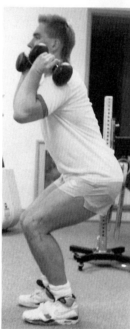

Fig. 8-4. Manual resistive exercise techniques. **(A)** Knee extension with linear hip extension. **(B)** Extension-abduction-internal rotation with knee extension-internal rotation. **(C)** Weight-bearing hip/knee extension.

Bracing

Posterolateral instability has been associated with an increase in varus, external tibial rotation, and hyperextension. Each of these components should be appropriately restrained by the brace selected. When the anterior and/or posterior cruciate ligaments are involved, appropriate constraint should be included as well. Few commercially available functional braces are designed specifically to restrain posterior tibial subluxation.

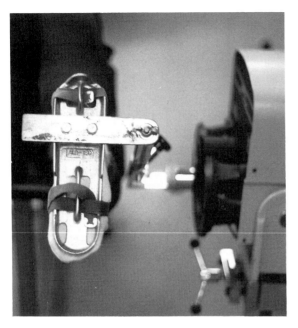

Fig. 8-5. Restraint of tibial external rotation for isokinetic knee flexion-extension.

Return to Activity

Return to functional athletic activity can begin when the patient no longer experiences any giving way of the affected knee while running, cutting, or jumping. Full neuromuscular function should be restored. Pain-free active and passive knee flexion-extension is important. There should be no effusion and an asymptomatic patellofemoral joint.

SUMMARY

Posterolateral knee instabilities continue to present difficult problems in both diagnosis and treatment. These instabilities result from injury to the popliteus (arcuate) ligament and lateral collateral ligament.[1,9,12] Increased varus rotation, tibial external rotation, and posterior translation have been documented by a variety of clinical tests.[1,8,9,12]

Operative approaches have been discussed in the literature.[3–7,10] To the best of our knowledge, nothing has been written on conservative approaches or rehabilitation. In addition, mild forms of posterolateral instability have not been discussed, although their con-

tribution to laxity in both the anterior and posterior cruciate ligament-deficient knees have been discussed.[1–7,9–14] We have presented an additional test for posterolateral instability and painful lesions associated with related structures that has been useful in diagnosis.[13]

Since injury to this region of the knee usually happens in conjunction with injury to other structures, mild to moderate instabilities are not appreciated acutely. Chronic cases in which a reversed pivot shift is present are often misdiagnosed as anterolateral problems.[9] On-going problems can include meniscal tears, degenerative joint changes, and progressive laxity.[9] Therefore, complete rehabilitation, with or without surgery, is required for adequate stabilization so that the patient can return to activity without further problems. More research is necessary to understand this complex, controversial, and challenging part of the knee.

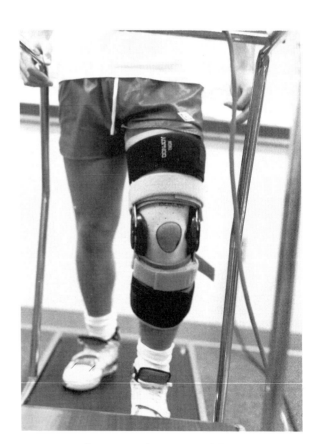

Fig. 8-6. Functional training with knee brace.

REFERENCES

1. Gollehan DL, Torzilli PA, Warren RF: The role of the posterolateral and cruciate ligaments in the stability of the human knee. J Bone Joint Surg 69:233, 1987

2. Hughston JC: The absent posterior drawer test in some acute posterior cruciate ligament tears of the knee. Am J Sports Med 16:39, 1988

3. Baker CL, Norwood LA, Hughston JC: Acute combined posterior cruciate and posterolateral instability of the knee. Am J Sports Med 12:204, 1984

4. Baker CL, Norwood LA, Hughston JC: Actue posterolateral rotatory instability of the knee. J Bone Joint Surg 65:614, 1983

5. DeLee JC, Riley MB, Rockwood CA: Acute straight posterolateral instability of the knee. Am J Sports Med 11:199, 1983

6. Fleming RE, Blatz DJ, McCarroll, JR: Posterior problems in the knee: posterior cruciate insufficiency and posterolateral rotatory insufficiency. Am J Sports Med 9:107, 1981

7. Hughston JC, Jacobson KE: Chronic posterolateral rotatory instability of the knee. J Bone Joint Surg 67:351, 1985

8. Hughston JC, Norwood LA: The posterolateral drawer test and external rotation recurvatum test for posterolateral instability of the knee. Clin Orthop Rel Res 147:82, 1980

9. Jakob RP, Hassler H, Staeubli H: Observations on rotatory instability of the lateral compartment of the knee. Acta Orthop Scand (suppl. 191) 152:1, 1981

10. Loos WC, Fox JM, Blazina ME et al: Acute posterior cruciate ligament injuries. Am J Sports Med 9:86, 1981

11. Hughston JC, Andrews JR, Cross MJ, Meschi A: Classification of knee ligament instabilities. Part II. The lateral compartment. J Bone Joint Surg 58:173, 1976

12. Grood ES, Stowers SF, Noyes FR: Limits of movement on the human knee. J Bone Joint Surg 70:88, 1988

13. Canner GC, Engle RP: The diagnosis of posterolateral laxity in the acutely injured knee, abstracted. Submitted.

14. Hughston JC, Andrews JR, Cross MJ, Meschi A: Classification of knee ligament instabilities. Part I. The medial compartment and cruciate ligaments. J Bone Joint Surg 58:159, 1976

15. Noyes FR, Grood ES, Butler DL, Paulos LE: Clinical biomechanics of the knee: ligament restraints and functional stability. p. 7. In Funk J. (ed): American Academy of Orthopaedic Surgeons Symposium on the Athlete's Knee. CV Mosby, St. Louis, 1981

16. Galway HR, MacIntosh DL: The lateral pivot shift: a symptom and sign of anterior cruciate ligament insufficiency. Clin Orthop Rel Res 147:45, 1980

17. Marshall JL, Gergis FG, Zelko RR: The biceps femoris tendon and its functional significance. J Bone Joint Surg 54:1444, 1972

18. Basmajian JV, Lovejoy JF: Function of the popliteus muscle in man. J Bone Joint Surg 53:557, 1971

19. Southmayd W, Quigley TB: The forgotten popliteus muscle. Clin Orthop Rel Res 130:218, 1978

20. Müller W: The Knee: Form, Function and Ligament Reconstruction. Springer-Verlag, New York, 1983

21. Voss DE, Ionta JK, Myers BJ: Proprioceptive Neuromuscular Facilitation. Harper & Row, New York, 1985

22. Beck JL, Wildermuth BP: The female athlete's knee. Clin Sports Med 4:345, 1985

23. Warren LF, Marshall JL: The supporting structures and layers on the medial side of the knee: an anatomical analysis. J Bone Joint Surg 61A:56, 1979

9

Nonoperative Anterior Cruciate Ligament Rehabilitation

ROBERT P. ENGLE

INTRODUCTION

Many patients who have experienced complete anterior cruciate ligament (ACL) tears prefer nonoperative treatment to operative ligament substitution. For these patients, the most effective method of management for functional knee stabilization with activity is a rehabilitation program.

Functional stability of the knee (as defined by Noyes et al.[1]) can be achieved essentially by compensation through the neuromuscular system for the resultant laxity. Each case presents a slightly different profile of instability, however, ranging from simple, low-grade anterior instability to more complex, multiplane instabilities. The degree to which musculotendinous structures can maintain stability in the unstable knee under functional conditions is largely unknown.

REVIEW OF THE LITERATURE

Several researchers have discussed nonoperative treatment.[2–18] In the vast majority of these studies, operative treatment is recommended as a long-term solution to patient care. Recurrent meniscal tears, advanced joint surface erosion, progressively increasing laxity, and chronic synovitis have all been documented in chronic ACL insufficiency.[5,12–14,18] These potential problems must all be considered when selecting rehabilitation techniques. Improper rehabilitation can easily elicit or accelerate further instability and symptoms.

In the literature, the key to successful treatment appears to be related to the level of hamstring function, proprioception, modification of activity in some patients, and the use of functional braces.[6,12–14,16,17,19] Unfortunately, however, no studies to date have documented the rehabilitation program in detail. Since rehabilitation is the cornerstone of nonoperative treatment, rehabilitation needs to be analyzed more critically for application by the physical therapist and physicians directing patient programs.

TREATMENT

The patient's course of treatment must be based on a thorough understanding of anatomy and biomechanics, diagnosis and examination, therapeutic exercise and rehabilitation, and the natural course of the ACL-deficient knee. This section addresses these areas in detail.

Diagnosis: History and Examination

Patients are seen following ACL disruptions both acutely and chronically. When taking the patient history, the initial onset of injury must be noted. When an acute injury occurs, patients often report a snapping or a popping sound, rapid onset of a hemarthrosis and/or the inability to bear weight normally, and range of motion restrictions. Weakness and giving way frequently follow.

Patients with chronic cases usually present with episodes of increasing giving way, pain, and/or effusion. Often their giving way may represent a meniscal tear or a change in activities rather than a true increase in the patient's instability. Reinjuries (with various pathomechanics of injuries) are common in this group, and each injury must be documented by the examiner as well as all treatment rendered. Reproducible symptoms are noted. Patients frequently complain of very specific activities that result in knee instability. These most commonly include pivoting and cutting in a specific direction. Understanding the biomechanics of this functional instability will lead the therapist to indicated treatment techniques.

Any surgical or examination under anesthesia (EUA) results should be obtained from the surgeon. Both acute and chronic insufficiency can have articular cartilage lesions. Acute injuries occur in some cases with osteochondral fractures of the tibiofemoral or patellofemoral articular surfaces. Chronic cases typically show wearing patterns through one or more compartments. In either case, articular cartilage lesions must be taken seriously since over time they will become the patient's greatest clinical problem.

Examination

Initial and on-going examinations are critical to understanding the patient's injury. Palpation can begin the process, with a thorough review of all the anterior, posterior, medial, and lateral structures mentioned in Chapter 3. Effusion, if present, can be an indicator of synovitis, range of motion limitation, and neuromuscular inhibition. Careful palpation of all capsuloligamentous structures is necessary since the pathomechanics of injury may also involve medial, lateral, and posterior ligaments.

Patellofemoral joint evaluation should include medial and lateral stability tests, compression and articular cartilage tests, and palpation of peripatellar structures. This joint is frequently involved in traumatic ligament injuries and tends to undergo a degradation process and chronic maltracking or instability.

Stability examination is the most effective method of diagnosing ligament tears. Torg et al.[20] described the Lachman examination as the most important indicator of ACL tears. Daniel et al.[21] have shown that acute ACL disruptions typically show 2 to 3 mm of increased anterior laxity relative to the uninvolved side. In time, the secondary restraints can be overstressed, allowing even greater anterior as well as mediolateral laxity.

The pivot shift phenomenon (typical of ACL insufficiency) develops as lateral complex laxity is increased when the joint axis of rotation shifts medially.[22-24] This shift in knee mechanics can represent a reproduction of the patient's symptoms of giving way. A variety of tests can be used to confirm, including the pivot shift, jerk, Lossee, Slocum, and flexion-rotation-drawer tests.[1,23,25-27]

In acute, isolated ACL ruptures without any injury to the mediolateral structures, the pivot shift phenomenon is not seen initially but develops over time. This time frame can vary greatly. Meticulous evaluation of the medial, lateral, and posterior compartments is necessary to diagnose ligament injuries, concomitant to the ACL tear.

Testing should include the valgus and varus stress tests for medial and lateral collateral ligaments, respectively, the rotation test for posterolateral instability, and the posterior tibial sag test for the posterior cruciate ligament (PCL) injury. Valgus-varus and rotation tests can be performed at the same 20- to 30-degree position of knee flexion used for the Lachman examination, as well as full extension if available. Tibial sag can be best be used for PCL assessment at 75 to 90 degrees of flexion, making it difficult in some acute cases in which range of motion is restricted and painful. Injuries to these structures are common and must not be overlooked.

Range of motion should be assessed for limitations compared with the uninvolved side, painful or painless end-feel, and/or symptomatic arc. Neuromuscular evaluation to assess quadriceps, hamstrings, and lower extremity neuromuscular function can begin with observation of atrophy, weight-bearing capabilities, and guarding in acute cases. The patient's knee can then be tested in ranges of motion that are deemed safe. With chronic cases (in which full range is generally not very painful), the knee should be tested with three-dimensional positioning, both weight bearing and non-weight bearing, to assess for insufficiencies to control specific pathomechanic instabilities for that patient.

Structural examination with the patient bearing weight will reveal valgus-varus alignment, pelvic asymmetries, and rearfoot/forefoot relationships that could accentuate or accelerate negative changes to the stabilizers and joint surfaces. A more dynamic functional evaluation can test this system further along with balance and proprioception, sports-specific deficiencies, and other components of the affected extremity.

The examination process must be completely understood before good, introspective treatment can begin. Be sure to consider all structures as well as the ACL. For example, both operatively and nonoperatively treated ACL patients often report patellofemoral pain on long-term follow ups. This needs to be considered on the patient's initial visit and planned into the program.

Therapeutic Exercise Techniques and Procedures

Initial emphasis in therapeutic exercise is placed on procedures that facilitate hamstring function for control of the excessive anterior tibial translation. These

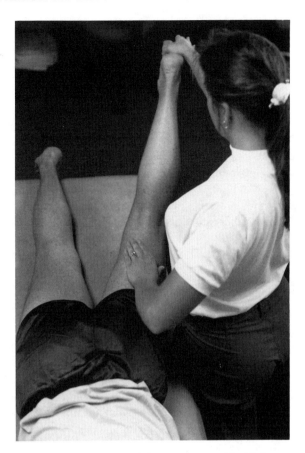

Fig. 9-2. D1 extension with knee maintained in 20 degrees of flexion prone.

can begin immediately in isolated proprioceptive neuromuscular facilitation and modified knee flexion or synergistic lower extremity patterns with isometric-isotonic knee flexion. In patients who present with a positive pivot shift, resisted tibial external rotation with knee flexion, especially eccentric, will be added immediately. Components of valgus-varus with these procedures must be avoided. Careful attention must be paid to the posterolateral corner when using resisted external rotation.[2,3]

Several procedures are important to hamstring recruitment including

Hip extension-abduction, extension-adduction, or linear extension with the knee isometrically maintained at 0 to 30 degrees of flexion, prone, supine, and/or sitting (Figs. 9-1 and 9-2).

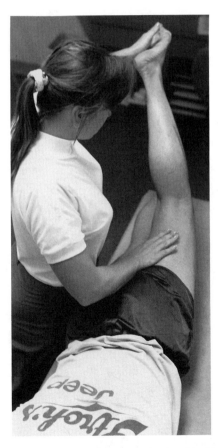

Fig. 9-1. D2 extension with knee maintained in 20 degrees of flexion prone.

Knee flexion with tibia neutral, internal or external rotation as indicated prone, supine, and/or sitting (Figs. 9-3 and 9-4).

Hip flexion-adduction-internal rotation, flexion-adduction-external rotation, or linear flexion with knee flexion and tibia neutral and isometrically or isotonically resisted rotation supine or sitting (Figs. 9-5 and 9-6).

Adjunctive progressive resistive exercises (PREs) with elastic cords, weights, or pulleys to augment the manual procedures

Concentric-eccentric isokinetic hamstring training as soon as the patient can tolerate the additional exercise

Balance board and bicycle exercises emphasizing hamstring function

Although antagonistic to the ACL-deficient knee, quadriceps facilitation must begin immediately, but in a manner that does not overstress the patellofemoral joint, synovium, or secondary restraints. Begin with isometric knee positions for quadriceps irradiation from a stronger proximal component. Then progress to knee flexion movement patterns, primarily using the modified or closed kinetic chain to reduce anterior translation. These patterns include

Hip flexion-adduction-internal rotation and flexion-adduction-external rotation with the knee isometrically maintained in one position from full extension to 55 degrees of flexion with patient supine or sitting (Figs. 9-7 and 9-8)

Hip extension-adduction-external rotation or linear hip extension with knee extension through full knee motion with patient supine or sitting (Fig. 9-9)

Isotonic reversal of both diagonal patterns for successive induction of quadriceps and hamstrings.

Isolated knee extension techniques avoiding 30 degrees to full extension to avoid repetitive overstress to the secondary restraints where anterior tibial translatory forces are highest.

Bridging techniques to emphasize quadriceps-hamstring cocontractions

Adjunctive PREs possibly including straight leg raises, squats, step-ups, and leg press (Figs. 9-10 and 9-11) (knee extension PREs are limited in extension to 45 degrees)

Wall pulley PREs to supplement the manual techniques; elastic cord or weights for same exercises on home basis

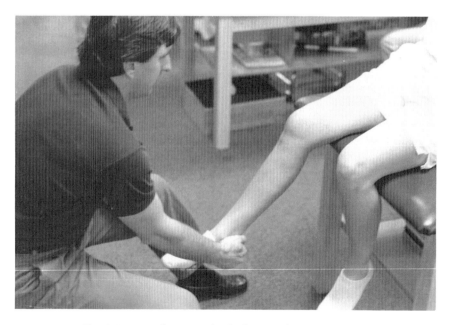

Fig. 9-3. Knee flexion with tibial internal rotation sitting.

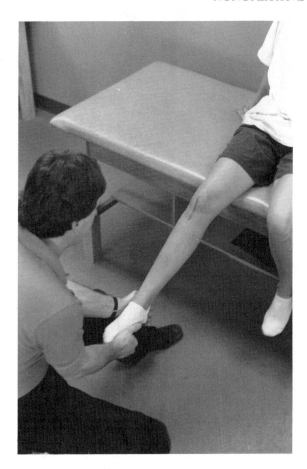

Fig. 9-4. Knee flexion with tibial external rotation sitting.

Functional training includes

Balance and proprioceptive functional activities that involve synergistic knee stabilization using all lower extremity muscle groups (Fig. 9-12)

Bicycle ergometer, cross-country ski equipment, stair climbers, forward, backward, sideways walking to running and others

Sports-specific training skills

Joint Mobilization

Acute cases of ACL disruption are often taken to arthroscopy and EUA. For secondary restraint protection, these patients are maintained in a knee immobilizer for 7 to 21 days until adequate neuromuscular stabil-

ization has been restored. Predictably, this immobilization and the ensuing postarthroscopy synovitis leaves the patient with restricted range of motion.

One component of joint mobility that is immediately affected is the patellofemoral joint. Patellar mobilization beginning the first week postsurgery is important for stretching the tight peripatellar structures. Knee flexion-extension is rarely a problem in acute cases and returns as synovitis and effusion recedes. Chronic cases commonly lack the end range of flexion.

Modalities

Electrical muscle stimulation is the modality most beneficial to restoring neuromuscular function. Repetitive stimulation of neural pathways aides re-education and recruitment. Vastus medialis oblique dysfunction and

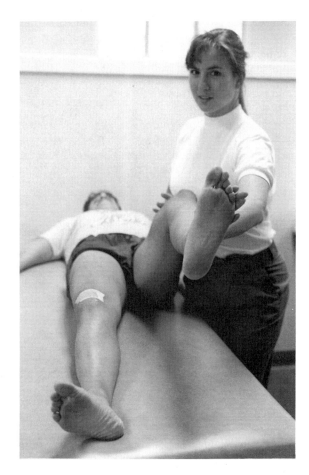

Fig. 9-5. D2 flexion with knee flexion supine.

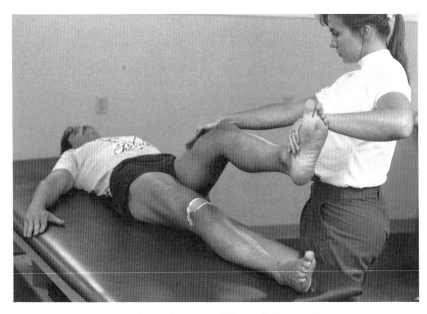

Fig. 9-6. D1 flexion with knee flexion supine.

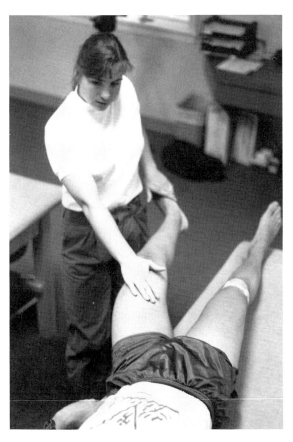

Fig. 9-7. D1 flexion with knee maintained in 20 degrees of flexion supine.

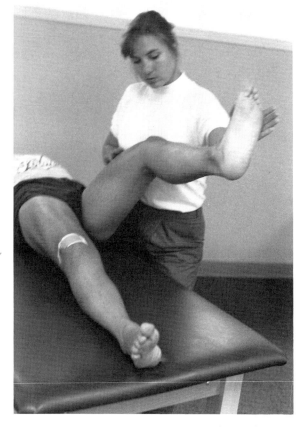

Fig. 9-8. D2 flexion with knee maintained in 20 degrees of flexion supine.

no clinical results have been reported. This interrelationship of the knee with other lower quarter components has been largely overlooked in the orthopaedic literature.

Return to Activity

Return to activity for the patient with acute or chronic ACL deficiency must be based on several factors. To begin return to activity, the patient should have

1. No effusion.
2. Full active and passive range of motion in functional weight-bearing positions without symptoms.
3. Full neuromuscular function on bilateral comparison, including strength, endurance, stabilization, balance, and proprioception.

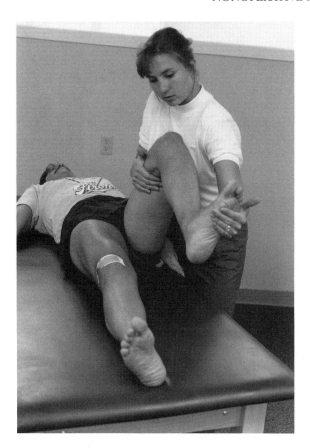

Fig. 9-9. D2 extension with knee extension-external rotation.

ACL instability are particular problems well suited for selective stimulation (Fig. 9-13).

Other modalities can be used for control of inflammation or healing of affected structures besides the ACL. Generally, the manual therapy and therapeutic exercise techniques are the most effective methods in controlling the resultant dysfunction.

Orthotic Devices

Despite the lack of strong scientific support, functional knee braces have been widely used for knee stabilization of both acute and chronic ACL instabilities (Fig. 9-14). Further investigation of each commercially available brace is necessary, as each has a unique design and features.

Orthotic device control of abnormal knee kinematics has drawn recent interest by clinicians, although

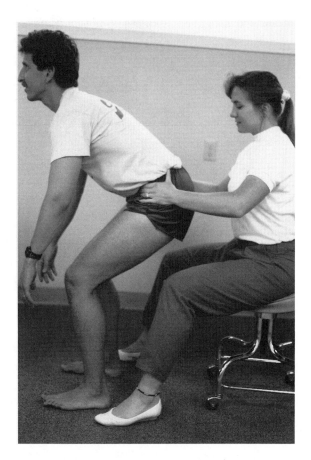

Fig. 9-10. Knee bends with manual resistance.

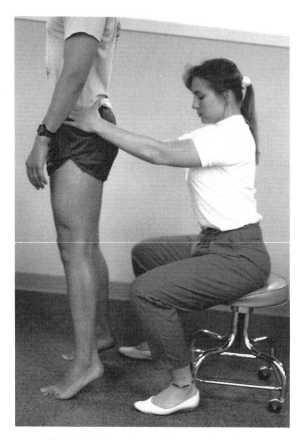

Fig. 9-11. Toe raises with manual resistance.

4. Full functional stability with sport- or task-specific tests. Several studies have discussed functional tests in the literature.[16,17,19,28]

Follow-up

Patients should be monitored closely for 2 years after an acute disruption. Instrumented knee ligament evaluations can document changes in the patient's stability, as can repeat clinical examinations. Some stabilization depends on the neuromuscular system. On-going functional testing is important. Patients often need to modify or discontinue activities in high-risk sports because of symptoms more closely related to joint surface erosion, as well as giving way.

SUMMARY

There are several key concepts that are important to remember in nonoperative management of the ACL-deficient knee. Each patient presents differently; therefore, each examination must be thorough and fully understood by the clinician. Some patients will have significant varus and posterolateral component with the mechanism of injury. Osteochondral fractures are common in knee trauma, and meniscal tears may or may not be present.

Consider the natural course of the ACL-deficient knee, that is, recurrent meniscal tearing, advanced joint surface erosion, progressively increasing instability, giving way, and synovitis. Plan immediately for

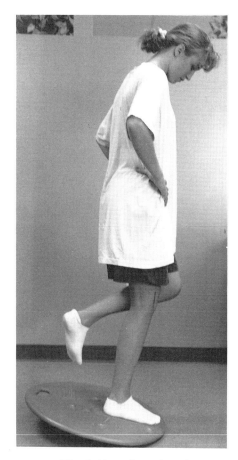

Fig. 9-12. Balance board.

possible future patellofemoral pain and dysfunction with treatment. Expect to see more complex laxity with time that can be more difficult to restrain dynamically.

ACL instability typically has a three-dimensional component. Rehabilitation techniques and procedures must attempt to restrain all these components for a successful outcome. Functionally, the abnormal kinematics must be controlled primarily via eccentric muscle action.

Resultant functional instabilities, that is, giving way, are usually position specific. Work the patient in these ranges with functional techniques that include eccentric control. Full range reciprocal flexion-extension

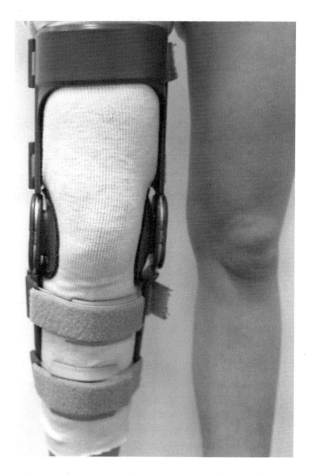

Fig. 9-14. Functional knee brace for ACL instability.

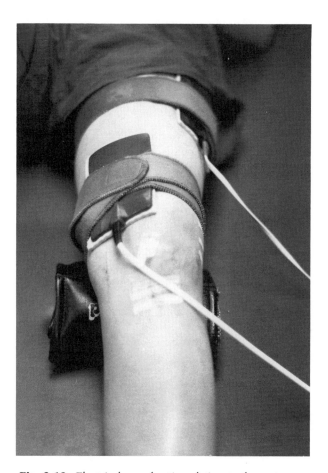

Fig. 9-13. Electrical muscle stimualation to the vastus medialis oblique.

bouts in a non-weight-bearing position are usually unnecessary and ineffective with these patients.

Consider the interaction between the dynamic musculotendinous and static capsuloligamentous structures when approving appropriate techniques. Consider the lower quarter biomechanics, ground reaction forces, and their influence as well.

Combined hands-on manual therapy and functional training approaches have proved highly effective. Proprioception, although difficult to measure objectively, may be most responsible for successful management of these patients. Continual re-evaluation is necessary to understand the effectiveness of treatment and patient progress.

REFERENCES

1. Noyes FR, Grood ES, Butler DL, Paulos LE: Clinical biomechanics of the knee: ligament restraints and functional stability. p. 7. In Funk J (ed), American Academy of Orthopaedic Surgeons Symposium on the Athlete's Knee. CV Mosby, St. Louis, 1981

2. Engle RP, Canner GC: Proprioceptive neuromuscular facilitation (PNF) and modified procedures for anterior cruciate ligament (ACL) instability. J Orthop Sports Phys Ther 11:230, 1989

3. Engle RP, Canner GC: Rehabilitation of symptomatic anterolateral knee instability. J Orthop Sports Phys Ther 11:237, 1989

4. Fetto JF, Marshall JL: The natural history and diagnosis of anterior cruciate ligament insufficiency. Clin Orthop 147:29, 1980

5. Fowler PJ, Regan WD: The patient with symptomatic chronic anterior cruciate ligament insufficiency. Results of minimal arthroscopic surgery and rehabilitation. Am J Sports Med 15:321, 1987

6. Giove TP, Miller SJ, Kent BE et al: Non-operative treatment of the torn anterior cruciate ligament. J Bone Joint Surg 65A:184, 1983

7. Hawkins RS, Missamore GW, Merritt TR: Follow-up of the acute nonoperative isolated anterior cruciate ligament tear. Am J Sports Med 14:205, 1986

8. Jokl P, Kaplan N, Stovell P et al: Non-operative treatment of severe injuries to the medial and anterior cruciate ligament injuries of the knee. J Bone Joint Surg 66A:741, 1984

9. Kannua P, Jarvinen M: Conservatively treated tears of the anterior cruciate ligament. J Bone Joint Surg 69A:1007, 1987

10. McDaniel WJ, Dameron TB: The untreated anterior cruciate ligament rupture. Clin Orthop 172:158, 1983

11. McDaniel WJ, Dameron TB: Untreated ruptures of the anterior cruciate ligament. A follow-up study. J Bone Joint Surg 62A:696, 1980

12. Noyes FR, Matthews DS, Mooar PA, Grood ES: The symptomatic anterior cruciate deficient knee. Part II. The results of rehabilitation, activity modification and counseling. J Bone Joint Surg 65A:163, 1983

13. Noyes FR, McGinniss GH, Grood ES: The variable functional disability of the anterior cruciate ligament-deficient knee. Orthop Clin North Am 16:47, 1985

14. Noyes FR, Mooar PA, Matthews DS, Butler DL: The symptomatic anterior cruciate deficient knee. Part I. The long-term functional disability in athletically active individuals. J Bone Joint Surg 65A:154, 1983

15. Pattee GA, Fox JM, DelPizzo W, Friedman MJ: Four to ten year follow-up of unreconstructed anterior cruciate ligament tears. Am J Sports Med 17:430, 1989

16. Shelbourne KD, Rettig AC, McCarroll JR et al: Functional ability in atheltes with an anterior cruciate ligament deficiency (abst). Am J Sports Med 15:628, 1989

17. Tibone JE, Antich TJ, Fanton GS, et al.: Functional analysis of anterior cruciate ligament instability. Am J Sports Med 14:276, 1986

18. Warren RF, Levy IM: Meniscal lesions associated with anterior cruciate ligament injury. Clin Orthop 172:32, 1983

19. Barber SD, Noyes FR, Mangine RE et al: Quantitative assessment of functional limitations in normal and anterior cruciate ligament deficient knees. Clin Orthop 255:204, 1990

20. Torg JS, Conrad W, Klein V: Clinical diagnosis of anterior cruciate ligament instability in the athlete. Am J Sports Med 4:84, 1976

21. Daniel DM, Stone ML, Sachs R, Malcolm L: Instrumented measurement of anterior knee laxity in patients with acute anterior cruciate ligament disruption. Am J Sports Med 13:401, 1985

22. Bach BR, Warren RF, Wickiewicz TL: The pivot shift phenomenon: results and description of a modified clinical test for anterior cruciate ligament insufficiency. Am J Sports Med 16:571, 1988

23. Galway HR, MacIntosh DL: The lateral pivot shift: a symptom and sign of anterior ligament insufficiency. Clin Orthop 147:45, 1980

24. Noyes FR, Grood ES, Butler DL, et al: Clinical laxity tests and functional stability of the knee: biomechanical concepts. Clin Orthop 147:84, 1980

25. Hughston JC, Andrews JR, Cross MJ, Moschi A: Classification of knee ligament instabilities. Part II. The lateral compartment. J Bone Joint Surg 58A:173, 1976

26. Lossee RE, Johnson TR, Southwick WO: The anterior subluxation of the lateral tibial plateau: a diagnostic test and operative repair. J Bone Joint Surg 60A:1015, 1978

27. Slocum DB, Janes SL, Singer KM: Clinical test for anterolateral rotatory instability of the knee. Clin Orthop 118:63, 1976

28. Daniel DM, Malcolm L, Losse G et al: Instrumented measurement of anterior laxity of the knee. J Bone Joint Surg 67A:720, 1985

10

Rehabilitation Following Arthroscope-Assisted Anterior Cruciate Ligament Reconstruction with Semitendinosus and Gracilis Tendon Autografts

LESLEY K. ROGAN
ALEXANDER A. SAPEGA

INTRODUCTION

The treatment of anterior cruciate ligament (ACL) injuries has recently evolved at an extraordinary pace. Only 4 or 5 years ago, patients were casted following reconstructive surgery. Now, most patients are placed in a hinged knee brace and allowed immediate motion postoperatively. While the patients of 5 years ago would just be coming out of their cast at week 7 or 8, today's patients are riding a stationary bike, doing squats, and working isokinetically to increase their strength at the same point in time after surgery.

Advances in surgical technique, bracing, and rehabilitation, as well as an increased awareness of the negative physiologic consequences of joint immobilization, have all fueled this recent revolution in treatment. The deleterious effects of joint immobility have been well documented.[1-3] Articular cartilage requires motion for nutrition and weight-bearing stresses to maintain its biomechanical health and material properties.[4] Knee immobilization predisposes the joint to arthrofibrosis and contracture, with potentially disastrous long-term effects and functional disability. The

evidence is now overwhelming that all synovial joints depend on motion for their optimal well-being, even immediately after surgery.

The ACL is responsible for providing 86 percent of the knee joint's passive restraint to anterior tibial translation.[5] An increase in anterior tibial laxity greater than 2 to 3 mm implies a complete loss of functional load-carrying capacity of this ligament. It is this loss of functional capacity, more than the disruption of physical continuity, that is the basis for the diagnosis of a third-degree ACL sprain.[6]

Recently, investigators have stated that neither conservative treatment nor primary (suture) repair of the ACL is the most efficacious treatment for young, athletically active patients with complete ACL tears.[7,8] Ligament reconstruction followed by appropriate rehabilitation is generally the treatment of choice in these cases.

Arthroscope-assisted ACL reconstruction using a combined semitendinosus-gracilis autograft is a procedure that offers several major advantages to the patient. It leaves the extensor mechanism undisturbed and therefore has no intrinsic patellofemoral morbidity. Without patellofemoral side effects, patients regain their mobility more easily and thus restore the health of their joint sooner and more completely. This procedure also avoids the risk of patellar tendon rupture or patellar fracture, which can occur following a patellar tendon autograft procedure.[9] Although using a cadaveric (allograft) patellar tendon substitute also avoids this risk, this is still an experimental procedure that is not yet recommended for general use by the orthopaedic community.

A combined semitendinosus-gracilis tendon graft provides strength and mechanical properties similar to those of a normal ACL, at least immediately (the ultimate mechanical properties of ACL grafts in humans are unknown). A fresh semitendinosus-gracilis autograft (combined single thickness approximately 6.5 to 7 mm in diameter) approximates 120 percent of the tensile strength of the normal ACL and is as strong as an 11-mm-wide patellar tendon graft.[9,10] In addition, the tensile strength per unit of cross-sectional area of these tendons is almost twice that of the patellar tendon.[9] This allows much smaller bone tunnels to be drilled when placing grafts of equal strength. It has also been demonstrated that the use of these tendons as grafts produces no detectable loss of lower extremity strength in either knee flexion or internal rotation.[11]

SURGICAL TECHNIQUE

In light of the above technical advantages, the current ACL reconstruction procedure of choice for all surgeons at the University of Pennsylvania Sports Medicine Center is the arthroscopically assisted semitendinosus-gracilis autograft. Each surgeon performs his or her own variation of the basic semitendinosus-gracilis procedure. The tendons are typically left attached to the tibia for a strong, natural fixation distally; they are routed across the knee joint either single thickness (full length) or double thickness (half length), or a combination of one single and one double thickness is used. Doubling the tendons increases the intra-articular tensile strength of the graft but leaves less tendon substance available for fixation externally on the femur. This can reduce the immediate overall load-

bearing capacity of the leg (until the graft becomes naturally fixed in the femoral bone tunnel) and may therefore delay full weight-bearing ambulation. Therapists working with patients who have had a semitendinosus-gracilis procedure should inquire of the surgeon the particular graft configuration and fixation technique employed, as this may influence the early postoperative rehabilitation regimen.

While this chapter is not meant to teach surgical technique, it is important that certain other aspects of the surgical procedure itself be understood. For that reason, what follows is a very abbreviated description of the basic arthroscopically assisted procedure. (Refer to reference 10 for a more detailed description.)

Generally, all required arthroscopic meniscal and articular surface procedures are completed before the intra-articular reconstruction is begun. If a delicate arthroscopic meniscal repair has been done that will require a period of postoperative immobilization, consideration is often given to deferring the ACL reconstruction until the knee has regained full mobility. The intercondylar notch of the femur is cleared of scar tissue and enlarged slightly to provide adequate spatial clearance for the ACL graft.

A 1½-inch extra-articular incision is made over the tibial insertion of the semitendinosus and gracilis tendons. They are identified and detached proximally from their musculotendinous junction in a closed fashion by a tendon stripper. Their distal tibial insertions are left intact. A 2-inch lateral femoral incision is made proximal to the joint, for access to drill the femoral bone tunnel. (No arthrotomy is necessary.) A drill guide system and isometry testing apparatus are then used to determine proper bone tunnel locations for isometric graft placement. The tendon grafts are drawn up through the tibial bone tunnel, across the joint, and out the femoral bone tunnel. The intra-articular span of the graft is observed arthroscopically while the knee is brought up through a full range of motion. There must be no impingement of the graft by the roof of the intercondylar notch in full knee extension and there should be no significant contact abrasion of the graft with the lateral wall of the intercondylar notch during knee motion. Under adequate tension to eliminate abnormal anterior tibial translation, the grafts are then fixed to the femur by the surgeon's preferred means. After the incisions are closed, a sterile electrical muscle stimulation (EMS) electrode pad is applied over the distal quadriceps prior to applying the dressing and protective hinged brace. The reconstruction is complete and a phased progressive rehabilitation program is now begun.

REHABILITATION PROGRAM

The design of a rehabilitation program is a combination of science and art. It requires, among other things, that healing tissue be stressed but not overloaded.[4] The newly reconstructed ligament must be protected, but the deleterious effects of immobility and disuse must be minimized and motion must be achieved as early as possible.[8,12] The art is in knowing how to balance sound scientific principles and many individual's desire to return to activity as soon as possible. While some feel that the specifics of rehabilitation following ACL surgery remain enigmatic,[13] there no longer appears to be any question that a safe, well-conceived rehabilitation program designed to return the individual to preinjury status is as important as the reconstruction itself.[14]

While variations in tendon graft configuration and fixation method will dictate certain modifications, what follows is a general discussion and description of the rehabilitation program we use following a combined semitendinosus-gracilis ACL autograft reconstruction. Patients who have had ancillary procedures such as meniscal repairs and/or articular surface procedures are not progressed as rapidly as patients who did not require these procedures.

Phase I (Preoperative Consultation)

Our rehabilitation program routinely begins *preoperatively*. The patient is seen in our physical therapy facility for evaluation and instruction. The patient's expectations, questions, and goals are discussed and the anticipated course of rehabilitation is explained. Patients are instructed in the exercises that they will perform in phase II (Table 10-1) of rehabilitation, im-

Table 10-1. Phase II (Long-Leg Brace): Weeks 1 and 2

Ambulatory status:	Heel-toe gait (do not toe-touch only) with crutches. Percentage of full weight bearing set by physician.
Knee bracing:	Hinged brace on at *all* times; range of motion (ROM) set by physician.
Muscle stimulation:	Begin immediately if sterile electrode has been placed under dressing, otherwise begin at first dressing change (stimulation protocol programmed at sports medicine clinic).
Starting modalities:	None.
Initial ROM (10 min):	**Flexion:** Start with *supine* (hip flexed 90 degrees) passive gravity flexion of knee, controlled by quadriceps. Leg supported by hands locked behind thigh; starting position is 30 degrees of knee flexion. Patient lowers foot and lower leg into knee flexion, lets gravity stretch-band knee a bit, then actively extends knee back to starting position. Repeat 20 times. Progress as tolerated to active knee flexion in *standing* position (all body weight on opposite leg).
	Extension: *No* active extension from *sitting* position; use only simple passive gravity extension (no added weight yet) while lying on table with heel propped. Do *not* allow knee to hyperextend.
	For all ROM exercises, work gradually to range limits set by post-operative brace.
Bikework:	None.
Quadriceps:	40 degrees *bent* leg raises (work up to 25 repeats × 3; no weights); sitting hip flexion with *proximal loading* (up to 20 lbs); 90-degree sitting isometrics.
Hamstrings:	Sitting isometrics at multiple angles within ROM of brace.
Abductors and adductors:	Side-raises (abduction only) with no weights.
Lower leg:	Instruct in sitting or supine unrestricted ankle/footpump exercises: 30 repeats per hour during waking hours.
Final ROM (5 min):	Same as initial.
Finishing modalities:	None.
Home program:	Same as above, done 1–2 times per day.

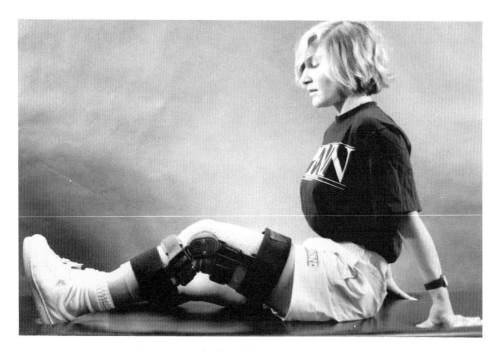

Fig. 10-1. Multiple ankle hamstring isometrics.

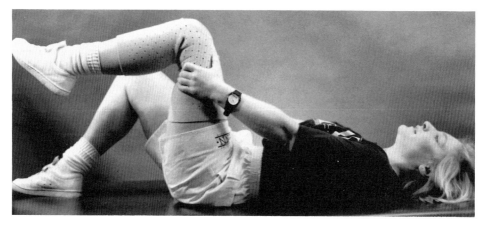

Fig. 10-2. Gravity-assisted passive range of motion.

mediately after surgery. These exercises include multiple-angle hamstring isometrics (Fig. 10-1), bent leg raises (knee flexed to 40 degrees), sitting hip flexion, gentle gravity-assisted passive range of motion (Fig. 10-2), and ankle pumps (deep venous thrombosis prophylaxis). Patients are also instructed in the use of the EMS unit they will be using immediately postsurgery.

The primary objective of this phase is to allow the patient to be as well-informed as possible about the upcoming surgery and what to do between hospital discharge and the first postoperative office visit. It is also hoped that this will encourage patients to become willing, active, and enthusiastic participants in their rehabilitation programs.

Phase II (Immediately Postoperative to 2 Weeks)

Phase II begins as soon as the patient leaves the operating room following surgery. The patient's programmable, portable EMS unit is made available, and its use is encouraged the first night after surgery.

While the use of immediate postoperative EMS is not universally advocated, there are several reported benefits. EMS at low pulse rates (i.e., those that cause observable muscle twitching) can be effective for de-creasing soft tissue swelling.[15] The postoperative quadriceps inhibition reflex is diminished with the use of EMS,[4] and postoperative EMS is also beneficial for the patellofemoral articulation when joint motion is limited.[16]

All the exercises used in phase II are designed to facilitate the early return of knee joint motion and encourage quadriceps activity within a range of motion that does not allow the patellar tendon to exert large anterior shear forces on the tibia. In most patients, the rehabilitation brace has been set in the operating room to allow motion from 5 to 120 degrees of flexion, and gentle active (flexion) and gravity-assisted (extension) range of motion exercise is encouraged up to the limits provided by the brace.

At their first postoperative visit (generally 1 week after surgery), patients are instructed in a few additional exercises that they can begin doing immediately. These include quadriceps isometrics with the knee at 90 degrees, standing hamstring isotonics, and active hip abduction with the involved knee flexed 40 to 60 degrees (Fig. 10-3). Patients are allowed to add light resistance, placed just proximal to their knee, when they work on their bent leg raises and sitting hip flexion (Figs. 10-4 and 10-5). They continue with all their other exercises as per their preoperative instructions.

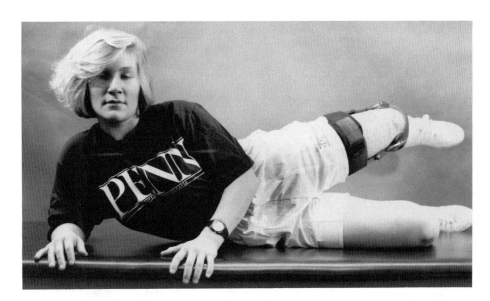

Fig. 10-3. Active hip abduction with the involved knee flexed 40 to 60 degrees.

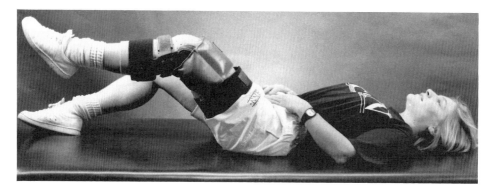

Fig. 10-4. Light resistance, placed just *proximal* to the knee, when working on bent leg raises.

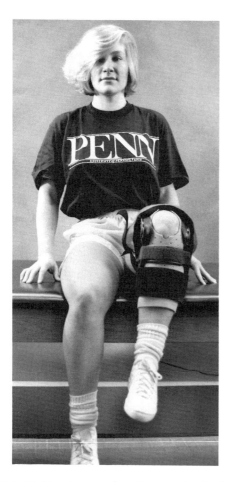

Fig. 10-5. Light resistance, placed just *proximal* to the knee, when working on sitting hip flexion.

Protected, partial weight bearing is begun on the operated extremity.

Phase III (3rd and 4th Postoperative Week)

At the beginning of phase III, the patient is transferred from the long-leg postoperative brace into a functional ACL brace. A more active rehabilitation program is now begun (Table 10-2). Patients usually progress to full weight bearing by the end of week 4. Crutches are discontinued, and a cane is used temporarily. During all partial weight-bearing ambulation, a normal heel-to-toe gait is encouraged, as it has been demonstrated that a toe-touch gait is more stressful to the ACL graft.[6]

Stationary bike work is initiated by week 3, primarily to facilitate recovery of joint motion. Patients begin at low speed (approximately 60 rpm) and very low loads. If a patient has insufficient range of motion to complete a revolution of the pedals, a simple back-and-forth motion is practiced until full range can be achieved. Very often, it is easier for patients to pedal backward rather than forward to initiate full rotational motion. As a general guideline, once a patient is able to ride the stationary bike for 5 minutes, EMS is discontinued.

Lower extremity strengthening work is advanced significantly during this phase. Squats are a time-honored, although poorly understood, way to strengthen the quadriceps and hamstrings. The recent work of Ohkoshi and Yasuda[17,18] has demonstrated that both double-legged and single-legged half-squats, when performed with a forward trunk lean of greater than

Table 10-2. Phase III (Functional ACL Brace; Partial Weight bearing): Weeks 2 through 4

Ambulatory status:	Gradually progress from initial (phase II) degree of weight bearing to full weight bearing *with crutches* over the course of phase III (no full weight bearing until very *end* of phase III).
Knee bracing:	Donjoy Super Sport Brace with 10-degree extension stop. Keep on at *all* times while exercising, ambulating, and sleeping (may be removed only for *flexion* ROM exercise).
Muscle stimulation:	Discontinue EMS when bike work begins.
Starting modalities:	Ice (10–15 min), until all swelling is gone, then heat if desired.
Initial ROM:	Same as phase II, but for flexion, patient may begin pulling tibia back into flexion manually. Continue simple, passive gravity extension stretch only (no added weight yet). Do *not* let knee hyperextend. Attempt to reach 5 to 120 degrees by end of week 3. Note: *No active, full extension efforts when out of brace* for showers, etc.
Bike work:	Begin and gradually advance as tolerated. Start with 5 min at *low* rpm and very *low* load, and progress. If ROM is not sufficient to pedal full cycle, simply start with gentle back-and-forth motion until complete 360 degrees is possible.
Quadriceps:	PRE, with weights placed on *thigh*; 40 degrees bent leg raises and sitting hip flexion; isometrics at 90 and 60 degrees; standing half-squats (50% weight bearing each leg, trunk flexed 45 degrees).
Hamstrings:	Sitting isometrics and standing isotonics as tolerated.
Abductors and adductors:	Side-lying abduction (knee flexed 30 degrees); ball squeeze for adduction and belt stretch for isometric abduction (resistance applied *proximal* to knee in all exercises).
Lower leg:	Discontinue ankle pumps. No toe raises yet.
Final ROM (5 min):	Same as initial.
Finishing modalities:	Ice (20 min).
Other:	Can take showers with brace off (sitting only). No standing on leg without brace.

30 degrees, produce a *posterior* tibial shear force through the knee joint range required for this exercise. This actually relaxes the ACL. When performed in this manner, half-squats are a safe, effective, and uncomplicated way to facilitate early cocontraction and strengthening of the hamstrings and quadriceps.[19,20]

Patients continue to work on fully restoring their range of motion. Active-assisted knee flexion exercises are begun. If indicated, the patient will be instructed in a gentle, passive knee extension and/or flexion stretching regimen.

All the exercises initially begun in phase II are continued and progressed. Quadriceps isometrics are done at multiple angles through a range of 90 to 60 degrees (Fig. 10-6). Resistance is added proximal to the knee as tolerated during bent leg raises, hip abduction, and especially sitting hip flexion. Resistance is also added to the standing knee flexion exercise (Fig. 10-7).

The new exercises initiated during phase III, in addition to the half-squats and stationary bike work, include hip adduction isometrics and isotonic hip extension (Fig. 10-8).

The thermal modality of choice during all phases of our rehabilitation program is ice. All patients use ice for at least 15 minutes after they have completed each workout session. Late in phase III and into phase IV, patients who are having difficulty regaining terminal motion may begin using moist heat prior to their exercise session to help facilitate motion.

Phase IV (Weeks 5 to 16)

Knowledge of the mechanical strain behavior of a reconstructed ACL during rehabilitation activity is essential to safely rehabilitate the knee.[13] Active knee extension in a sitting position begins to strain the ACL at 45 degrees, with progressively increasing ACL strain occurring as the knee approaches full extension.[4,13,20,21]

With that knowledge as the basis for governing rehabilitative treatment, isokinetic work is begun on our patients when they reach the end of postoperative week 4. Patients work only on a Cybex unit with the Johnson antishear device in place.[22] Initially, range of motion is allowed from full flexion to 45 degrees from full extension. Slower speeds (up to 60 degrees per second) are used initially, as patients are generally unable to generate sufficient force to work at higher speeds. Work is gradually progressed so that by the

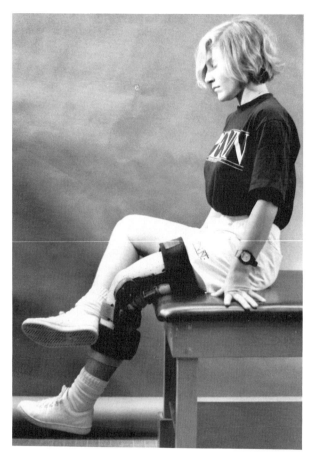

Fig. 10-6. Quadriceps isometrics are done at multiple angles through a range of 90 to 60 degrees.

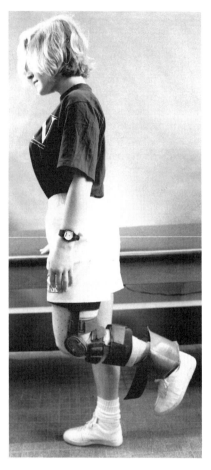

Fig. 10-7. Resistance added to the standing knee flexion exercise.

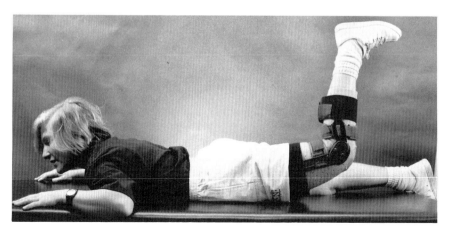

Fig. 10-8. Isotonic hip extension.

end of week 16, the patient is working isokinetically at speeds from 60 to 210 degrees per second from full flexion through full extension, with the antishear device still in place.

Phase IV (Table 10-3) progresses as a continuum of increasing exercise intensity. Patients enter this phase and continue working on all their previous exercises with the number of sets, repetitions, and resistance increased.

During phase IV, patients begin to work on selected isotonic weight-lifting equipment. Patients begin working on the leg press machine, beginning with a limited range and progressing over 12 weeks to full range. Patients also continue performing hip abduction and adduction but on an isotonic machine that applies resistance proximal to the knee. Hamstring

work is progressed slowly from the initial standing isotonics to Nautilus and then to Cybex isokinetic work.

Half-squat training becomes more demanding as the patients progress to using more and more resistance (weight) (Fig. 10-9). Patients also begin doing toe raises, progressing from double-legged toe raises to single-legged toe raises with added resistance.

Late in phase IV, patients begin work on improving proprioception through various balancing exercises. They should have achieved close to full range of motion sometime between weeks 7 and 12 (0 to 3 degrees through 130 degrees). If patients are having difficulty restoring normal joint motion, then more specific flexion and/or extension stretching regimens are added to their programs. We have found that a kneeling

Table 10-3. Phase IV (ACL Brace; Full Weight Bearing): Weeks 5 through 16

Ambulatory status:	Switch from crutches to cane; gradually wean away from cane over 1–2 weeks.
Knee bracing:	Brace can come off (for sleep only) by end of week 6; extension block as per physician.
Muscle stimulation:	Only if full-range bike work not yet possible.
Starting modalities:	Heat/ice as preferred, 10–15 min (use heat if passive gravity stretch is going to be performed next).
Initial ROM:	Gentle prolonged (10–30 min) passive gravity stretch into extension (5–15 lbs), only if not yet at desired ROM; otherwise same as phase III (goal is 0–3 degrees by 7–12 weeks). After week 8, all ROM exercises can be done without brace or range limits, but *never* push knee into hyperextension.
Bike work:	*Gradually* advance rpm, time, and work load to arrive at 20+ min, 90 rpm, 12–1,500 kmp workout by end of phase IV.
Quadriceps:	Discontinue isometrics and bent leg raises; brace on for *all* exercises except Cybex. Most resistive exercises should be three sets of 10 repeats, or similar routine.

	Beginning of Phase IV	Gradual Progression	By End of Phase IV
Sitting or Semisupine Hip Flexion (proximal loading):	Should be 10+ lbs	→	Up to 30 lbs
Standing squats (trunk flexed 45 degrees):	Simple, standing half-squats (no weight)	→	Body weight +40 lbs half-squats
Cybex (*only with antishear device*):	60 degrees/sec with extension limited to 35 degrees	→	Up to 210 degrees/sec through full ROM
Leg press (sitting):	20 lbs, 30-degree extension limit	→	No weight limit, full ROM allowed by brace
Isotonic knee extensions:	Lifts from 100–60 degrees only, resistance as tolerated	→	May lift from 120 to 30 degrees. No terminal extension yet

Hamstrings:	Standing isotonics or Nautilus (prone) as tolerated and same Cybex routine (i.e., rpm, repeats) as quadriceps. Hamstrings do *not* have to be pushed hard until after 12th week.
Abductors and adductors:	Can begin isotonic machine work with *proximal* loading *only*.
Lower leg:	Toe raises; gradually progress from 50% weight bearing to 100% with 20–40 lbs extra weight.
Final ROM:	Repeat initial only as needed.
Finishing modalities:	Direct ice application for 20–30 min.
Other:	Shower in sitting position until end of week 8, then standing OK.

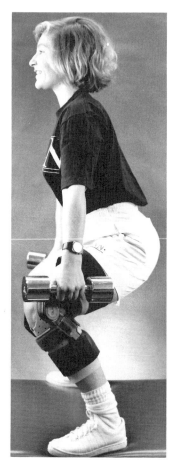

Fig. 10-9. Half-squat training becomes more demanding as the patient progresses to using more and more resistance (weight).

At the end of phase IV, 16 weeks after surgery, the patient undergoes a formal isokinetic evaluation for quadriceps and hamstring strength. Standard isokinetic test procedures are followed with the only modification being that the patient is tested through a limited range (95 to 40 degrees). These test results are then used as the basis for future exercise prescriptions.

If functional deficits greater than anticipated still exist in either strength or range of motion, then a continuing remedial program is designed to address those specific deficits. Patients who have progressed as anticipated move on to phase V.

Phase V (17 Weeks and Onward)

Patients who have achieved adequate range and strength by the end of phase IV now begin working toward the more specific skills they will require to return to their desired activity (Table 10-4).

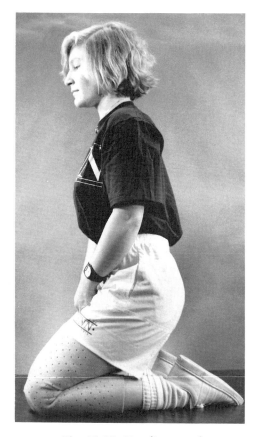

Fig. 10-10. Kneeling stretch.

stretch, as demonstrated in Figure 10-10, is an extremely effective way to safely acquire full flexion. The patient bears the weight of the body on the tibial tubercle during this stretch. This pushes the tibia posteriorly, thus relaxing tension on the ACL graft. If patients are having difficulty obtaining full extension, we will use the Temple protocol[23] (see Ch. 17) to help achieve full end-range extension.

Stationary biking moves from an adjunctive range of motion technique to a method of building muscle endurance and cardiovascular fitness (Fig. 10-11). The patient advances from 5 minutes at low speed and low load to 30+ minutes at 90 rpm and a 1,200 to 1,500 kpm (kilo pound meter) workload.

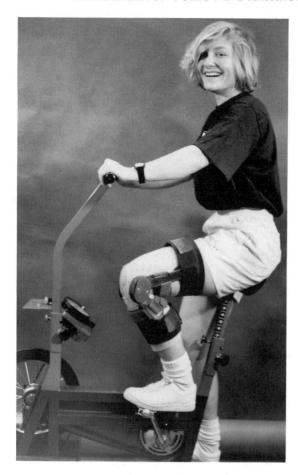

Fig. 10-11. Stationary biking moves from an adjunctive range of motion technique to a method of building muscle endurance and cardiovascular fitness.

Table 10-4. Phase V (Brace Off for Activities of Daily Living): Week 17 Onward

Ambulation/bracing:	ACL brace off for activities of daily living. Wear only for weight lifting or ambulation on slippery or uneven surfaces.
Starting modalities:	Usually none; use heat if passive stretch is still needed.
Initial ROM:	Passive gravity stretch (extension) or kneeling stretch (flexion) only if behind desired ROM. Use formal Temple protocol[23] for resistant contractures: 1. Heat entire knee joint for 15 min. 2. Passive gentle stretch for 15–30 min while heat continues. 3. Cool entire knee in maximally stretched position (10 min).
Bikework:	20–30 min 90 rpm minimum 1,200–1,500 kpm
Quadriceps:	Cybex can continue (optional) with antishear device. Continue leg presses and half-squats. Isotonic knee extension PRE program begins with 30-degree extension limit and progresses to full range by 20 weeks.
Hamstrings:	Full program. No restrictions.
Abductors and adductors:	Full program. No restrictions, but maintain proximal resistance application.
Lower leg:	One-leg toe raises, holding 20+ lbs.
Final ROM:	Repeat initial only as needed.
Other:	None.
Finishing modalities:	Direct ice application for 20 to 30 min.

Isokinetic work is generally discontinued, as patients continue to progress to a full isotonic workout. The isotonic knee extension progressive resisted exercise (PRE) program begins with a 30-degree extension limit and progresses to full range by 20 weeks.

At 20 to 24 weeks, patients generally begin a running program. In preparation for their return to full activity, sport-specific skills are incorporated into the last 3 to 4 weeks of the running program as indicated.

Most participants in the rehabilitation program are able to return to physically demanding employment (i.e., manual trades, construction work, etc.) at 6 months. Return to competitive athletics is usually accomplished by 8 to 10 months after surgery.

SUMMARY

Rehabilitation is a combination of science and art. While science constitutes the technical basis for rehabilitation protocols, the latter are just guidelines and not dictums. The art is in individualizing those protocols to each patient, so rehabilitation is both fun and dynamic and an enjoyable experience. It is imperative that each patient be recognized as an individual with a special set of priorities and goals. Our experience has repeatedly demonstrated that patients who have had the arthroscopically assisted semitendinosus-gracilis autograft recover their strength and range of motion much faster than patients who have had a patellar tendon autograft. Our patients do not have the patellofemoral pain and complications seen in most other autografts. We are able to progress rapidly through the rehabilitation program. One of the most common difficulties we face is trying to restrain our patients from overdoing their rehabilitative exercises and daily physical activities. Somewhere between 6 and 12 weeks postoperation, they start to feel better than they have in a long time. Some patients tend to forget that they have had a major joint reconstruction and may reactivate a synovitis from overactivity.

Rehabilitation is a dynamic process. It evolves on a daily basis. New research and improved techniques are constantly sought and incorporated into treatment regimens. Changes in surgical techniques can stimulate entirely new methods of rehabilitation.

Patient, therapist, doctor, trainer, coach, rehabilitation nurse—everyone's final goal is the same: to return the individual to work or athletic activity as safely and quickly as possible. In our experience, an arthroscope-assisted, semitendinosus-gracilis ACL reconstruction followed by the rehabilitation protocol described accomplishes that goal reliably and efficiently.

REFERENCES

1. Johnson RJ: The effect of immobilization on ligaments and ligamentous healing. Contemp Orthop 2:237, 1980
2. Noyes FR: Functional properties of knee ligaments and alterations induced by immobilization, a correlative biomechanical and histological study in primates. Clin Orthop Rel Res 123:210, 1977
3. Tipton CM, Matters RD, Maynard JA et al: The influence of physical activity on ligaments and tendons. Med Sci Sports 7:165, 1975
4. Silfverskoild JP, Steadman JR, Higgins RW et al: Rehabilitation of the anterior cruciate ligament in the athlete. Sports Med 6:308, 1988
5. Butler DL, Noyes FR, Grood ES: Ligamentous restraints to anterior-posterior drawer in the human knee. J Bone Joint Surg 62A:259, 1980
6. Noyes F, Butler DL, Grood ES et al: Biomechanical analysis of human ligament repairs and reconstructions. J Bone Joint Surg 66A:344, 1984
7. Kannus P, Jarvinen M: Conservatively treated tears of the anterior cruciate ligament: long term results. J Bone Joint Surg 69A:1007, 1987
8. Zarnis B, Adams M: Medical progress knee injuries in sports. N Engl J Med 318:950, 1988
9. Noyes FR, Keller CS, Grood ES et al: Advances in the understanding of knee ligament injury, repair and rehabilitation. Med Sci Sports Exerc 16:427, 1984
10. Sapega AA: Arthroscopically assisted reconstruction of the anterior cruciate ligament. p. 292. In Walsh P, Torg JS (eds): Current Therapy in Sports Medicine. 2nd Ed. BC Decker, Philadelphia. 1989
11. Lipcomb AB, Johnston RK, Snyder RB et al: Evaluation of hamstring strength following use of semitendinosus and gracilis tendons to reconstruct the anterior cruciate ligament. Am J Sports Med 10:340, 1982
12. Paulos LE, Payne FC III, Rosenberg TD: Rehabilitation after anterior cruciate ligament surgery. p. 291. In Jackson DW, Drez D (eds): The Anterior Cruciate Deficient Knee. CV Mosby, St. Louis, 1987
13. Arms SW, Pope MH, Johnson R et al: The biomechanics of anterior cruciate ligament rehabilitation and reconstruction. Am J Sports Med 12:8, 1984
14. Seto JL, Brewster CE, Lombardo J et al: Rehabilitation of

the knee after anterior cruciate ligament reconstruction. J Orthop Sports Phys Ther 8 July, 1989

15. Antich TJ, Brewster CE: Rehabilitation of the non-reconstructed anterior cruciate ligament deficient knee. Clin Sports Med 7:813, 1988

16. Anderson AF, Lipscomb, AB: Analysis of rehabilitation techniques after anterior cruciate reconstruction. Am J Sports Med 17:154, 1989

17. Ohkoshi Y, Yasuda K: Biomechanical analysis of shear force exerted on anterior cruciate ligament during half squat exercises. p. 193. 35th Annual Meeting of the Orthopaedic Research Society, 1989

18. Ohkoshi Y, Yasuda K: Shear force on the knee joint and muscle tension of the quadriceps and hamstrings during muscle exercise in standing. p. 499. 36th Annual Meeting of the Orthopaedic Research Society, 1990

19. Sapega AA, Moyer RA, Schneck C et al: The biomechanics of intra-operative "isometry" testing during anterior cruciate ligament reconstruction. Trans Orthop Res Soc 13:130, 1988

20. Henning E, Lynch MA, Glick KR: An in vitro strain guage study of elongation of the anterior cruciate ligament. Am J Sports Med 13:22, 1985

21. Grood EF, Suntay WJ, Noyes FR et al: Biomechanics of knee extension exercises. J Bone Joint Surg 66A:725, 1984

22. Johnson D: Controlling anterior shear during isokinetic knee extension exercise. J Ortho Sports Phys Ther 4:23, 1982

23. Sapega AA, Quedenfeld TC, Moyer RA et al: Biophysical factors in range-of-motion exercise. Physician Sportsmed 12:57, 1981

11

Anterior Cruciate Ligament Reconstruction Rehabilitation

ROBERT P. ENGLE
DANIEL P. GIESEN

INTRODUCTION

Reconstructive surgery for the anterior cruciate ligament (ACL)-deficient knee requires a long, carefully planned postoperative rehabilitation. The following have all been discussed in the published literature: strength, healing, and remodeling of substituted structures; period of immobilization or progressive mobilization; weight bearing; biomechanics of quadriceps, hamstrings, and other exercises; and the return to activity.[1–40]

Before beginning the rehabilitation process in ACL reconstruction, both physician and physical therapist should understand the stresses that they will be introducing to the patient's knee. Since each patient presents with a slightly different clinical profile, there can be no standard rehabilitation protocol. However, several important concepts and guidelines must be understood and used. These include: (1) acute versus chronic ACL insufficiency; (2) materials used for substitution and other associated procedures; (3) weight bearing; (4) range of motion guidelines; (5) neuromuscular considerations, including specific therapeutic exercise techniques; (6) progression to activity; (7) return to previous activity and maintenance. Each will be discussed relative to the bone-patellar tendon-bone autograft and allograft in this chapter.

REVIEW OF ACL REHABILITATION LITERATURE

Several common problems were encountered in postoperative ACL rehabilitation prior to the work of Paulos et al.[35] Immobilization following knee ligament surgery was a common practice. Extensive research, however, clearly demonstrated the negative impact of immobilization on articular cartilage.[1–7,29,33,40] This research quickly led to a trend toward early motion. Allowing range of motion was not without problems, however. Extension, primarily through the final 30 degrees of knee extension, was shown to increase ACL stress dramatically, jeopardizing surgical grafts.[35] Of the autogenous materials available to surgeons, only a bone-patellar tendon-bone graft was considered to have sufficient strength to allow immediate full passive extension and flexion.[13,30,31] Since then, the development of allografts and synthetic materials has provided an alternative to autograft procedures. The stiffness of these materials is inherently high, and their use eliminates the need to sacrifice a portion of the extensor mechanism.

At the time of surgery, biologic grafts are avascular. Their revascularization takes place during the first 6 weeks and is then followed by the formation of collagen, which remodels the necrotic graft into a functional ligament. This remodeling of healing autograft or allograft materials takes place slowly over 12 months or more. Research has shown that the grafted structures never reach their pretransplanted strength levels. During the first 6 weeks following surgery, graft strength is at its highest levels, followed by gradual weakening.[8,14,16,21,26,28,36]

Excessive stresses placed on the ACL during healing and an early return to activity can cause partial or full failure. Early quadriceps work has proved to be stressful, especially over the terminal portion of knee extension.[9,19,22,24,35,37] Quadriceps facilitation is clearly necessary, however, because of the intimate relationship between the quadriceps and the patellofemoral joint, and because the quadriceps undergo extensive disuse atrophy.

Although there are those who advocate very early resistive quadriceps exercise, others do not encourage a quadriceps program until several months after surgery.[10–12,24,25,27,35,38,39,41,42] Results of comparative rehabilitation protocols relative to ACL stability with fairly aggressive quadriceps activity do not exist in the literature. A standard quadriceps prescription based simply on the number of weeks since surgery is often inadequate, since each case is different and should be approached on an individual basis. Daniel et al.[19] found that the quadriceps actually translated the tibia posteriorly from 70 to 90 degrees of flexion, thereby decreasing ACL stress. This was also seen in the work of Arms et al.[10] and Renstrom et al.[37] Renstrom's study further documented the increased ACL stress during quadriceps contraction with tibial internal and neutral rotation. External rotation showed relatively lower ACL stress.[37] Quadriceps cocontraction with the hamstrings decreases ACL strain from full flexion to approximately 55 to 60 degrees of flexion and increases in further extension.[9]

These studies are important in understanding quadriceps and hamstring biomechanics, specifically on the ACL. Recent studies, unlike those previously cited, have investigated the effect of specific weight-bearing or functional, closed chain exercises on anterior translation and ACL rehabilitation. Knee stability should be enhanced by tibiofemoral compression in this position, especially at full extension, where the knee is in a closed packed or locked position.[10,18,23,25,34,38,39,41,42]

Most surgeons begin their patients on a non-weight-bearing or limited weight-bearing program with crutches. Early weight-bearing has recently been advocated by several investigators.[25,38,39] Progression can be either time based or dependent on variable, objective criteria such as instrumented examination, neuromuscular function, or range of motion measurements. Graft fixation must obviously be secure to allow early weight bearing. If fixation is considered weak, weight bearing should be delayed. Return to activity before the 12 months necessary for good graft remodeling and maturation has generally been contraindicated by several researchers.[16,18,35,38] Recent work has shown that a select group of patients can be safely returned to full activity in sports by 7 months, with no detrimental long-term effects.[25,38] Running and other activities can be permitted earlier provided good muscular support has been established.

POSTOPERATIVE REHABILITATION PROGRAM

Postoperative rehabilitation of bone-patellar tendon-bone ligament substitution is centered around components of the rehabilitation program already mentioned. Each of these is addressed separately with this program.

Acute Versus Chronic Insufficiency

Acutely reconstructed ACL ruptures typically rehabilitate differently from those that have chronic insufficiency. Relatively low levels of anterior displacement are elicited in the acute group since stretching of the secondary restraints has not had time to begin. The integrity of these secondary restraints leads to enhanced joint stability and less ACL stress postoperatively.

Chronic ACL insufficiency commonly leads to progressive secondary restraint stretching and instability, advanced joint surface erosion, chronic synovitis, and recurrent meniscal tears and surgeries.[43,44] These may all have been present before surgery, representing potential complications to normal rehabilitation.

Early weight bearing in these chronic patients may overstress the remaining menisci, lax secondary restraints, and articular surfaces that have already begun the degenerative process. Restoring range of motion quickly will be important, as these patients tend to lose motion more easily after surgery, especially if their own patellar tendons are sacrificed for autograft procedures. Quadriceps input to the patellofemoral joint must be established early, especially for preventing patella infera, a common postoperative complication.[45–47]

Comprehensive history taking and discussions with the surgeon following surgery will alert the physical therapist to some of these problems.

Associated Surgical Problems

Although this discussion is primarily limited to bone-patellar tendon-bone autograft and allograft, it is worthwhile mentioning other procedures that commonly accompany ACL reconstruction. Meniscus, medial collateral ligament, lateral collateral ligament, posterolateral capsular, patellofemoral, and osteochondral injuries can be associated with both acute and chronic ACL insufficiency. Reflex sympathetic dystrophies seen with traumatic knee injuries and surgical procedures must be recognized early.[48]

These can be dealt with in a number of ways, both surgically and conservatively. It is important to know what, if anything, has been done in conjunction with the ACL reconstruction. Weight bearing, range of motion limitations, and neuromuscular training will need to be altered accordingly.

Range of Motion Guidelines

We favor a program of immediate, controlled progressive mobilization over rigid immobilization. Full passive range of motion is permitted immediately with use of a high-strength graft such as bone-patellar tendon-bone. Continuous passive motion (CPM) devices and self range of motion exercises are used initially, without stress to the graft, to restore motion both with extension and flexion.[32,49,50]

Patients are initially maintained in a postoperative cast brace system with limitation of the final 20 degree extension and flexion to 90 degree or greater. These or other specially designed postoperative braces can be set to maintain the knee at full extension for flexion contracture management. The patient is placed in a functional knee brace between 2 and 4 weeks after surgery when swelling and comfort permit. Flexion is unlimited, but an extension limit with progressive increases to full extension can be used. Extension restrictions are dependent on graft function as measured by instrumented examination.

Patellar mobilization is a vital aspect of the rehabilitation program. These manual techniques to restore patellar gliding and prevent contractures of peripatellar structures, such as the patellar tendon, are critical.[51,52] They should begin as soon after surgery as possible and be augmented by quadriceps setting exercises and electrical muscle stimulation.

Weight Bearing

ACL graft strength is highest immediately following surgery and should be minimally affected by weight bearing forces. Weight bearing is important for stimulating mechanoreceptors that assist with proprioception and neuromuscular recruitment. Articular cartilage nourishment and function is also stimulated. Antero-posterior translation is decreased in the weight-bearing position, which in turn decreases ACL stress.

During the first 4 weeks, patients are limited to partial weight bearing on crutches with their postoperative cast brace or functional brace systems. After week 4, patients can progress to full weight bearing without crutches, using the functional knee brace for control of anterior translatory and ACL forces. Tolerance to unrestricted ambulation without crutches varies from patient to patient, so each case should be handled individually. Cases in which significant articular cartilage defects or meniscal repairs are present will require a more conservative timetable. Patient grafts should be monitored carefully during this period.[53]

Neuromuscular Training: Specific Therapeutic Exercise Techniques and Procedures

Extensive disuse atrophy affecting the entire lower extremity, including the quadriceps and hamstrings, results from ACL reconstructive procedures. Not only is strength in the muscle groups diminished, but endurance, stabilization, balance, coordination, and proprioception are greatly decreased. These, in turn, effect gait, synergistic patellofemoral and tibiofemoral dynamic stability, and range of motion.

Reflex inhibition mechanisms begin immediately following surgery from the synovitis, harvesting of the patellar tendon in autografts, effusion, and pain. As arthroscopic surgical techniques have evolved, the need to dissect through the synovium and its mechanoreceptor system has decreased. Early motion has been shown to decrease effusion, pain, and inhibition.[32] Weight bearing, as mentioned previously, provides early input to the mechanoreceptors, also enhancing neuromuscular response.

Since disuse atrophy is a neuromuscular and not simply a muscular problem, an innovative neurophysiologic approach is necessary for facilitating return of full neuromuscular function. The techniques and procedures of Voss et al.[54] and Johnson and Saliba[55] work the entire extremity and their synergistic components in functional, diagonal, and spiral patterns, both weight bearing and non-weight bearing. These exercises must be applied and modified within the orthopaedic constraints of individual surgical procedures. Readers are encouraged to review the work of these and other investigators for a clearer understanding of their approaches.

Generally, therapeutic exercise procedures progress from those that are the least stressful to the healing graft to those that must be more cautiously applied. Manual techniques afford many advantages for the physical therapist and patient. Specific input can be directed more effectively to elicit a more specific motor output and avoid substitution patterns. Resistance can be applied to points in the range of motion where the patient is most deficient, using isometric, concentric, and eccentric techniques. The joint can be taken to end range to increase and reinforce range of motion gains. Proprioception can be enhanced through manual contacts and other stimuli.

Knowing these and other techniques is not enough, however. A clear understanding of the biomechanics of the musculotendinous structures and weight-bearing forces across the knee is necessary. Quadriceps and hamstring function at the knee has already been briefly described.

The hamstrings act to restrain anterior translation of the tibia relative to the femur, thereby decreasing

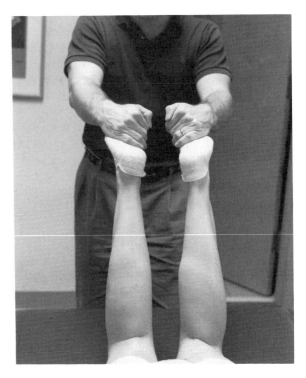

Fig. 11-1. Knee flexion prone using bilateral technique.

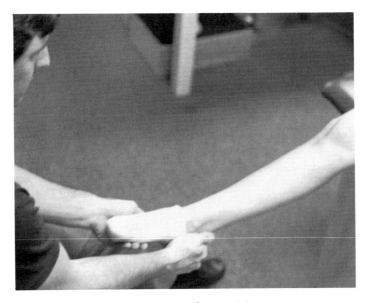

Fig. 11-2. Knee flexion sitting.

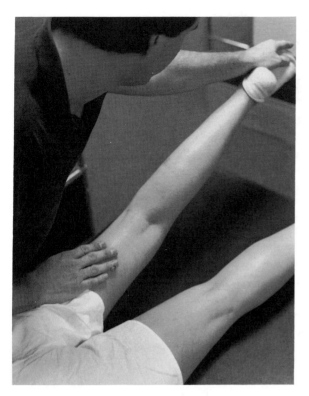

Fig. 11-3. D1 extension with knee maintained in 20 degrees of flexion prone.

ACL stress throughout knee range of motion. Furthermore, the semimembranosus and pes anserinus stabilize the medial and the biceps femoris and popliteus stabilize the lateral components posteriorly. Functionally, they assist in control of knee extension eccentrically in gait and provide a compressive force of the femur on the tibia. They can be emphasized during the initial stages of rehabilitation.

Conversely, the quadriceps anteriorly translate the tibia relative to the femur (except beyond 70 to 75 degrees) into further flexion. Research has documented the negative effects on ACL grafts by the quadriceps, primarily in isolated knee extension.[9,19,20,22,24,35,37] Functionally, however, the quadriceps work synergistically with the hamstrings and other muscle groups in weight bearing or a closed kinetic chain manner. Much less is known about quadriceps' effect on these positions. These closed and modified closed chain techniques provide a better alternative to the open kinetic chain training approaches for the quadriceps, although more research is necessary.

Integration of open, modified closed, and closed kinetic chain procedures with manual techniques are preferable. Adjunctive procedures are supplemented by machines and other resistive or proprioceptive de-

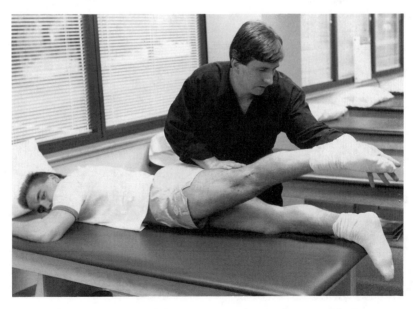

Fig. 11-4. D2 extension with knee maintained in 20 degrees of flexion prone.

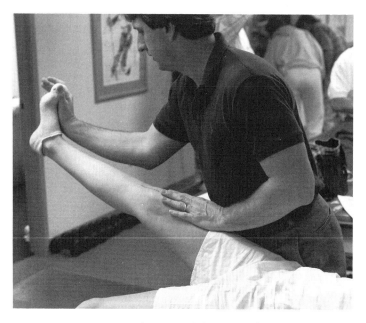

Fig. 11-5. D1 flexion with knee straight supine.

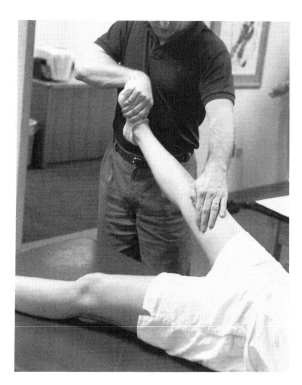

Fig. 11-6. D2 flexion with knee straight supine.

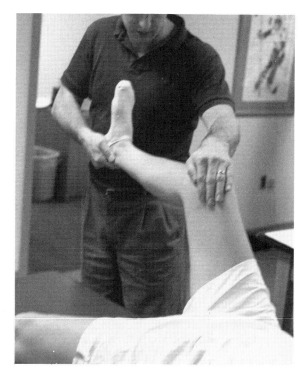

Fig. 11-7. D1 flexion with knee flexion supine.

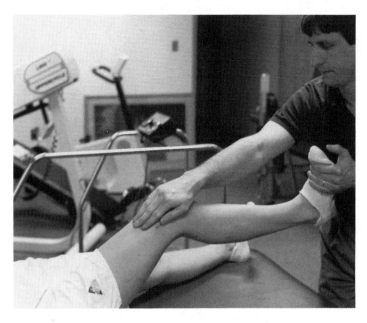

Fig. 11-8. D2 flexion with knee flexion supine.

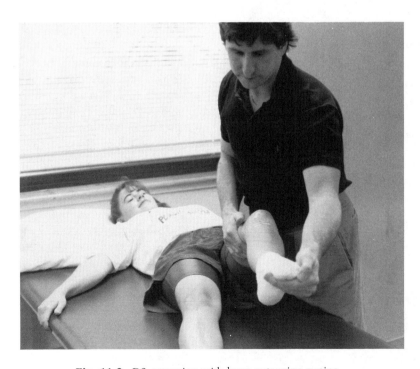

Fig. 11-9. D2 extension with knee extension supine.

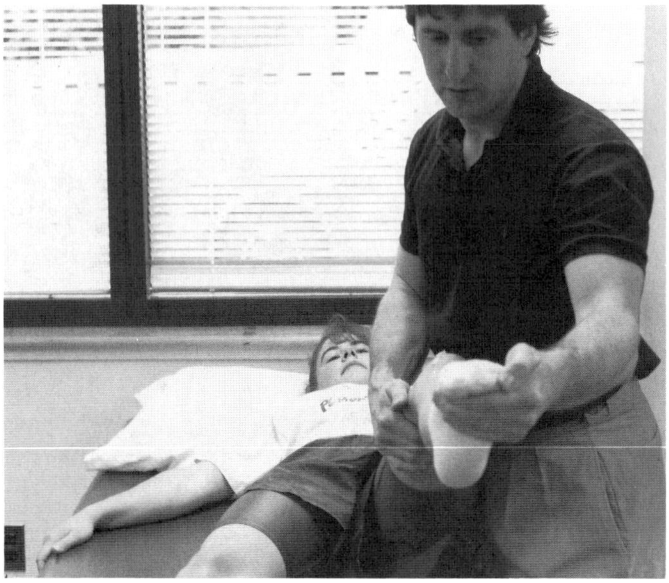

Fig. 11-10. Linear hip-knee extension.

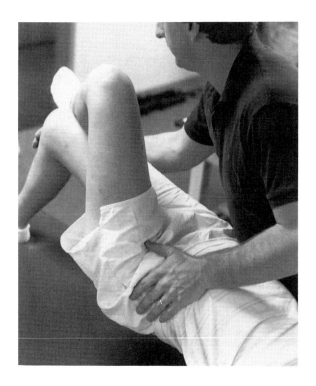

Fig. 11-11. Bridging bilateral with 90 degrees of knee flexion.

vices. Each time an exercise is selected, its effect on the ACL and other components of the knee (menisci, articular surfaces, and other capsuloligamentous structures) must be considered. Continual, ongoing re-evaluation of the patient is necessary to avoid negative effects. Instrumented ligament examination is helpful in assessing ACL stability.

Neuromuscular facilitation can be broken down into a progression of levels as follows.

Level I

In immediate ACL reconstruction rehabilitation, several open and modified closed chain procedures are important. These include knee flexion through the available range of motion with the patient prone, sitting, or supine (Figs. 11-1 and 11-2). Both lower extremity extension diagonals with the patient prone and/or supine and the knee isometrically maintained in end-range extension or other positions by the hamstrings can be used (Figs. 11-3 and 11-4). These patterns primarily recruit the hamstrings and decrease ACL stress. They also begin stretching of the tight anterior structures and facilitate components of trunk rotation and extension.

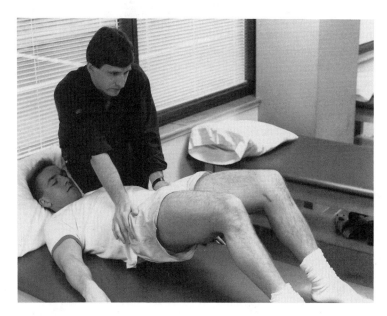

Fig. 11-12. Bridging unilateral with tibial external rotation.

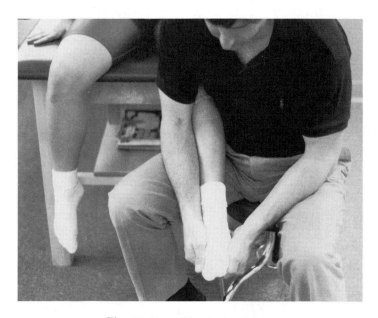

Fig. 11-13. Ankle plantar flexion.

Next, the therapist must pay attention to the quadriceps through the lower extremity patterns that create quadriceps irradiation from a stronger proximal component without inducing high forces on the ACL. Both flexion-adduction and flexion-abduction diagonal patterns can be used. The knee can be maintained in flexion from 30 degrees or greater, with the patient supine or sitting, using a combination of isotonic techniques (Figs. 11-5 and 11-6). With autograft procedures, in which full knee extension is often lost, we prefer to maintain the knee in full extension when graft fixation is secure. This helps glide the patella superiorly at full extension, preventing patella infera. Isotonic reversal techniques with reciprocal flexion-extension components of the pattern are also used.

Flexion-adduction and flexion-abduction with knee flexion isotonically recruits the hamstrings (Figs. 11-7 and 11-8). Tibial rotation accompanying these patterns can be resisted isometrically initially. Movement into external rotation depends on the specific procedure and should be discussed with the surgeon. Internal rotation must be avoided.

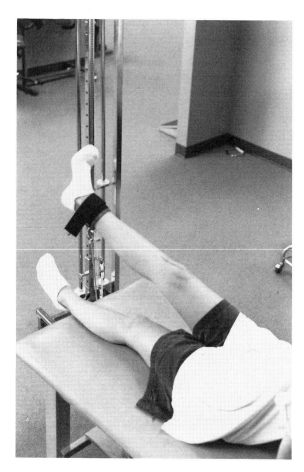

Fig. 11-15. Wall pulley progressive resisted exercises in D1 flexion with knee straight sitting.

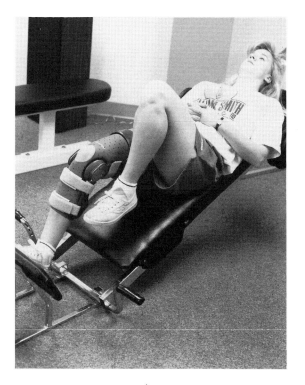

Fig. 11-14. Leg press.

Extension-adduction-external rotation with knee extension increases facilitation of the vastus medialis oblique while decreasing ACL stress (Fig. 11-9). However, the posterolateral complex undergoes stresses that may be contraindicated. Linear hip with knee extension patterns can be substituted to decrease ACL stress (Fig. 11-10). Manual contacts on the foot can simulate weight-bearing forces or contact to a limited degree, making these procedures modifications of a closed kinetic chain.

Bridging is an early partial weight-bearing technique (Figs. 11-11 and 11-12). The knee can be isotonically or isometrically resisted with one or both feet contacting the ground through a selected range of motion. Pelvic and trunk components can be facilitated synergistically with the quadriceps and hamstrings. Dorsi and plantar flexion can also be worked from this position, as well as within the other patterns already mentioned (Fig. 11-13).

Adjunctively, several techniques reinforce neuromuscular recruitment without direct, hands-on intervention by the physical therapist. Leg press or squat exercises on a Total Gym (EMI Engineering, San Diego, CA) offer various degrees of incline for more or less weight bearing, with the capability of adding weighted resistance (Fig. 11-14).

Wall pulleys in the patterns described supplement the manual techniques (Fig. 11-15).[56] Knee flexion or hamstring concentric-eccentric training on resistive exercise and isokinetic training equipment can follow initial manual sessions. Isolated resisted knee extension in deep flexion (75 to 95 degrees) can be included. Stationary bicycling is permitted when knee flexion is adequate. Partial range or unaffected leg cycling can begin earlier.

Balance and proprioception can be assisted through training on a platform system, beginning with minimal and progressing to eventual full unilateral weight bearing (Fig. 11-16). Electrical muscle stimulation has been helpful in augmenting the rehabilitation program by providing increased input to both the quadriceps and hamstrings.[57,58] This is especially helpful in conjunction with quadriceps isometrics at full extension to avoid disassociation.

Level II

Patient rehabilitation can progress to a higher, more stressful level at 3 to 6 weeks if the instrumented examination remains negative. Aggressive patellar mobilization is generally still necessary to stretch the tight inferior and lateral structures in conjunction with quadriceps facilitation (Fig. 11-17). Procedures already presented continue to be useful during this period.

Weight-bearing exercises are added with resistance through manual contacts with other methods. These include toe raises, squats, step-ups, resisted gait, and reciprocal lower extremity extension (Figs. 11-8 to 11-21). Squats and step-up exercises have recently been shown to decrease ACL stress.[15,18,34,38] Treadmill walking, stair climbing, and several other closed chain activities were safer than performing a simple Lachman examination in Henning's work (Figs. 11-22 and 11-

23).[24] The joint must be stressed cautiously with these exercises, however, and monitored closely for effusion, laxity, and joint surface irritation. As surgical fixation has improved, weight-bearing exercises have been added much sooner in the rehabilitation program.

Level III

Hamstring, hip-pelvic, and lower leg neuromuscular function is typically restored in our patients within 3 months of surgery. Full active and passive knee extension and flexion, an asymptomatic patellofemoral joint, and no effusion should also be seen at this point. Quadriceps function, balance, and proprioception, however, are often still deficient. More aggressive re-

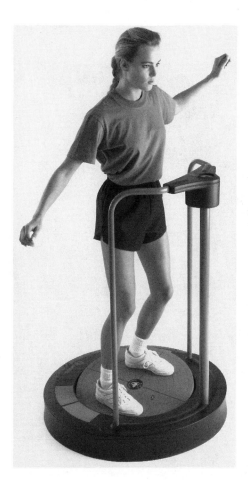

Fig. 11-16. Balance training. (Courtesy of BREG, Inc., Vista, CA.)

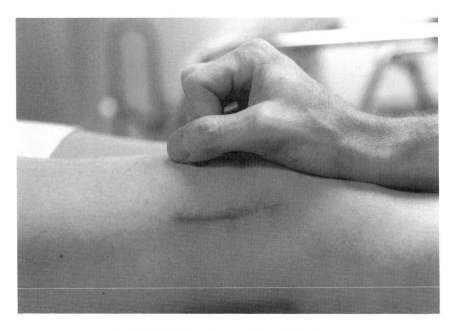

Fig. 11-17. Superior patellar mobilization.

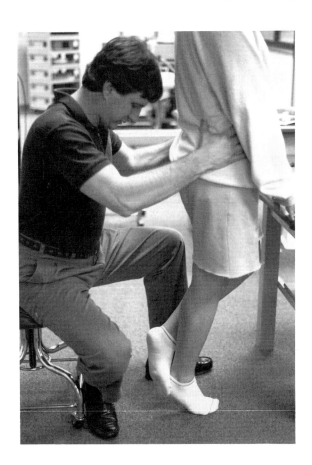

Fig. 11-18. Ankle plantar flexion weight bearing.

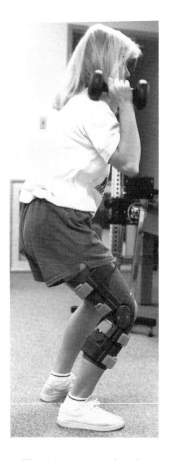

Fig. 11-19. Knee bends.

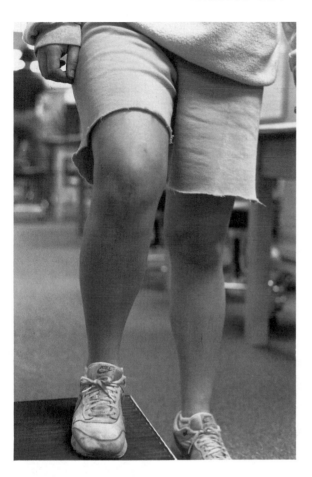

Fig. 11-20. Step-ups.

Progression and Return to Activity

Each patient presents for surgery with individual goals and activities. As the rehabilitation program unfolds, selected components of their desired activity can be incorporated into their exercise bouts or periods. The most common components involve simple walking and running, which are introduced early (within 3 to 5 months) in uncomplicated cases. Activities requiring turning, pivoting, jumping, and cutting are generally not introduced until 5 months after surgery.

Return to full and unrestricted activity, without instability or other signs and symptoms, is the ultimate goal of surgery. Rehabilitation must be complete to allow patients to risk graft function in stressful activities. Several criteria must be met by patients in our program.

First, graft strength and stability must be within 3 mm with full instrumented and manual maximal anterior translation tests. Compliance index measurements should be equal bilaterally. This will be monitored closely during the progression to activity. De-

sistance, endurance, and proprioceptive training is continued. The specific neuromuscular deficits are addressed without jeopardizing graft or patellofemoral function. Very low level plyometric or functional training activity in the weight-bearing position can progress between 6 and 12 weeks after surgery. These exercises are designed to stimulate the mechanoreceptor system (Figs. 11-24 to 11-26).

Repeat clinical examination continues over the initial 12 weeks (including instrumented stability and neuromuscular testing). At 12 weeks, patients can usually decrease formal therapy and follow an independent functionally oriented program. Appropriate monitoring is necessary to ensure compliance and effectiveness of progression toward the goals of rehabilitation.

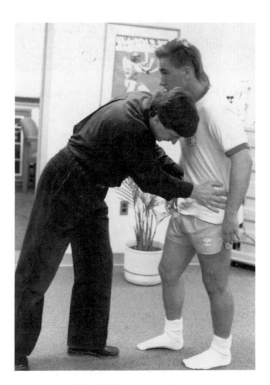

Fig. 11-21. Resisted gait.

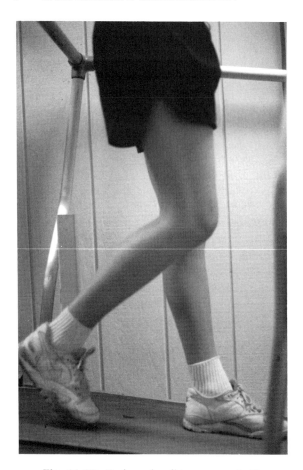

Fig. 11-22. Backward walking on treadmill.

creases in graft strength make early return a contraindication.

Second, adequate lower extremity neuromuscular function must be restored. Equal hamstring function on bilateral manual, and isokinetic comparisons under concentric and eccentric conditions is necessary. The quadriceps complex should be within 10 percent of the uninvolved side in terms of strength and endurance. Clinical and functional tests in which the quadriceps are working synergistically with other muscle groups must be critically assessed on a sport- or activity-specific test.

Third, patellofemoral function should be cleared for maximal stress. Good vastus medialis support to patellofemoral joint stability and tracking is vital. Retropatellar symptoms, including crepitus and pain, should be monitored during progression to activity and symptoms should be considered under control. Many ACL reconstruction patients experience patellofemoral symptoms in follow-up with no compromise of ACL stability.

Fourth, adequate range of motion should be present for the chosen activity. Our preference is to have full active-passive knee flexion-extension on bilateral comparison before allowing full activity. Concentrated joint surface stresses, particularly at the patellofemoral joint, occur with limited extension and activities that repetitively stress the knee at end range.

Fifth, patients should be free from effusion during the period when activity levels are increasing. Recurrent effusion and synovitis lead to advanced articular cartilage erosion, reflex neuromuscular inhibition mechanisms, and negative effects on the ACL graft.

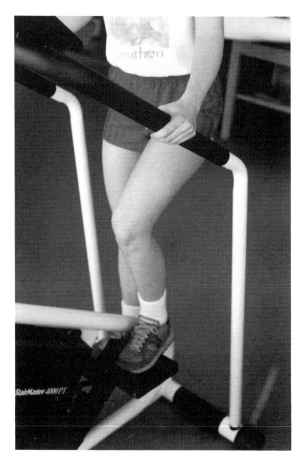

Fig. 11-23. Stair climbing. (Stairmaster 400PT, Randal Sports Medical Products, Kirkland, WA.)

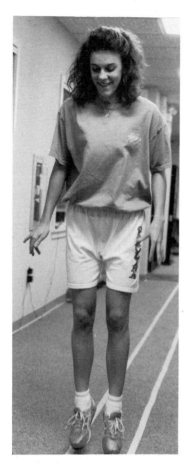

Fig. 11-24. Forward/backward hopping.

Maintenance

It is not unusual for a patient to be told following ACL surgery that rehabilitation will be a lifelong project. Unfortunately, the injuries that cause the rupture usually involve significant damage to the joint, compromising its long-term function.

Extensive surgery that involves a relatively high morbidity can contribute further to the joint's and patient's ultimate demise. Fortunately, surgery is becoming less traumatic to the joint with the increased technical skills of arthroscopic surgeons and the movement toward early and complete rehabilitation.

Patients in our program are encouraged to follow a conditioning program that specifically addresses the patellofemoral joint, any residual instabilities, specific neuromuscular deficiencies, and the patient's individual demands and activities. This can be a continuous program, although patient compliance is better on a periodic basis that coincides with their sports seasons.

Sixth, the affected knee should be free of pain or instability both during and after activities. We believe these criteria should be met in all postoperative ACL reconstruction patients before permitting return to full activity.

Finally, a general timetable must be considered for sufficient healing to have occurred. Twelve months or longer has been the standard time until full activity is permitted secondary to adequate ACL graft maturation. Some patients fail to meet the criteria outlined above within that time period and should be held back. At this time, however, there is some hope of safely returning a group of ACL reconstruction patients to activity sooner than the traditional 12 months.[25,58] Further research is necessary to determine whether or not graft maturation can occur more rapidly in some patients.

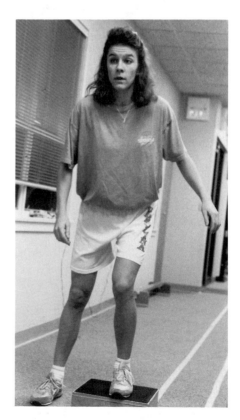

Fig. 11-25. Side to side box jumping.

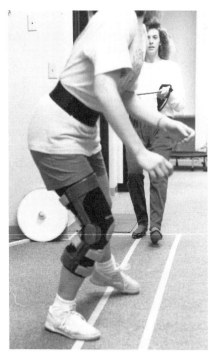

Fig. 11-26. Resisted running laterally with elastic cords (Sportcord, SPORT, Vail, CO).

We hope that, through early diagnosis, rapid and effective surgical treatment, and complete rehabilitation, patients will not be engaged in a lifelong struggle with their knees.

FOLLOW-UP

Patients are seen by the physician for follow-up every 2 to 3 weeks until 4 months after surgery. Re-evaluations to monitor knee stability, range of motion, neuromuscular, and other components of joint function are performed at 6, 9, 12, 18, and 24 months.

SUMMARY

ACL surgical reconstruction and rehabilitation techniques have advanced dramatically over the past several years. Research has expanded our knowledge of anatomy, biomechanics, diagnosis, surgical techniques, remodeling of biomaterials, synthetic substitutes, effects of immobility on articular cartilage, weight bearing, range of motion, therapeutic exercise and adjunctive procedures, return to activity, and complications. Physical therapists and physicians need to understand all these components for successful management of the patient with ACL problems.

Rehabilitation following bone-patellar tendon-bone autograft and allograft substitution for ACL insufficiency has been discussed. As clinical experience and basic science advance, both surgery and rehabilitation will continue to change in a positive direction. The result will be improved patient care.

REFERENCES

1. Akeson WH: An experimental study of joint stiffness. J Bone Joint Surgery 43A:1022, 1961
2. Akeson WH, Amiel D, LaViolette D: The connective tissue response to immobility: a study of chondroiton-4 and -6 sulfate and dermation sulfate changes in periarticular connective tissue in control and immobilized knees of dogs. Clin Orthop 51:183, 1967
3. Akeson WH, Amiel D, LaViolette D et al: The connective tissue response to immobility: an accelerated aging response? Exp Gerontol 3:289, 1968
4. Akeson WH, Amiel D, Mechanic GL et al: Collagen cross-linking alteration in joint contractures. Changes in the reducible cross-links in periarticular connective tissue collagen after nine weeks of immobilization. Connect Tissue Res 5:15, 1977
5. Akeson WH, Amiel D, Woo SL: Immobility effects on synovial joints. The patheomechanics of joint contracture. Biorheology 17:95, 1980
6. Akeson WH, Woo SL, Amiel D et al: The connective tissue response to immobility: biochemical changes in periarticular connective tissue of the immobilized rabbit knee. Clin Orthop 93:356, 1973
7. Akeson WH, Woo SL, Amiel D, Frank CB: The biology of ligaments. p. 93. In Hunter LY, Funk FJ (eds): Rehabilitation of the Injured Knee. CV Mosby, St. Louis, 1984
8. Alm A, Ekstrom H, Gillquist J et al: The anterior cruciate ligament—a clinical and experimental study on tensile strength, morphology and replacement by patellar ligament. Acta Chir Scand, suppl. 445, 1974
9. Arms SW, Pope MH, Johnson RJ et al: The biomechanics of anterior cruciate ligament rehabilitation and reconstruction. Am J Sports Med 12:8, 1984
10. Begnnon BD, Pope MH, Fleming BC et al: An in-vivo study of the ACL strain biomechanics in the normal knee. Orthrop Trans 13:361, 1989

11. Blackburn TA: Rehabilitation of anterior cruciate ligament injuries. Orthop Clin North Am 16:241, 1985

12. Brewster CE, Moynes DR, Jobe FW: Rehabilitation for anterior cruciate reconstruction. J Orthop Sports Phys Ther 5:121, 1983

13. Butler DL, Noyes FR, Grood ES et al: Mechanical properties of transplants for the anterior cruciate ligament. Trans Orthop Res Soc 4:81, 1979

14. Cabaud HE, Rodkey WG, Feagin JA: Experimental studies of acute anterior cruciate ligament injury and repair. Am J Sports Med 7:18, 1979

15. Chandler TJ, Wilson GD, Store MH: The effects of the squat exercise on knee stability. Med Sci Sports Exerc 21:299, 1989

16. Clancy WG, Nanechania RG, Rosenberg TD et al: Anterior and posterior cruciate ligament reconstruction in rhesus monkeys. J Bone Joint Surg 63:1270, 1981

17. Clancy WG, Nelson DA, Reider B, Narechania RG: Anterior cruciate ligament reconstruction using one-third of the patella ligament augmented by extra-articular tendon transfers. J Bone Joint Surg 64A:353, 1982

18. Collins C, Yack J, Whieldon T: A case for using closed kinetic chain activities in the rehabilitation of ACL deficient knees, abstracted. Athl Train 24:120, 1989

19. Daniel D, Lawler J, Malcom L et al: The quadriceps-anterior cruciate interaction. Orthop Trans 6:199, 1982

20. Delsman PA, Lasse GM: Isokinetic shear forces and their effect on the quadriceps active drawer, abstracted. Med Sci Sports Exerc 16:151, 1984

21. Gelberman RH, Menon J, Gonslaves M et al: The effects of mobilization on the vascularization of healing flexor tendons in dogs. Clin Orthop 153:283, 1980

22. Grood ES, Suntay WJ, Noyes FR, Butler DL: Biomechanics of the knee extension exercise. Effect of cutting the anterior cruciate ligament. J Bone Joint Surg 66A:725, 1984

23. Haggmark T, Ericksson E: Cylinder or mobile cast brace after knee ligament surgery: a clinical analysis and morphological and enzymatic studies of changes in the quadriceps muscle. Am J Sports Med 7:48, 1979

24. Henning CE, Lynch MA, Glick K: An in vivo strain gauge study of elongation of the anterior cruciate ligament. Am J Sports Med 13:22, 1985

25. Higgins RW, Steadman JR: Anterior cruciate ligament repairs in elite skiers. Am J Sports Med 15:434, 1987

26. Hirsch EF, Morgan RH: Causal significance of traumatic ossification in tendon insertions. Arch Surg 39:824, 1939

27. Heugel M, Indelicato PA: Trends in rehabilitation following anterior cruciate ligament reconstruction. Clin Sports Med 7:801, 1988

28. Kennedy JC, Weinberg HW, Wilson AS: Anatomy and function of the anterior cruciate ligament. J Bone Joint Surg 56A:223, 1974

29. Noyes FR: Functional properties of knee ligaments and alterations induced by immobilization. Clin Orthop 123:210, 1977

30. Noyes FR, Butler DL, Grood ES et al: Biomechanical analysis of human ligament grafts used in knee-ligament repairs and reconstructions. J Bone Joint Surg 66:344, 1984

31. Noyes FR, Butler DL, Paulos LE, Grood ES: Intra-articular cruciate reconstruction. I. Perspectives on graft strength, vascularization and immediate motion after replacement. Clin Northop 172:71, 1983

32. Noyes FR, Mangine RE, Barber S: Early knee motion after open and arthroscopic anterior cruciate ligament reconstruction. Am J Sports Med 15:149, 1987

33. Noyes FR, Torvik PJ, Hyde WB et al: Biomechanics of ligament failure. II. An analysis of immobilization, exercise and reconditioning effects in primates. J Bone Joint Surg 56:1406, 1974

34. Ohkoshi Y, Yasuda K: Biomechanical analysis of shear force exerted to anterior cruciate ligament during half squat exercise. Orthop Trans 13:310, 1989

35. Paulos L, Noyes FR, Grood E, Butler DL: Knee rehabilitation after anterior cruciate ligament reconstruction and repair. Am J Sports Med 9:140, 1981

36. Paulos LE, Payne FC, Rosenberg TD: Rehabilitation after anterior cruciate ligament surgery. p. 291. In Jackson DW, Drez D (eds): The Anterior Cruciate Deficient Knee. CV Mosby, St. Louis, 1986

37. Renstrom P, Arms SW, Stanwyck TS et al: Strain within the anterior cruciate ligament during hamstring and quadriceps activity. Am J Sports Med 14:83, 1986

38. Shelbourne KD, Nitz P: Accelerated rehabilitation following anterior cruciate ligament reconstruction. Am J Sports Med 18:292, 1990

39. Steadman JR, Foster RS, Silferskiold JP: Rehabilitation of the knee. Clin Sports Med 8:605, 1989

40. Woo SLY, Matthews JV, Akeson WH et al: The connective tissue response to immobility: a correlative study of the biomechanical and biochemical measurements of the normal and immobilized rabbit knee. Arthritis Rheum 18:257, 1975

41. Engle RP, Lauchle LE, Canner GC, Meade TM: Immediate post-operative anterior cruciate reconstruction: quadriceps facilitation in full knee extension, abstracted. Presented at the American Physical Therapy Association Annual Meeting, 1990

42. Jonsson H, Karrholm J, Elmquist LG: Kinematics of active knee extension after tear of the anterior cruciate ligament. Am J Sports Med 17:796, 1989

43. Noyes FR, Matthews DS, Mooar PA, Grood ES: The symptomatic anterior cruciate deficient knee. Part II: The results of rehabilitation, activity modification and counseling in functional disability. J Bone Joint Surg 65A:163, 1983

44. Noyes FR, Mooar PA, Matthews DS, Butler DL: The symptomatic anterior cruciate-deficient knee. Part I: The long-term functional disability in athletically active individuals. J Bone Joint Surg 65A:154, 1983

45. Paulos LE, Rosenberg TD, Drawbert J et al: Infrapatellar contracture syndrome. Am J Sports Med 15:336, 1987

46. Roberts TS, Drez D, Banta CJ: Complications of anterior cruciate ligament reconstruction. p. 169. In Sprague NF (ed): Complications in Arthroscopy. Raven Press, New York, 1989

47. Wojtys EM, Noyes FR: Patella infera syndrome. Presented at the 53rd Annual Meeting of the American Academy of Orthopaedic Surgeons. New Orleans, LA, February 1986

48. Poehling GC, Koman LA, Pollock FE: Reflex sympathetic dystrophy of the knee. p. 53. In Sprague NF (ed): Complications in Arthroscopy. Raven Press, New York, 1989

49. Anderson AF, Lipscomb AB: Analysis of rehabilitation techniques after anterior cruciate reconstruction. Am J Sports Med 17:154, 1989

50. Burks R, Daniel D, Losse G: The effect of continuous passive motion on anterior cruciate ligament reconstruction stability. Am J Sports Med 12:323, 1984

51. Kattenborn FM: Mobilization of the Extremity Joints. p. 149. Olaf Norlis Bokhandel, Oslo, 1985

52. Maitland GD: Peripheral Manipulation. p. 252. Butterworth, Boston, 1977

53. Torg JS, Vegso JJ, Torg E: Rehabilitation of Athletic Injuries: An Atlas of Therapeutic Exercises. Year Book Medical Publishers, Chicago, 1987

54. Voss DE, Ionta JK, Myers BJ: Proprioceptive Neuromuscular Facilitation. Harper & Row, New York, 1985

55. Johnson G, Saliba V: Proprioceptive Neuromuscular Facilitation I and II. Course Manual. Institute of Physical Art, San Anselmo, CA, 1988

56. Engle RP: Knee ligament rehabilitation. Clin Manage Phys Ther 10:36, 1990

57. Arvidsson I, Eriksson E: Counteracting muscle atrophy after ACL injury: scientific basis for a rehabilitation program. p. 451. In Feagin JA (ed): The Crucial Ligaments. Churchill Livingstone, New York, 1988

58. Kain CC, McCarthy JA, Arms S et al: An in vivo analysis of the effect of transcutaneous electrical stimulation of the quadriceps and hamstrings on anterior cruciate ligament deformation. Am J Sports Med 16:147, 1988

12

Postoperative Anterior Cruciate Ligament Synthetic Reconstruction Rehabilitation

T. J. ANTICH

INTRODUCTION

Development of the Gore-Tex polytetrafluoroethylene (PTFE) prosthetic ligament (Fig. 12-1) began in 1979 by W. L. Gore & Associates in Flagstaff, AZ. Several criteria would have to be met for the final product to be considered orthopaedically successful as well as acceptable to the United States Food & Drug Administration (FDA). Bruckman et al.[1] reviewed the requirements of a prosthetic ligament graft, which included

1. the need for an easy surgical placement;
2. the need for sturdy fixation with subsequent early joint mobilization;
3. the need for proper anatomic and biomechanical placement to prevent excess wear and tear at extremes of motion;
4. the need for in vivo longevity greater than or equal to that of other available ligament grafts whether autografts or allografts; and
5. the need for graft acceptance and tissue compatability within the human knee joint.

One main reason for the development of this synthetic ligament is its ultimate tensile strength with respect to other autogenous tissues (Table 12-1).[2,3] During its laboratory testing, the PTFE prosthesis demonstrated elongation of only 3 percent following 20 million cycles at a 285-newton (N) load (63.6 lbs).[3]

The main reasons for utilizing a synthetic ligament graft are

1. to spare the body's autogenous tissue, especially in cases in which small patellar tendon might result in the harvesting of a narrow graft;
2. to avoid tampering with the extensor mechanism graft site and to avoid the potential for patellofemoral joint symptoms and long-term quadriceps weakness; and
3. to accelerate rehabilitation and return to function via a stronger graft early on in the postoperative period.

At present, the Gore-Tex PTFE synthetic ligament is approved by the FDA for implantation only in the knees of patients who have failed intra-articular reconstruction. One would obviously have to expect less impressive results in a patient who has had a prior failed surgical procedure than in a patient with a "virgin knee."

The role of the physical therapist cannot be underestimated in the patient's rehabilitation and how it will effect the overall outcome of the surgery. In the ideal model, the therapist works closely with the attending orthopaedic surgeon. As a team, the two evaluate the patient pre- and postoperatively as they continue to monitor the patient through follow-up visits.

PREOPERATIVE EVALUATION

The patient meets with the therapist prior to surgery for an evaluation as outlined in Figure 12-2. The answers to specific questions provide data against which postoperative responses can be matched.

135

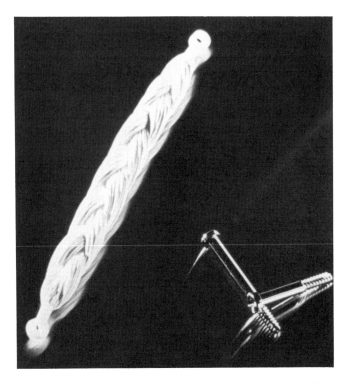

Fig. 12-1. Gore-Tex polytetrafluorethylene (PTFE) prosthetic ligament. (Courtesy of W. L. Gore and Associates, Flagstaff, AZ.)

A very important question in the preoperative evaluation is the overall functional rating. This is explained by the therapist as including pain, motion, strength, ability, and disability, both with daily activities and with recreational and competitive sports. When answered as a definite number, these data are then quantified and can be utilized statistically in comparisons.

Discussion of present complaints is extremely important, as the patient is telling you why the surgery is being performed. This then allows the therapist to determine whether the patient's goals have been met.

Objective evaluation includes range of motion and limb girth measurements for assessment of muscle atrophy as well as joint swelling. The KT-1000 arthrometer is utilized for documentation of increased anteroposterior (AP) laxity. Isokinetic quadriceps and hamstrings testing is performed at slow and fast speeds on both the uninjured and the preoperative sides.

SURGICAL TECHNIQUE

Following ligamentous examination under anesthesia, the arthroscope is introduced for evaluation of meniscal, capsular, or other articular lesions. A notchplasty is performed (Fig. 12-3), making sure that adequate bone is removed posteriorly to minimize possibilities of graft impingement and ultimate failure.[4]

A 2-inch vertical tibial incision is made medial to the patellar tendon, and the tibial drill hole aims toward the lateral femoral condyle. This is followed by a 3.5-inch cut over the distal lateral femur, with the femoral hole being drilled from superolaterally. Umbilical tape is utilized to measure for the appropriate

Table 12-1. Ultimate Tensile Strengths of the Human Anterior Cruciate Ligament and Other Structures

Structure	Newtons
Gore-Tex PTFE ligament	4,900
Patellar tendon graft	2,900
Human anterior cruciate ligament	1,725
Semitendinosus tendon	1,216

(Modified from Noyes et al.[2] and Bolton and Bruchman,[3] with permission.)

Table 12-2. Key Surgical Points for Optimal Results

Adequate notchplasty

Tunnels in line with graft to prevent angulation as it exits drill holes

Deepen bone trough over lateral femoral condyle to improve isometric placement

Burr edges of tunnels to reduce sharp edges

Pretension ligament graft prior to screwing in tibial end (50 repeats)

graft size, and the Gore-Tex graft is then pulled through from the tibial hole superiorly through the femur. A bicortical screw fixes the femoral eyelet to the lateral femur approximately 4 inches cephalad to the drill hole (Fig. 12-4) in a transverse lateral-to-medial fashion.

Twenty pounds of pressure is applied to the tibial end of the graft as the knee is taken through 20 arcs of full flexion and extension. This serves to take out all the slack that exists in the synthetic ligament. Up to 5 mm of unwanted laxity (Fig. 12-5) can result if the ligament is not pretensioned properly.[5]

Table 12-2 lists the key surgical points for optimal results.

POSTOPERATIVE HOSPITAL CARE

The patient arrives in the recovery room, where the operated knee is placed in a continuous passive motion unit to begin early range of motion (ROM). Since many patients undergoing Gore-Tex reconstruction will have had failed intra-articular reconstructions with associated other joint degenerative changes, it is imperative that motion begin early to prevent joint contractures.

A Jackson-Pratt drain is kept in the joint the first night to minimize fluid accumulation. The patient remains in the hospital usually for 2 nights and is discharged on postoperative day 2 as long as no other complications arise. Patients leave the hospital ambulating under their own power with the assistance of axillary crutches. Physical therapy starts in the first postoperative week, with the therapist recording ROM and joint girth measurements bilaterally on patient arrival.

Table 12-3 compares postoperative care and rehabilitation at different clinics.

FIRST 2 WEEKS AFTER SURGERY

The therapist's primary function is to accurately document motion and decrease of swelling. ROM exercises with no restrictions on terminal flexion or extension are started and performed at home as well. Isometric hamstring sets are performed at angle of 60 degrees of flexion to maximize electromyographic (EMG) and torque output. Quadriceps sets are performed with a bolster under the knee as this usually enables the patient to generate a more forceful contraction.

Hip abduction (side leg raise) exercises are utilized to maintain the strength of the gluteus medius while the patient continues to use crutches for gait. Isotonic

Table 12-3. Differences in Postoperative Care and Rehabilitation

	Ferkel[a]	Tibone[b]	Steadman[c]	Ahlfeld[d]
Hospital stay	50% 1 Night 40% 2 Nights			
Crutches	5–10 days as needed	For comfort (1 week)	3 days to 3 weeks	Up to 6 weeks
Weight bearing	Night of surgery	Immediate	Immediate	10% weight bearing immediately
Bracing	High-stress sports	None	Custom brace for cutting sports	Custom brace 4 months postsurgery
Running	6–12 weeks	3 months	When ROM and strength will allow	6 months with 75% strength
Full sports	3–6 months; contact sports not recommended	6 months	4–6 months; must pass functional test	9 months with 90% strength

[a] SCOI, 15211 VanOwen Street, Suite 300, Van Nuys, CA 91405-3603.
[b] Kerlan-Jobe Orthopaedic Clinic, 501 E. Hardy St., Inglewood, CA 90301.
[c] Steadman-Hawkins Clinic, 181 W. Meadow Drive, Suite 400, Vail, CO 81657.
[d] 1815 N. Capitol Avenue, Suite 560, Indianapolis, IN 46202.

NAME _____ DATE _____

SURGERY _____ EVAL _____

Circle any of the following which bother your knee.

JOINT NOISES OR SENSATIONS:

Clicking	Grating
Snapping	Crunching
Popping	Shifting
Clunking	Crackling
Catching	Locking

No joint noises or sensation

INSTABILITY:

Only after vigorous sports
With mild athletic activity
With activities of daily living
Rolling over in bed
No joint instability at all

OTHER SENSATIONS:

Knee feels numb
Knee tires easily
Knee feels weak
Leg feels heavy

PAIN AND DISCOMFORT:

Sharp	Stiffness
Dull	Soreness
Aching	Shooting
Throbbing	Burning
Radiating	Where? _____

No pain or discomfort at all

LOCATION:

Anterior
Lateral
Posterior
Medial
Deep inside joint

PAIN:

None at all
Only after vigorous sports
With mild athletic activity
All the time

OVERALL FUNCTION:

On a scale from 0–100%, how would you presently rate your knee. Please remember that this is an overall rating, and should include pain, motion, strength, abilities, and disabilities.

Overall knee rating: _____ %

CONTINUED COMPLAINTS:

Please be as specific as possible and outline for us what types of pain or problems you continue to have with different activities. Also include any activities you are still unable to perform.

1. _____

2. _____

3. _____

FOR POSTOPERATIVE PATIENTS ONLY:

Comparing your present condition to your condition prior to surgery, how would you rate each of the following:

Pain levels:	Better	Worse	No different
Range of motion:	Better	Worse	No different
Overall strength:	Better	Worse	No different

Fig. 12-2. Knee evaluation form. (*Figure Continues.*)

	RIGHT	LEFT	DIFFERENCE
I. RANGE OF MOTION			

II. GIRTH
- 20 UP
- 5 UP
- JT LN
- 15 DN

III. KT–1000
- POST–20
- ANT–15
- ANT–20
- ENDPOINT
- MAX PASSIVE
- ACTIVE

IV. FUNCTIONAL INDEX QUESTIONNAIRE

	WNL	P/P	U/A	DNP
UPSTAIRS				
DOWNSTAIRS				
JOG 1 MILE				
WLK 4–5 BLKS				
MOVIE SIGN				
SQUATTING				
KNEELING				
CUT SPORTS				
WTB ALL DAY				
OTHER _____				
SPORTS _____				
_____				

V.   STRENGTH TESTING (CBE/BDX)

- Quadriceps pct.   _____
- Hamstrings pct.   _____
- TOTAL TORQUE
- Right Quadriceps   _____
- Left Quadriceps   _____
- Right Hamstrings   _____
- Left Hamstrings   _____

Fig. 12-2. (*Continued*).

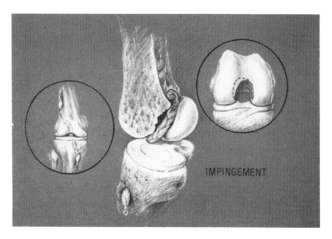

Fig. 12-3. Notchplasty revision of lateral femoral condyle. (From Ferkel et al.[7], with permission.)

hamstring exercises can be started utilizing free weights or machines. Short-arc quadriceps exercises (Fig. 12-6) are performed from 45 degrees of flexion to full extension because

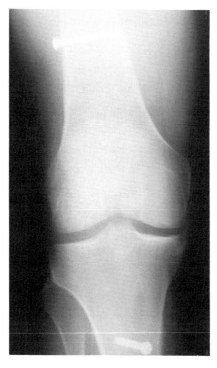

Fig. 12-4. AP radiograph following implantation of Gore-Tex graft.

1. terminal extension is the part of the ROM where the extensor mechanism is most mechanically disadvantaged;
2. terminal extension provides the greatest stress to the fibers of the vastus medialis oblique as the patella rides proximally out of the intercondylar groove;
3. terminal extension is the functional part of the arc of knee motion; and
4. terminal extension is, in our clinical experience, where patients suffer the least patellofemoral joint pain during exercise.

Despite the objection of some physical therapists to open kinetic chain exercises and terminal extension based on excessive anterior shear stress on the graft, we feel that due to the greater tensile strength of the Gore-Tex graft along with the technologic advances concerning graft isometricity, the clinician is safe in the utilization of this exercise without fear of adverse effects to the patient.

WEEKS 3 AND 4 AFTER SURGERY

Patients are weaned from the ambulation aids first by walking unaided in the familiar grounds of their homes. This will usually occur with a concomitant normalization of joint girth, ROM, and postoperative pain.

Stationary cycling is begun and resistance increased to the patient's tolerance as long as pain and swelling do not increase.

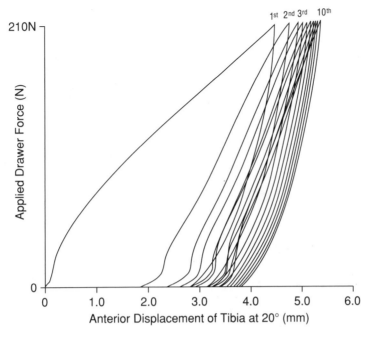

Fig. 12-5. Increased anterior excursion (5.4 mm) following 10 applications of 45-lb. force at 20 degrees of flexion after implantation of Gore-Tex ligament in cadaver knee. Prosthetic ligament grafts must be "pre-tensioned" prior to final fixation in order to minimize this unwanted laxity. (Redrawn from Stonebrook et al.,[5] with permission.)

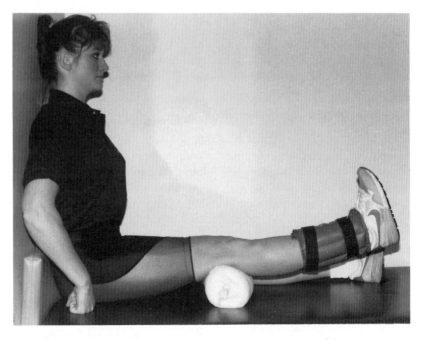

Fig. 12-6. Short arc quadriceps exercises emphasizing terminal knee extension.

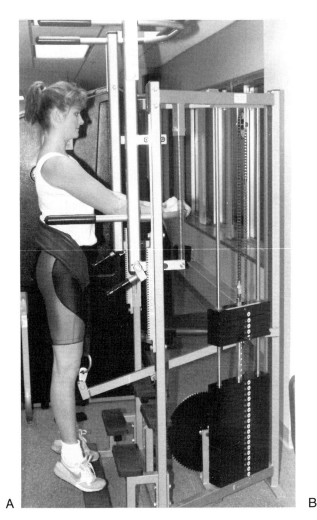
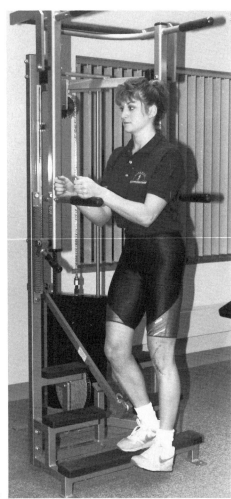

A   B

Fig. 12-7. (A) Calf-raising exercises utilizing Nautilus equipment in closed kinetic chain method. **(B)** Step-up exercises to generate quadriceps-hamstring co-contraction.

Closed kinetic chain (foot-fixed) exercises including calf raises and step-up exercises (Fig. 12-7) are incorporated. The latter exercise works the hamstrings and quadriceps together, similar to functional activities.

ONE MONTH AFTER SURGERY

At 1 month after surgery, knee ROM and a full thigh, joint, and calf girth series are measured and recorded. This information serves as feedback to the patient on progress made to date and also what deficits remain. KT-1000 arthrometer testing is performed to docu-

ment knee stability for progression to running activities. If the patient is able and the surgeon's consent is obtained, isokinetic testing can be performed. In our experience, this 1-month postoperative interval is too early for strength testing.

The running progression program is started as long as the patient progresses without increased pain or swelling. A mini-trampoline is utilized since this decreases the compression stresses on the knee. The first stage of trampoline work is *bouncing* (Fig. 12-8A), in which the patient maintains forefoot contact with the trampoline surface. This may progress to *jumping* activities in which the patient leaves the trampoline sur-

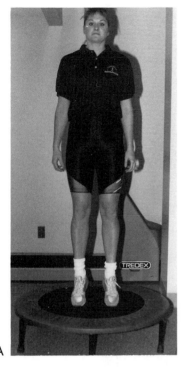
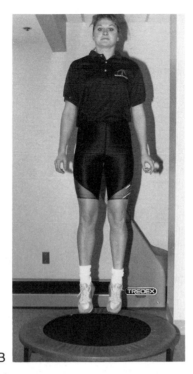
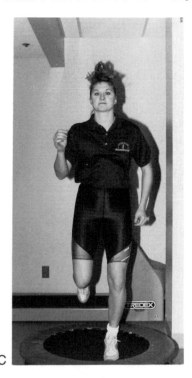

A   B   C

Fig. 12-8. (A) Trampoline bouncing—light compression joint loads. **(B)** Trampoline jumping—medium joint compression loads. **(C)** Trampoline jogging—greater joint compression loads.

face only to land back on both limbs simultaneously (Fig. 12-8B) and finally to *jogging* in place (Fig. 12-8C), when each foot strikes the surface sequentially.

Treadmill running is then incorporated, and the patient progresses with regard to speed and grade as the therapist continues to monitor knee joint pain and swelling.

TWO MONTHS AFTER SURGERY

The 2-month follow-up evaluation is again performed with regard to ROM and thigh and calf girth gains. KT-1000 testing is again performed to document graft stability. Patients are now more likely able to withstand isokinetic strength testing. Results of testing are discussed in detail with the patients as their progress is charted.

Outdoor running may begin at the 2-month post-surgery mark with progression to agility drill training including side-shuffling activities, cariocas, zig-zag running, and finally straight and cross-cutting maneu-

vers. Athletes practice the skills of their general sport as well as the specific maneuvers related to their position.

THREE MONTHS AFTER SURGERY

Follow-up evaluation at 3 months is performed using the same form as preoperatively, and a comparison is made. Key questions again relate to the overall percentage of normal knee function as rated by the athlete. Each preoperative complaint is discussed and continuing complaints are noted. Objective evaluation including ROM, girth, KT-1000 testing, and strength is performed, and discussion among the surgeon, therapist, athlete, and family determines the athlete's readiness for return to competition.

Use of a postoperative functional brace is a very individual decision. However, we believe that the athlete who has returned to acceptable muscle girth and strength scores and fluent, asymptomatic skill performance is at no greater risk than normal.

LONG-TERM RESULTS

Glousman and colleagues[6] reported on 82 patients who underwent Gore-Tex prosthetic ligament replacement with an average follow-up of 18 months. Patient subjective results were 89 percent improved, 9 percent unchanged, and 2 percent worse. Knee ROM returned to full extension and a 3-degree lack of full flexion at 18 months and AP laxity decreased from a side-to-side difference of 4.8 mm preoperatively to 2.4 mm at 18 months postoperation. Isokinetic quadriceps strength measured at 180 degrees/sec was 89 percent of the contralateral side at the 18-month point. Complications included four knees with complete graft rupture (5 percent) and four knees with partial rupture or attenuation with sterile effusion (5 percent).

Ferkel and associates[7] performed arthroscopy on 21 knees of 103 an average of 11 months postoperatively for a variety of reasons including painful screw removal, giving way, and recurrent effusions. The overall complications present are reported by the manufacturer as indicated in Table 12-4.

Indelicato et al.[8] reported on 41 patients who had undergone Gore-Tex implantation with a minimum of 2 years of follow-up of whom 9 (22 percent) had had one or more episodes of sterile effusion. This was somewhat higher than the national average.

Ahlfeld et al.[9] placed Gore-Tex ligaments in the knees of 30 patients with failed, multiply operated knees, with 87 percent demonstrating a reduction in anterior excursion, 67 percent experiencing an improvement in pain, and 30 percent having total pain relief for an overall 83 percent satisfactory rate.

Results have also been reported by the manufacturer.[10]

Table 12-4. Complications Related to Gore-Tex Surgery

	Ahlfeld[9]	Glousman[6]	Indelicato[8]	Ferkel[7]
No. of patients	30	82	41	103
Follow-up	2 years	1.5 years	2 years	2 years
Graft failure	3%	5% complete 5% partial	10%	1%
KT-1000 >4 mm	NL[a]	NL	7%	4%
Sterile effusion	NL	5%	22%	5%
Screw removal	NL	4%	7%	7%
Infection	3%	1%	2.4%	1%

[a] NL, Not listed.

REFERENCES

1. Bruchman WC, Bolton CW, Bain JR: Design considerations for cruciate ligament prosthesis. p. 254. In Jackson, Drez, Jr (eds): The Anterior Cruciate Deficient Knee: New Concepts in Ligament Repair. CV Mosby, St. Louis, 1987
2. Noyes FR, Butler DL, Grood ES et al: Biomechanical analysis of human ligament grafts used in knee ligament repairs and reconstructions. J Bone Joint Surg 66A:344, 1984
3. Bolton WC, Bruchman CW: The Gore-Tex™ expanded polytetrafluoroethylene prosthetic ligament. Clin Orthop Rel Res 196:202, 1985
4. Friedman MJ: Gore-Tex anterior cruciate ligament reconstruction. Tech Orthop 2:36, 1988
5. Stonebrook SN, Berman AB, Bruchman WE et al: Functional biomechanics of the Gore-Tex cruciate-ligament prosthesis: effects of implant tensioning. p. 140. In Friedman MJ, Ferkel RD (eds): Prosthetic Ligament Reconstruction of the Knee. WB Saunders, Philadelphia, 1986
6. Glousman RE, Shields CL, Kerlan RK et al: Gore-Tex™ prosthetic ligament in anterior cruciate deficient knees. Am J Sports Med 16:321, 1988
7. Ferkel RD, Fox JM, Wood D et al: Arthroscopic "second look" at the Gore-Tex™ ligament. Am J Sports Med 17:147, 1989
8. Indelicato PA, Pascale MS, Heugel MO: Early experience with the Gore-Tex polytetrafluoroethylene anterior cruciate ligament prosthesis. Am J Sports Med 17:55, 1989
9. Ahlfeld SK, Larson RL, Collins HR: Anterior cruciate reconstruction in the chronically unstable knee using an expanded polytetrafluoroethylene (PTFE) prosthetic ligament. Am J Sports Med 15:326, 1987
10. Gore-Tex™ cruciate ligament prosthesis: 3 year clinical results. W.L. Gore & Associates, Inc., Flagstaff, AZ, 1987 (brochure)

13

Nonoperative Posterior Cruciate Ligament Rehabilitation

ROBERT P. ENGLE

INTRODUCTION

The posterior cruciate ligament (PCL) provides the central axis of rotation of the knee joint. In cases of PCL injury, the loss of this structure has been associated with significant long-term joint surface erosion and functional disability.[1,2] Unlike the anterior cruciate ligament-deficient knee, these injuries result in a much lower incidence of functional instability.[1]

Controversy, at present, continues to exist regarding operative versus nonoperative management of this problem. There are advocates of both, although critical analysis of the published literature reveals various observations on the instabilities present with a torn PCL.[1-21] These resulting instabilities obviously depend on the mechanism of injury and other structures involved besides the PCL.

Hughston,[22] for example, noted that acute PCL injuries can present with a negative posterior drawer test, the most commonly accepted sign of a complete rupture. He believes this occurs with isolated PCL injury as opposed to chronic cases and combined injury of the PCL and medial or lateral ligament complex structures. In his experience, confirmed by other investigators, a portion of these patients can go on to do well functionally without surgical repair or reconstruction.[1,2,4,5,9,15,19,22] He, however, advocates surgery for combined instabilities that are causing functional disability.[2]

Clancy et al.[1] acknowledge the success of some patients in achieving acceptable results with nonoperative treatment of isolated PCL injuries. In their experience, most patients progress in time to medial compartment and patellofemoral joint arthrosis, which would be negated by early surgical intervention.[1] Clancy et al. stress the need, however, for effective postoperative PCL graft function, that is, 5 mm or less resultant posterior translation on follow-up examination to reconstruction.

Reviewing the literature is beneficial in understanding PCL anatomy, biomechanics, diagnosis, and surgery. Some researchers already cited discuss postoperative rehabilitation superficially. Nothing can be found that discusses in detail specific techniques used in nonoperative or operative PCL rehabilitation.

This chapter presents a rationale for rehabilitation of the PCL-deficient knee in patients referred to the physical therapist for a nonoperative course of treatment. Clinical diagnosis and examination and acute and chronic rehabilitation are presented.

CLINICAL DIAGNOSIS AND EXAMINATION

Diagnosis of PCL tears begins with the patient history. Acute mechanisms of injury may include a direct blow to the anterior tibia driving it posteriorly. This occurs from falls, motor vehicle, and athletic trauma.[2] Hyperextension mechanisms of injury have also been associated with PCL ruptures.

The PCL is also torn with a posterolaterally directed force at the anterior tibia that first tears the arcuate complex and then the PCL.[3] Valgus and varus injuries with the knee in full extension have also been reported with PCL and associated medial or lateral ligament tears.[3,23]

145

Following acute injury to the PCL, patients typically do not experience the tense hemarthrosis seen in ACL tears. Patients also will not necessarily experience giving way or severe pain with the initial injury, although weight bearing may be difficult. If medial or lateral ligament complex injuries or osteochondral injuries accompany the PCL tear, more pain and swelling may be present at the respective compartment.

Patients with chronic PCL deficiency commonly present with no prior knowledge of PCL injury. A large number of these patients were previously seen but the diagnosis was missed. Many recall their mechanism of injury but after the initial episode elected not to seek treatment. Patellofemoral or medial compartment discomfort, instability with stairs and inclines, and recurrent swelling are the main complaints that bring these patients to the clinic. Increasing laxity of secondary restraints, primarily the posterolateral structures, makes the laxity more perceptible to the patient.

Contusions to the subcutaneous peripheral nerves must be considered with the traumas typically causing PCL disruption. Saphenous nerve injury and reflex sympathetic dystrophy (RSD) is difficult to diagnose and treat but must be considered with a blow to the anterior tibia.

Major range of motion limitations are not common in this PCL-deficient patient group. End-range flexion may be painful. Extensor lags can be present secondary to quadriceps and extensor mechanism dysfunction or RSD.

Several clinical laxity tests have been used to determine PCL integrity. These include the tibial sag or drop-off test, posterior drawer with tibia neutral, anterior drawer with tibia internally rotated, and valgus and varus stress tests in full extension.[2,3,22,24-27]

With the knee flexed 75 to 90 degrees in the drawer test position, a posterior gravity-aided sagging of the tibia is present on bilateral comparison. The examiner can palpate this posterior dropback using the tibial condyle's posterior shift relative to the femur, confirming the instability. This sag can also been demonstrated by holding the hips and knees in 90 degrees of flexion with the patient supine to increase gravity's effect on the tibial subluxation posteriorly.

From the 75- to 90-degree drawer position, a quadriceps active displacement test as described by Daniel et al.[28] can be used. In this test, quadriceps isometric contraction translates the tibia anteriorly from a posteriorly subluxed to a neutral, reduced position. Posterior drawer testing from this position passively translates the tibia. The magnitude of displacement can vary from 1 to 2 mm in acute deficiencies to greater than 15 mm in chronic deficiencies (relative to the uninvolved side).

External rotation with the posterior drawer test, or posterolateral drawer, is positive with lesions of the arcuate complex and are markedly increased with PCL instability.[29] This combination of posterior and posterolateral instability is typically unappreciated in the diagnostic process but very important in both conservative and operative treatment.[3,22,24,25,29] Other important tests for accompanying posterolateral instability include the extension/recurvatum, rotation, dynamic posterior shift and reverse pivot shift tests.[25,29-31] Hughston and co-workers,[26,27] discuss positive valgus and varus stress test findings with PCL and accompanying medial and lateral ligament tears at full extension as well.

Meticulous patellofemoral assessment should include positioning, tracking, static and dynamic stability, and functional tests. An accompanying lower quarter functional and structural examination from the lumbopelvic complex to the feet is essential to understand the patellofemoral and tibiofemoral joint function within its synergistic lower extremity function components.

Because of the quadriceps' intimate relationship to the PCL and patellofemoral joint, evaluation and ongoing re-evaluation will be important. Testing can be done in a combination of ways including open chain, isolated knee extension with the tibia internally or externally rotated or neutral, various closed chain techniques such as knee bending on one or both legs, functional tests, and simple observation and patient history. It is important to test the quadriceps qualitatively as well as quantitatively with considerations for its effect on the patellofemoral joint, specific resultant instabilities, and functional demands of the patient. Exercise approaches and procedures will be much more effective with this in mind.

Neuromuscular examination and re-examination for proprioception, balance, coordination, flexibility, and strength of components other than the quadriceps is also necessary. Among these are the gluteals, adductors, gastrocsoleus, and others.

REHABILITATION

Acute and chronic PCL-deficient patients must be approached differently in the rehabilitation process and are discussed separately. Examination will determine treatment in both acute and chronic rehabilitation since no two injuries seem to be the same. Involvement of a myriad of structures can make rehabilitation complex and challenging.

Acute PCL Deficiency

Many variables make up the patient's history and examination, as mentioned previously. These can lead to a wide variation of treatment. For example, the acute patient with an RSD accompanying a combined PCL and posterolateral insufficiency will have significantly more pain and disability than the patient with an isolated PCL rupture with a barely perceptible posterior tibial sag.

Usually, the acute patient's rehabilitation can be divided into three sections, initial, intermediate, and late rehabilitation, before return to activity.

Initial Rehabilitation

Initial rehabilitation can be defined as the first 3 to 4 weeks from the date of injury. During this period the patient is non- or partial weight bearing on crutches with either a knee immobilizer or a cast brace system to allow secondary restraint and articular cartilage healing. Reflex inhibition mechanisms and proprioceptive deficits occur immediately, reducing the effective dynamic component to stability in a joint already faced with loss of a major static restraint.

Specific exercise procedures are introduced to begin recruitment and re-education of the quadriceps, the key dynamic restraint to posterior instability. Other techniques for the affected lower extremity are important as well. These include the following.

1. Quadriceps setting exercises at full extension begin basic recruitment, prevent extensor lag, mobilize or glide the patella, and decrease effusion. Patients should be educated to visualize the contraction and compare the involved to the normal side. Electrical muscle stimulation (EMS) is an important adjunct.

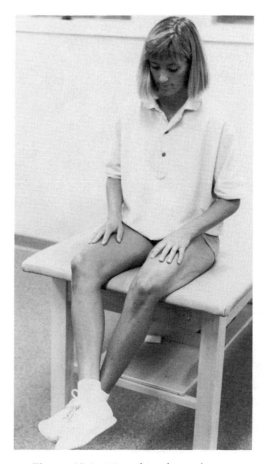

Figure 13-1. MR multiangle quadriceps.

2. Quadriceps isometrics can be performed in three different ways: manual resistance (MR) open chain, MR closed chain, and proprioceptive neuromuscular facilitation (PNF) and modified patterns with the knee isometrically maintained in one position.[32]
   a. *MR Open Chain:* The knee is isometrically resisted in isolated knee extension at various angles from 0 to 70 degrees with the tibia neutral or internally or externally rotated depending on patient's stability examination (Fig. 13-1).
   b. *MR Closed Chain:* The patient is isometrically resisted in the full weight-bearing position on both legs at various angles beginning at end-range extension and progressing gradually to 70 degrees (Fig. 13-2). Facilitory input is given through the pelvis including approximation and

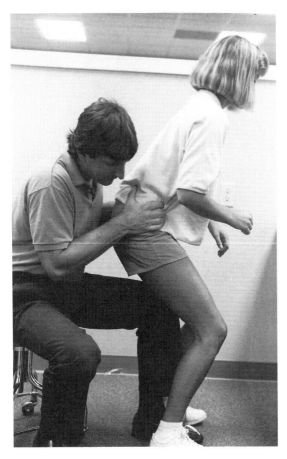

Figure 13-2. MR squats at 30 to 45 degrees of knee flexion.

stabilizing isometrics. Full trunk flexion must be avoided because anterior shifting of the femur will occur.[33] Rotation can be used to protect the secondary restraints.

c. *PNF and Modified Techniques and Procedures:* The knee is isometrically maintained at various angles from full extension to 60 degrees of flexion during lower extremity flexion diagonal patterns supine, sitting, or prone (Fig. 13-3). Irradiation from the stronger proximal components assists in quadriceps recruitment as well as strengthening the hip and distal lower extremity. Adduction and external rotation of the hip facilitates the vastus medialis oblique (VMO). Hamstring stretch at end ranges further decreases the patellofemoral compressive forces. A linear hip

adduction pattern with the hip externally rotated and quadriceps contracted is also effective.

3. Other PNF and modified techniques and procedures include the following exercises. The knee can be isometrically resisted in other patterns such as extension diagonals avoiding posterior tibial sag actively or passively. Pelvic techniques are important in preparation for weight bearing (Fig. 13-4).

4. Lower leg-isolated MR techniques in both the closed and open chain with special emphasis on the gastrocnemius, a key dynamic restraint, can be used.

5. Adjunctive therapeutic exercise techniques include hip progressive resisted exercises (Fig. 13-5), toe raises, plantar-dorsi flexion isokinetics, knee bends with modified weight bearing on Total Gym (EFI, San Diego, CA), straight leg raises, short-arc quads

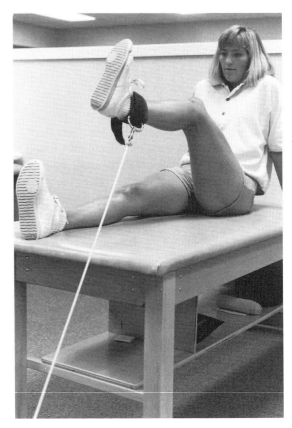

Figure 13-3. Flexion-adduction with patient sitting and knee maintained at 20 degrees of flexion.

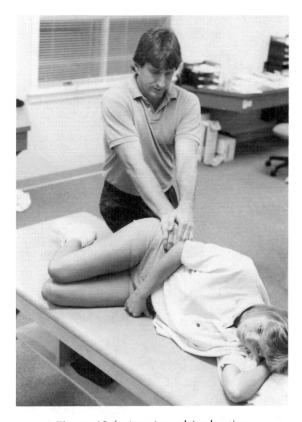

Figure 13-4. Anterior pelvic elevation.

in terminal extension, and basic balance board exercises.

6. Other rehabilitation techniques including patellar mobilization, continuous passive motion (CPM), or static stretch are effective for resolution of joint contractures; and cryotherapy and compression wrap and other modalities decrease synovitis and effusion.

Intermediate Rehabilitation

An intermediate period follows initial rehabilitation at approximately weeks 3 to 4 continuing to weeks 6 to 8. At this point, the patient can discontinue crutches and a cast brace system unless a significant articular cartilage lesion is present and/or the patient has a severe quadriceps shutdown such as seen with RSD. Functional knee braces specifically designed to control posterior instabilities can be applied to further control

posterior tibial displacement, although the effectiveness of these devices is unproved.

Clinical stability tests will dictate the status of healing secondary restraints. Complete medial and posteromedial and lateral and posterolateral ligament tears may require further protective motion in their cast brace to ensure their optimal healing. Good early quadriceps tracking and control of the patellofemoral and tibiofemoral joints should be established. Restoration of quadriceps function can occur slowly in many patients. These patients must be identified early and progress through rehabilitation more cautiously when there is decreased dynamic support to the PCL instability and patella.

Important therapeutic exercise procedures at this point include the following.

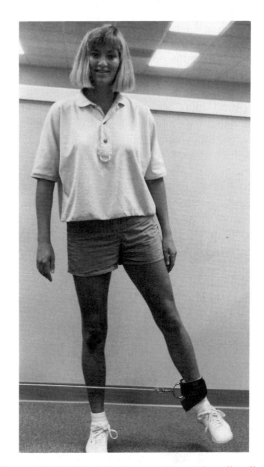

Figure 13-5. Hip abduction standing with wall pulleys.

1. Techniques and procedures from the initial period may still be beneficial, especially in the presence of synovitis or patellofemoral symptoms. Isometric quadriceps facilitation via the PNF and modified techniques will provide strong recruitment without synovial or patellar stresses inherent in isotonic procedures.

2. Hip-knee extension procedures with the patient supine, sitting, or sidelying offer several important patterns for quadriceps facilitation: extension-adduction-external rotation or extension-abduction-internal rotation with the tibia externally or internally rotated, respectively, or isometrically maintained at neutral, and linear hip with knee extension with the tibia neutral.

3. Bridging with the knees flexed provides mechanoreceptor input for proprioception, articular cartilage stimulation, and cocontractions of the dynamic restraints. Patients can progress from bilateral to unilateral weight bearing.

4. Knee extension MR techniques in the open chain enhance quadriceps recruitment, but they must be applied with patellofemoral precautions. Patients can be positioned sitting or supine and resisted as isolated patterns or pivots of lower extremity diagonals. Tibial internal, neutral, or external rotation can add mechanical and neuromuscular emphasis to the various patellar and quadriceps components (Fig. 13-6).

5. Knee flexion MR techniques in the open chain enhance hamstring recruitment. Since the hamstrings posteriorly translate the tibia, these exercises must be limited to terminal extension (0 to 20 degrees).[19] Internal tibial rotation with flexion brings the popliteus into the pattern, protecting the posterolateral corner. External rotation, conversely, will pull the tibia into posterolateral subluxation, stretching this complex of structures.

6. Adjunctive therapeutic exercise techniques include knee bends, with partial weight bearing as described earlier using slight hip adduction for increased VMO input progressing to full weight bearing with weights or elastic cords (Fig. 13-7); step-ups; toe raises; more advanced bilateral and unilateral full weight-bearing balance board exercises; bicycling; stair climbing; treadmill walking; cross-country ski tracks; proprioceptive boards; knee ex-

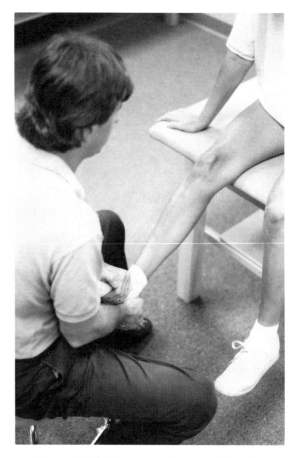

Figure 13-6. Knee extension-external rotation.

tension PREs (0- to 70-degree arc of motion); knee flexion PREs (0 to 20 degrees, avoiding tibial external rotation), and wall pulley PREs corresponding to PNF and modified patterns introduced to this point.

7. Important correlated techniques include lower quarter (lumbopelvic to foot-ankle complexes) manual therapy and biomechanical techniques to correct imbalances or compensatory changes; gait training including MR techniques; taping for patellar stabilization; joint mobilization, static stretch, and/or CPM if joint contracture is still present; and sport- or skill-specific exercises consistent with these techniques already introduced. Functional knee bracing can be used with all the exercises presented if desired.

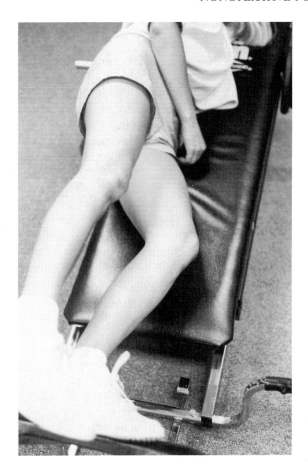

Figure 13-7. Leg press sidelying with slight adduction.

Late Rehabilitation

By 6 weeks, the rehabilitation process is complete for these uncomplicated cases. However, most PCL-deficient patients will probably never be entirely asymptomatic, making complete and thorough rehabilitation essential to good joint function. Patients may need to accept some limitation in function and pain or elect to undergo reconstructive surgery.

Entering late rehabilitation, the patient will typically exhibit 85 to 90 percent qualitative and quantitative quadriceps and lower extremity neuromuscular function including proprioception, optimal stability from the secondary restraints, and good lower quarter biomechanical function for return to activities.

The most advanced MR and adjunctive techniques from the earlier periods are emphasized for resolution of the most major neuromuscular and biomechanical deficits still present. Weight-bearing, plyometric, and functional training exercises are important in progressing toward restoration of normal activities (Fig. 13-8). Precautions must be followed for articular cartilage, however.

Discharge criteria include the following.

1. Full qualitative and quantitative quadriceps function assessed by manual, instrumented, clinical, and functional evaluation in both the open and closed kinetic chain must be achieved.
2. Ligamentous healing must be judged to be complete by manual, instrumented, and functional stability examination.
3. The patellofemoral joint should be asymptomatic. There should be full dynamic function (especially VMO) and support (stability, tracking, mobility).

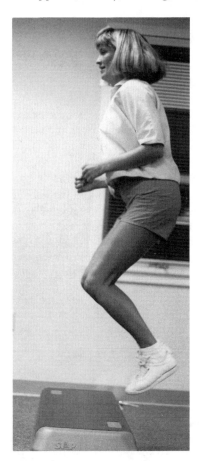

Figure 13-8. Plyometric training for jumping sports.

4. Lower quarter examination should be negative for abnormalities that may lead to future repetitive microtrauma at the knee and elsewhere through the lower kinetic chain.
5. Patients must have progressed through appropriate activity training without symptoms.

Patients are seen for follow-up re-evaluation at 3, 6, 9, and 12 months to ensure that they are following an appropriate independent course.

Chronic PCL Deficiency

Patients present for treatment with chronic PCL deficiencies secondary to new macrotrauma or repetitive microtrauma that typically produce medial compartment and patellofemoral arthrosis and pain. They may have combinations of posterior, lateral, and posterolateral instabilities, patellar dysfunction including patellar tendonitis and maltracking, biomechanical lower quarter compensatory changes, chronic synovitis, and RSD. Each of these components must be fully investigated and treatment directed toward them through techniques presented above.

Those who are highly symptomatic or reinjured may need a period of protected weight bearing and mobilization to decrease stresses on the articular cartilage and remaining secondary restraints. Quadriceps procedures must be introduced gradually to protect the patellofemoral joint but aggressively to control the posterior instability that is the patient's chief underlying problem. Bracing and taping the patella or tibiofemoral joint may be necessary.

Progression to activity and discharge criteria follow from the goal-directed rehabilitation program similar to acute patients. Patients are observed after discharge to monitor progress and resolve on-going deficits. Independent programs are given at discharge and updated on follow-up.

SUMMARY

Nonoperative PCL rehabilitation presents the clinician with interesting and challenging treatment choices. Long-term PCL deficiency has been associated with articular surface arthrosis of the medial compartment and patella. These result from the altered center of motion and increased patellar shear forces created through quadriceps function. Good quadriceps function is necessary to control anterior displacement of the femur, however.

Long-term degenerative changes further lead to recurrent synovitis. This recurrent synovitis accelerates articular cartilage breakdown, which, in turn, sets up reflex inhibition mechanisms of the quadriceps. Quadriceps dysfunction not only results in poor control of the PCL instability but also compromises patellar tracking with functional activities. Some patients have patellofemoral problems (chondromalacia, maltracking, instability) before they ever injure their PCL, making their rehabilitation more difficult.

PCL ruptures, depending on the mechanism of injury, can be accompanied by medial and lateral ligament complex, osteochondral, and meniscal injuries. In those patients with relatively isolated PCL-only injury, there is a natural tendency toward stretching of the important posteromedial and posterolateral secondary restraints. Tibial varum with gait can develop as these structures are stretched. At this time, operative approaches are far from perfected. PCL grafts are generally less stable than anterior cruciate grafts in the long term with the residual PCL laxity controlled by the quadriceps. If the patellar tendon is sacrificed for use as a ligament graft, this important dynamic component to PCL restraint is permanently weakened. Patellofemoral function is compromised as well. However, with the right indications and with improved arthroscopic techniques with lower morbidity, surgery can be an effective long-term solution.

Considering the severe disruption of normal joint function following a PCL tear and the limitations of surgical reconstruction, it is clear that rehabilitation is a critical component to patient management. This chapter attempts to present an approach to PCL rehabilitation when the patient and/or physician elects a nonoperative course of treatment. Effectiveness centers around the patient's initial and ongoing examinations as each case presents a myriad of problems that must be understood for a satisfactory patient outcome.

REFERENCES

1. Clancy WG, Shelbourne KD, Zoellner GB: Treatment of knee joint instability secondary to rupture of the posterior cruciate ligament. Report of a new procedure. J Bone Joint Surg 65A:310, 1983

2. Hughston JC, Degenhardt TC: Reconstruction of the posterior cruciate ligament. Clin Orthop 164:59, 1982

3. Baker CL, Norwood LA, Hughston JC: Acute combined posterior cruciate and posterolateral instability of the knee. Am J Sports Med 12:204, 1984

4. Cross MJ, Powell JF: Long-term followup of posterior cruciate ligament rupture: a study of 116 cases. Am J Sports Med 12:292, 1984

5. Dandy DJ, Pusey RJ: The long term results of unrepaired tears of the posterior cruciate ligament. J Bone Joint Surg 64B:92, 1982

6. Eriksson E, Haggmark T, Johnson RJ: Reconstruction of the posterior cruciate ligament. Orthopedics 9:217, 1986

7. Fleming RE, Blatz DJ, McCarroll JR: Posterior problems in the knee: posterior cruciate insufficiency and posterolateral rotatory insufficiency. Am J Sports Med 9:107, 1981

8. Fowler PJ, Messich SS: Isolated posterior cruciate ligament injuries in athletes. Am J Sports Med 15:553, 1987

9. Hughston JC, Bowden JA, Andrews JR et al: Acute tears of the posterior cruciate ligament. Results of operative treatment. J Bone Joint Surg 62A:438, 1980

10. Insall JN, Hood RW: Bone-block transfer of the medial head of the gastrocnemius for posterior cruciate insufficiency. J Bone Joint Surg 64A:691, 1982

11. Lipscomb AB, Anderson AF: Surgical reconstruction of both the anterior and posterior cruciate ligaments. Am J Knee Surg 3:29, 1990

12. Longenecker SL, Hughston JC: Long-term followup of isolated posterior cruciate injuries, abstracted. Am J Sports Med 15:628, 1987

13. Loos WC, Fox JM, Blazina ME et al: Acute posterior cruciate ligament injuries. Am J Sports Med 9:86, 1981

14. McCarroll JR, Ritter MA, Schrader J, Carlson S: The isolated posterior cruciate ligament injury. Physician Sportsmed 11:146, 1983

15. Parolie JM, Bergfeld JA: Long-term results of nonoperative treatment of isolated posterior cruciate ligament injuries in the athlete. Am J Sports Med 14:35, 1986

16. Roth JH, Kennedy JC, Best TM et al: Medial gastrocnemius tendon transfer to manage chronic posterior cruciate ligament insufficiency, abstracted. Am J Sports Med 15:628, 1987

17. Stanish WD, Rubinovich M, Armason T, Lapenskie G: Posterior cruciate ligament tears in wrestlers. Can J Appl Sport Sci 11:173, 1986

18. Strand T, Molster AO, Engesacter LB et al: Primary repair in posterior cruciate ligament injuries. Acta Orthop Scand 55:545, 1984

19. Tibone JE, Antich TJ, Perry J, Moynes D: Functional analysis of untreated and reconstructed posterior cruciate ligament injuries. Am J Sports Med 16:217, 1988

20. Trickey EL: Injuries of the posterior cruciate ligament: diagnosis and treatment of early injuries and reconstruction of late instability. Clin Orthop 147:76, 1980

21. Wirth CJ, Jager M: Dynamic double tendon replacement of the posterior cruciate ligament. Am J Sports Med 12:39, 1984

22. Hughston JC: The absent posterior drawer test in some acute posterior cruciate ligament tears of the knee. Am J Sports Med 16:39, 1988

23. Shelbourne KD, Mesko JW, McCarroll JR, Rettig AC: Combined medial collateral ligament-posterior cruciate rupture: mechanism of injury. Am J Knee Surg 3:41, 1990

24. Gollehon DL, Torzilli PA, Warren RF: The role of the posterolateral and cruciate ligaments in the stability of the human knee. J Bone Joint Surg 69A:233, 1987

25. Grood ES, Stowers SF, Noyes FR: Limits of movement in the human knee: effect of sectioning the posterior cruciate ligament and posterolateral structures. J Bone Joint Surg 70A:88, 1988

26. Hughston JC, Andrews JR, Cross MJ, Moschi A: Classification of knee ligament instabilities. Part II: The lateral compartment. J Bone Joint Surg 58A:173, 1976

27. Hughston JC, Andrews JR, Moschi A, Cross MJ: Classification of knee ligament instabilities. Part I: The medial compartment and cruciate ligaments. J Bone Joint Surg 58A:159, 1976

28. Daniel DM, Stone ML, Barnett P, Sachs R: Use of the quadriceps active test to diagnose posterior cruciate ligament disruption and measure posterior laxity of the knee. J Bone Joint Surg 70A:386, 1988

29. Hughston JC, Norwood LA: The posterolateral drawer test and external rotational recurvatum test for posterolateral rotary instability of the knee. Clin Orthop 147:82, 1980

30. Jackob RP, Hassler H, Stacubli HUI: Observations on rotary instability of the lateral compartment. Acta Orthop Scand 52, suppl. 191, 1981

31. Shelbourse KD, Benedict F, McCarroll JR, Rettig AC: Dynamic posterior shift test: an adjuvant in evaluation of posterior tibial subluxation. Am J Sports Med 17:275, 1989

32. Johnson G, Saliba VJ: Proprioceptive Neuromuscular Facilitation I & II. Course Notes. The Institute of Physical Art, San Anselmo, CA, 1990

33. Ohkoshi Y, Yasuda K: Biomechanical analysis of shear force exerted to anterior cruciate ligament during half squat exercise. Orthop Trans 13:310, 1989

14

Posterior Cruciate Ligament Reconstruction

KEVIN A. MANSMANN

DIAGNOSIS

Hughston et al.[1] in 1980 described the clinical presentation and physical findings noted with acute tears of the posterior cruciate ligament (PCL). They noted the clinical signs of an acute tear of the PCL to be most consistently (1) a positive abduction or adduction stress test in full extension, (2) a positive anterior drawer test in internal rotation, and (3) a positive posterior drawer test. The many instances of a negative posterior drawer test in a documented acute PCL rupture were explained by an intact arcuate ligament complex and/or intact posterior oblique ligament restricting this motion.

Grood et al.[2] through biomechanical testing of cadaver knees, challenged the clinical observations of Hughston et al.[1] They noted that there was greater varus-valgus laxity with a PCL-deficient knee in 90 degrees of flexion than in full extension. They determined, in the same study, that a positive posterolateral drawer test in 90 degrees of flexion was indicative of an arcuate ligament complex laxity and a PCL laxity. They also noted that the most sensitive position to test for complete rupture of the PCL is in flexion. This position relaxes the secondary restraints that can block posterior tibial translation.

More recently, Daniel and Stone[3,18] have described a quadriceps active test to aid in this diagnosis. That test incorporates an appreciation of the posterior sag sign and the active quadriceps firing to reduce this posterior sag. This is more useful in the chronically lax knee. Utilizing the KT-1000 arthrometer, Daniel and Stone[3] reported an anterior translation of 4 to 10 mm with a quadriceps contraction in the chronic PCL-de-

ficient knee. This is compared with the 2- to 6-mm translation with an acute PCL disruption, with both groups having normal varus and valgus laxity. The resting posteriorly subluxated position is frequently only 2 to 3 mm different from normal and hence is not clinically obvious. This may account for the frequent misinterpretation of this as an anterior laxity when the knee is tested and may explain Hughston's high incidence of positive anterior drawer tests in his series of acute knee PCL injuries. A posterolateral sag and the reverse pivot shift are also helpful in evaluating and diagnosing the ligamentous laxity of the chronic PCL-deficient knee. In the acutely injured knee, unless the patient is extremely stoic or examined under anesthesia, these tests are much less reliable.

Also of diagnostic value are radiographs to ascertain any fractures or growth plate injuries (with stress views if necessary) and magnetic resonance imaging (MRI). MRI would be of assistance in evaluating the integrity of the cruciate ligaments as well as associated meniscal lesions. The value of the MRI study is in large part related to the experience and expertise of the imaging center. These fortunately are steadily improving. MRI is a noninvasive study that can significantly help guide therapeutic decisions.

For those injuries that cannot be evaluated in the immediate postinjury period, after which the knee becomes increasingly swollen and painful, an examination under anesthesia and arthroscopic examination may be necessary. This is particularly true if the above diagnostic measures have been inconclusive. The patient should understand the potential options and courses that could be taken. An arthroscopic examination should be done with a prior understanding by the patient of the measures that would be taken as a result of the findings. This would afford the surgeon the preoperative consent to do the definitive procedure once the diagnosis is confirmed.

TREATMENT APPROACHES

The clinical approach to the isolated PCL injury is still controversial. This controversy centers around the natural history of the PCL-deficient knee. Clancy et al.[4] reported a 90 percent incidence of medial femoral condylar articular injury in those patients who had a symptomatic PCL-deficient knee for longer than 4 years. There was a 71 percent incidence in the 2- to 4-year group. They therefore advocated reconstruction of a PCL-deficient knee.[4]

Parolie and Bergfeld[5] confirmed the findings of Dandy and Pusey[6] by reporting an 80 percent satisfaction rate among their patients treated nonoperatively for an isolated PCL tear. They had a mean follow-up of 6.2 years. They reported that those patients who fully returned to sports and were satisfied with their knees had a quadriceps strength on the involved side greater than 100 percent that of the uninvolved quadriceps. They emphasized the need for appropriate rehabilitation of the quadriceps for unrestricted return to activities. They could not relate the amount of knee instability to the patient's satisfaction or successful return to sports.

The decision to reconstruct an acutely torn PCL must be individualized and discussed at length with the patient. A trial course of rehabilitation focused on regaining range of motion and then quadriceps strength could help clarify the options and the most fruitful therapeutic approach. The active individual who is physiologically young and anticipates a continued interest in sports or is a heavy laborer has clearer surgical indications. It is for these individuals that reconstruction of the PCL would be of most benefit, especially after a failed course of appropriate physical therapy.

The PCL injury associated with an ipsilateral, medial, or lateral compartment ligament injury is much less controversial. With these associated injuries, the best reported results are obtained with surgical treatment.[7] The PCL must be reconstructed or repaired with augmentation. Repair of either of the cruciate ligaments alone, without augmentation, has met with limited success, unless the injury is a bony avulsion that permits anatomic bone-to-bone fixation. Reconstruction of the associated ligamentous injuries, although acceptable and still practiced in many centers, is less absolute owing to the good results obtained with conservative early mobilization of these knees after the primary cruciate ligament injuries have been reconstructed or repaired with augmentation.[8,19] This has been supported by some recent experimental work.[20–22] This mobilization must be done with the added protection of a rehabilitation orthosis and integrated into the cruciate ligament rehabilitation protocol.

SURGICAL TREATMENT
Anatomy

Prior to the reconstruction of any ligament or ligamentous complex, a thorough appreciation of the anatomy and biomechanics of the ligamentous structure must be firmly grasped. Hughston et al.[1] and others[9] emphasized the importance of the PCL because of its relative size, tensile strength, and orientation along the central longitudinal axis of the knee joint. Girgis et al.[10] in 1975 nicely described the femoral and tibial attachments of the PCL (Figs. 14-1 and 14-2). The femoral origin of the PCL is on the posterior aspect of the lateral surface of the medial femoral condyle. The insertion of the PCL is located in the depression on the posterior aspect of the tibia in the midline just posterior to the articular surface of the tibia. The meniscal femoral ligaments of Wrisberg and Humphry make a variable contribution to the substance of the PCL.[10] The anterior meniscal femoral ligament (ligament of Humphry) courses anterior to the PCL, arising from the posterior aspect of the lateral meniscus. It has a significant variance in size, up to one-third the size of the PCL. The posterior meniscal femoral ligament (ligament of Wrisberg) courses posterior to the PCL and also extends from the posterior aspect of the lateral meniscus. This ligament may be one-half the diameter of the PCL. Either the anterior or posterior meniscal femoral ligament is present in approximately 70 percent of knees.[11]

The course of the PCL is directed posteriorly, laterally, and distally in its path from the femur to the tibia. It is centered along the central longitudinal axis

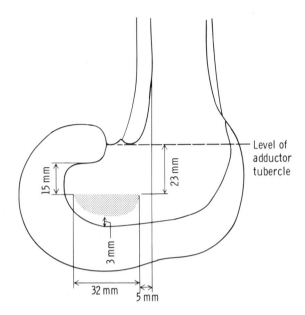

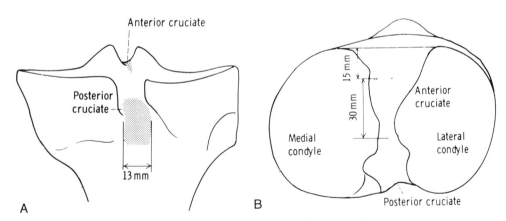

components in flexion and extension. The PCL was therefore arbitrarily divided into fascicles. The anterior component, which represents the largest portion of the ligament, tightens in flexion (Fig. 14-3). The posterior portion tightens in extension and is smaller than the anterior bundle. As Arnoczy and Warren[12] have noted, these two bundles merely represent an oversimplification of an actual continuum of fascicles. These fascicles are differentiated into bundles by the variable tension that is placed through this ligament through the arc of motion.

It is therefore a surgical goal to center the replacement or augmentation graft along the anatomic course of the PCL to maximize the isometricity of the course of the PCL graft. This is an idealized goal, for as Sapega et al.[13] and others[11,14–16] have shown, no fascicles are truly isometric in the anterior cruciate ligament and presumably the PCL is analogous in this regard.

Surgical Technique

After appropriate discussion with the patient regarding the therapeutic options, an appropriate course of action must be taken. The surgical approach to an acute PCL rupture with associated medial or lateral ligamentous injuries would be, in many surgeon's hands, an open procedure. Hughston et al.[1,23] described a medial hockey-stick incision used for the surgical repair of medial ligamentous injuries as well as the PCL injury (Figs. 14-4 and 14-5). The skin flaps are developed to

Fig. 14-1. Drawing of the lateral surface of the medial condyle of the femur showing the average measurements and bony relations of the femoral attachment of the PCL. (From Girgis et al.,[10] with permission.)

of the knee joint. Due to the breadth of the femoral and tibial attachments of this ligament, a kinematic analysis reveals that the functional course of this ligament is not truly isometric. Girgis et al.[10] noted this through the change of shape and tension of the PCL

Fig. 14-2. Drawing of **(A)** the posterior surface of the tibia and **(B)** the upper surface of the tibial plateau to show average measurements and relations of the tibial attachments of the ACL and PCL. (From Girgis et al.,[10] with permission.)

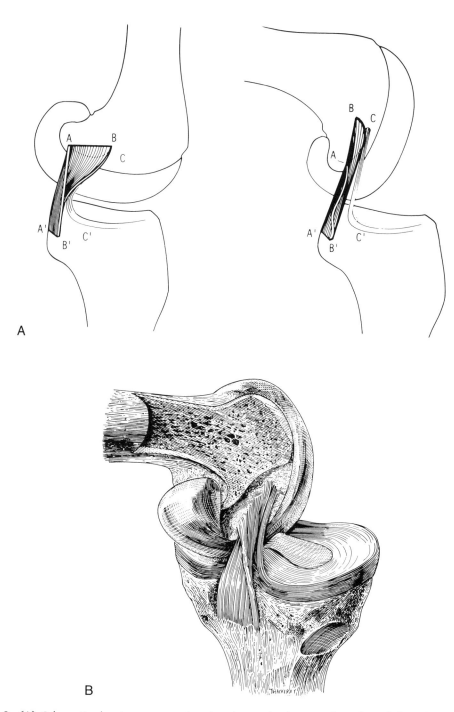

Fig. 14-3. (A) Schematic drawing representing the change in shape and tension of the PCL components in extension and flexion. In flexion there is lengthening of the bulk of the ligament (B-B′) and shortening of a small band (A-A′). C-C′ is the anterior meniscofemoral ligament (ligament of Humphrey) attached to the lateral meniscus. **(B)** Drawing of the PCL with the knee in flexion. Note that most of the ligament is taut while a small posterior band of fibers becomes loose. (From Girgis et al.,[10] with permission.)

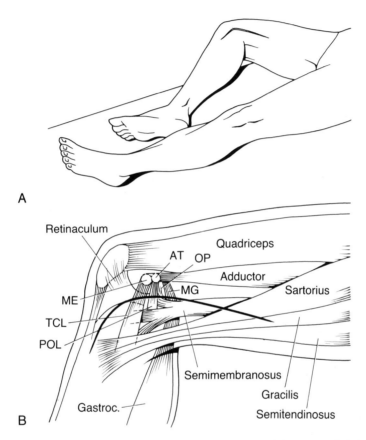

Fig. 14-4. (A & B) At surgery, the lower limb is positioned in external rotation and abduction at the hip with the knee flexed approximately 90 degrees. A medial hockey-stick incision is made along the line of the hamstrings and the joint line, almost to the patellar tendon. The incision then curves distally onto the anteromedial aspect of the tibia **(A)**. This approach allows access to the anterior and posterior intercondylar regions, the medial ligaments, and the medial femoral condyle **(B).** ME, medial epicondyle; AT, adductor tubercle; TLC, tibial collateral ligament; OP, oblique popliteal ligament; MG, medial head of gastrocnemius; POL, posterior oblique ligament. (From Hughston et al.,[1] with permission.)

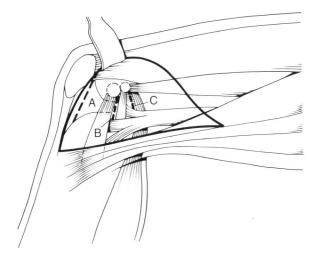

Fig. 14-5. When the medial ligaments and anterior retinaculum are not torn severely, or when there are no tears of the medial ligament associated with an injury to the lateral ligament, then the knee joint is examined through a longitudinal anteromedial retinacular incision along the medial border of the patella and patellar tendon **(A).** The posterior half of the medial meniscus and the tibial attachment of the PCL are visualized through a longitudinal retinacular incision between the tibial collateral ligament and the posterior oblique ligament **(B).** The posterior attachment of the PCL is made accessible through a longitudinal incision along the medial border of the medial head of the gastrocnemius, going transversely through the fibers of the oblique popliteal ligament and posterior capsule **(C).** (From Hughston et al.,[1] with permission.)

permit both anteromedial and posteromedial arthrotomies under the elevated flaps. Lateral ligamentous injuries require an additional incision laterally for repair, with the approach to the PCL again being made through the posteromedial and anteromedial arthrotomies.

Rosenberg et al.[17] have described an arthroscopic technique for cruciate repair and reconstruction. The advantages of arthroscopy include a less traumatic exposure of the anatomy necessary to anatomically reconstruct the PCL. This has been most useful for isolated ligamentous PCL injuries. Meniscal and osteochondral lesions could also be more readily addressed with arthroscopic techniques than with open procedures. With the increasing success rates associated with conservative care of collateral ligament injuries,

arthroscopic techniques can also be applied to combined ligament injuries. Extreme care must be taken in the acutely injured knee to minimize extravasation of irrigation fluid. This could cause popliteal neurovascular compression or a compartment syndrome. Undue extravasation of fluid may limit the arthroscopy to diagnostic purposes.

Clancy et al.,[4] using the open Hughston approach as described above, reconstructed the PCL utilizing the medial one-third of the patellar tendon together with its patellar and tibial bone attachments. Other autografts could be utilized, including combined semitendinosus and gracilis tendons or a doubled semitendinosus, as well as allograft substitutes for the reconstruction. Clancy et al.[4] recognized the importance of reconstructing the normal anatomic orientation of the graft substitute. They therefore emphasized the correct placement of the bone tunnels through which the graft substitute was passed for fixation.

The tibial tunnel poses special problems due to the extremely posterior site of insertion of the PCL. This site is just proximal to the tibial shelf, formed by the insertion of the posterior joint capsule. Adequate arthroscopic visualization may necessitate a posteromedial portal. With a 70-degree scope, the tibial PCL insertion site may be visualized from an anterolateral portal. The posteromedial portal could then be used for the instrumentation to prepare the tibial site. If inadequate visualization is obtained, a posteromedial arthrotomy should be performed. Utilizing an anteromedial or posteromedial portal, arthroscopic rasps and curettes are used to prepare the tibial site for drilling. Arthroscopic PCL drill guides, passed through the anteromedial portal, are utilized for accurate drilling of the desired tunnels. The popliteal neurovascular structures are coursing just posterior to the joint capsule and are closely adherent to it. This is why the K-wire placement for the drilling of this tunnel is done utilizing a stop on the guide wire to prevent posterior penetration of the popliteal neurovascular structures. The tunnel is overreamed to the size determined by the diameter of the graft substitute. The actual overreaming of the tunnel should be done under either arthroscopic or direct visualization and should also be done with a stop on the drill. If any question is still present regarding the location of the K-wire or drill bit, a radiograph should be obtained. In addition, a curette can be placed over the K-wire while the tunnel is being overdrilled to prevent inadvertent posterior migration of the K-wire. It is also possible to drill the tunnel directly, without the use of a K-wire, preventing the possibility of K-wire migration.

Clancy et al.[4] described the location of the ideal exit site for this tunnel posteriorly. It should be located such that the superomedial circumference of the tunnel lies in the anatomic center of the tibial insertion of the PCL. Rosenberg et al.[17] clearly indicated the need to initiate the tibial tunnel 1 to 2 cm below and medial to the tibial tubercle (Fig. 14-6A). This starting point is necessary due to the possible double penetration of the posterior cortex of the tibia if the starting point is too distal. If too proximal a starting point for the tibial tunnel is used (Fig. 14-6B), there would be inadequate bone between the proximal posterior tunnel aperture and the tibial plateau and insufficient fixation would be obtained. Subsequent tunnel drift could then occur with loading of the PCL.

The femoral attachment of the PCL is located on the lateral aspect of the medial femoral condyle in the notch at the 10 o'clock (left) or 2 o'clock (right) position, anterior and superior to the original femoral insertion of the PCL. The tunnel is overdrilled such that its infralateral circumference coincides with the anatomic center of the PCL. In the chronic PCL-deficient knee, where the PCL remnants are less identifiable, this would be approximately 7 to 8 mm proximal to the margin of the articular surface of the medial femoral condyle. The femoral extra-articular opening of the tunnel must be placed to minimize tunnel diversions through the complete range of motion. At 90 degrees of knee flexion, this site is midway between the medial femoral epicondyle and the medial articular margin of the femoral sulcus on a line between the medial epicondyle and the upper third of the patella (Fig. 14-7). Rasps and curettes are used to bevel and smooth the intra-articular margins of both the fem-

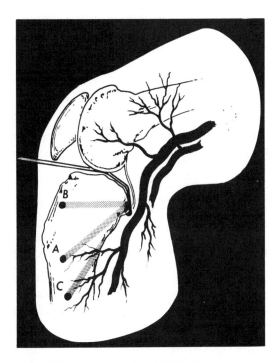

Fig. 14-6. To ensure that the drill bit does not penetrate beyond the tibial guide, the guide must be freely positioned without bending, and a drill point stop must be used. Point A is the desired drill hole starting point. (From Rosenberg et al.,[17] with permission.)

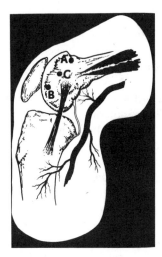

Fig. 14-7. Point A results in minimal tunnel divergence in full extension and in maximal tunnel divergence in flexion. Point B, conversely, results in maximal tunnel divergence in full extension and minimal tunnel divergence in flexion. Point C represents the ideal extra-articular opening of the femoral tunnel to minimize tunnel divergence through the complete range of motion. (From Rosenberg et al.,[17] with permission.)

oral and tibial tunnels to minimize any fraying of the graft substitute on these edges.

A suture passer is then passed from distal proximally through the tibial tunnel into the joint and through the femoral tunnel proximally. The graft is fed through the tibial tunnel into the joint and then out the femoral tunnel. The knee is then put through its range of motion with the graft under tension to assess any impingement in the intercondylar notch and to assess acceptable isometricity of the graft placement. As the knee is flexed beyond 20 degrees, the graft should tighten and loosen as the knee is extended.

Fixation of the graft is dependent on the graft substitute used. With a bone-patellar tendon-bone graft, interference screw fixation could be utilized. With the hamstring graft substitute, a screw with a spiked washer for fixation should be utilized. Care should be taken to bring the femoral fixation site proximal to the medial epicondyle to prevent an unacceptable prominence. After the femoral attachment is secure, the knee is again put through its range of motion with tension applied to the graft substitute to assess acceptability of the femoral and tibial tunnel placements. The knee should be able to move through a full arc of motion without undue tension on the graft. The intra-articular femoral hole, if placed too far proximal, will cause undue tension in extension or, if too distal, undue tension in flexion. This should be noted at this time and adjustments made through tunnel modification.

The knee is then brought to 30 to 40 degrees of flexion while an anterior drawer force is applied to the tibia. At this time the graft substitute is tensioned and fixed to the tibia. Again, either an interference screw fixation or screw with spiked washer is utilized.

At this time the integrity of the extra-articular and secondary capsular ligamentous restraints should be reassessed. If these are adequate the knee should be immobilized in 25 to 35 degrees of flexion. Alternatively, a femoral tibial transfixion pin could be used for stabilization of the femoral tibial joint in the reduced position. Another option is olecranization of the patella utilizing a smooth Steinmann pin from the patella into the anterior tibia. This permits early limited range of motion of the knee, while preventing any posterior subluxation of the tibia on the femur.

Appropriate dressings are applied. The postoperative course and rehabilitation protocol are determined by the integrity of the reconstruction and associated injuries. The fixation pins, if used, should be removed at approximately 6 weeks to permit progression of mobilization.

SUMMARY

In conclusion, it must be appreciated that the approach to the PCL-deficient knee is controversial. Care for any one patient must be individualized to suit the needs of that patient. The persistence of a symptomatic knee after an appropriate course of physical therapy is the most universally accepted criterion for PCL reconstruction. The argument for PCL reconstruction to prevent intra-articular degenerative changes is reasonable. There is as yet, though, no proof that PCL-reconstructed knees do not degenerate, as do symptomatic PCL-deficient knees. There is also the controversy of the role of therapeutic exercise to compensate for the PCL-deficient performance, symptoms, and possibly also the subsequent degeneration. As these issues are settled, the therapeutic approach to the PCL-deficient knee should become clarified.

ACKNOWLEDGMENT

The author would like to express appreciation for the efforts of Cari Cervantes for her secretarial services.

REFERENCES

1. Hughston JC, Bowden JA, Andrews JR, Norwood LA: Acute tears of the posterior cruciate ligament. Results of operative treatment. J Bone Joint Surg 62A:438, 1980

2. Grood ES, Stower SF, Noyes FR: Limits of movement in the human knee. J Bone Joint Surg 70A:88, 1988

3. Daniel DM, Stone ML: Diagnosis of knee ligament injury: tests and measurements of joint laxity. p. 287. Feagin JA (ed): The Crucial Ligaments. Churchill Livingstone, New York, 1988

4. Clancy WG, Jr, Shelbourne KD, Zoellner GB et al: Treatment of knee joint instability secondary to rupture of the posterior cruciate ligament. Report of a new procedure. J Bone Joint Surg 65A:310, 1983

5. Parolie JM, Bergfeld JA: Long-term results of nonoper-

ative treatment of isolated posterior cruciate ligament injuries in the athlete. Am J Sports Med 14:35, 1986

6. Dandy DJ, Pusey RJ: The long term results of unrepaired tears of the posterior cruciate ligament. J Bone Joint Surg 64B:92, 1982

7. Baker CL, Jr, Norwood LA, Hughston JC: Acute combined posterior cruciate and posteroskeletal instability of the knee. Am J Sports Med 12:204, 1984

8. Sandberg R, Balkfors B, Nillson B, Westlin N: Operative vs. nonoperative treatment of recent injuries to the ligaments of the knee. J Bone Joint Surg 69A:1120, 1987

9. Kennedy JC, Grainger RW: The posterior cruciate ligament. J Trauma 7:367, 1967

10. Girgis FG, Marshall JL, Al Monajem ARS: The cruciate ligaments of the knee joint. Anatomical, functional and experimental analysis. Clin Orthop 106:216, 1975

11. Heller L, Langman J: The menisco-femoral ligaments of the human knee. J Bone Joint Surg 46B:307, 1964

12. Arnoczy SP, Warren RF: Anatomy of the cruciate ligaments. p. 179. Feagin JA (ed): The Crucial Ligaments. Churchill Livingstone, New York, 1988

13. Sapega AA, Moyer RA, Schneck C, Komala-Hiranya N: Testing for isometry during reconstruction of the anterior cruciate ligament. Anatomical and biomechanical considerations. J Bone Joint Surg 72A:259, 1990

14. Dorlot JM, Christel P, Meunier A, Witvoet J: The displacement of the bony insertion sites of the anterior cruciate ligament during flexion of the knee. pp. 185. In Huiskes R, Van Campen D, DeWijn Boston J (eds): Biomechanics: Principles and Applications. Martinus Nijhoff, Dordrecht, The Netherlands, 1982

15. Hoogland T, Hillen B: Intra-articular reconstruction of the anterior cruciate ligament. An experimental study of length changes in different ligament reconstructions. Clin Orthop 185:197, 1984

16. Meglan D, Zuelzer W, Buck W, Berme N: The effects of quadriceps force upon strain in the anterior cruciate ligament. Trans Orthop Res Stockholm 11:55, 1986

17. Rosenberg TD, Paulos LE, Abbott PJ: Arthroscopic cruciate repair and reconstruction: an overview and description of technique. p. 409. In Feagin JA (ed): The Crucial Ligaments. Churchill Livingstone, New York, 1988

18. Daniel DM, Stone ML, Barrett P, Sachs R: Use of quadriceps active test to diagnose posterior cruciate-ligament disruption and measure posterior laxity of the knee. J Bone Joint Surg 70A:386, 1988

19. Sisk DT: Knee injuries. p. 2234. In Crenshaw AH (ed): Campell's Operative Orthopedics. CV Mosby, St. Louis, 1987

20. Hart DP, Dahners LE: Healing of the medial collateral ligament in rats. J Bone Joint Surg 69A:1194, 1987

21. Woo S, Young EP, Ohland J et al: The effects of transection of the anterior cruciate ligament on healing of the medial collateral ligament. A biomechanical study of the knee in dogs. J Bone Joint Surg 72A:382, 1990

22. Woo S, Gomez MA, Sites TJ et al: The biomechanical and morphological changes in the medial collateral ligament of the rabbit after immobilization and remobilization. J Bone Joint Surg 69A:1200, 1987

23. Hughston JC, Degenhardt TC: Reconstruction of the posterior cruciate ligament. Clin Orthop 164:59, 1982

15

Postoperative Posterior Cruciate Ligament Reconstruction Rehabilitation

ROBERT E. MANGINE
MARSHA A. EIFERT-MANGINE

INTRODUCTION

The posterior cruciate ligament (PCL) is often referred to as the primary stabilizer of the knee. The PCL controls motion in 4 of the 6 degrees of freedom of the knee; posterior translation, external rotation, hyperextension and varus rotation. PCL insufficiency may alter the biomechanics of both the tibiofemoral and patellofemoral joints. Conservative management of the PCL-insufficient knee offers limited success and is often associated with increased articular cartilage changes in the above-mentioned joints. Surgical management is quite controversial as acute and chronic procedures have varying results of success. Postsurgical management will be as demanding as conservative management. The long-term result in a variety of surgical techniques is still pending.

ANATOMY

The cruciate ligaments lie in the region of the intracondylar space of the femur and the tibia. The PCL, as its name implies, is situated behind the anterior cruciate ligament (ACL). The PCL has a broad proximal attachment on the lateral surface of the medial femoral condyle. The distal attachment on the tibia is posterior to the ACL on the posterior intracondylar fossa and on the posterior aspect of the tibial plateau. The PCL also extends along the posterior surface of the proximal tibia (Fig. 15-1).

The fibers of the PCL can be divided into two major bundles: (1) posteromedical and (2) anteromedial. An oblique reinforcing band has also been described to function along with the posteromedial bundle. Fiber direction runs lateral to medial at the tibial attachment and anterior to posterior at the femoral attachment. As the knee moves into full extension the posteromedial and oblique reinforcing bundles come under tension. In flexion the anteromedial bundle is tense.

The anatomic dimensions of the PCL differ from those of the ACL. A constant length ratio is present between the ACL and the PCL, the PCL being three-fifths the length of the ACL. The PCL as a whole is narrowest in the middle section and fans both superiorly and inferiorly (more so superiorly).

BIOMECHANICS

With motion at the knee, the cruciate ligaments function as the basis of control. This is achieved due to placement and shape of their anatomic attachment, influence on the roll-glide kinematics in both the sagittal and transverse planes, and length variances of the ligaments to accommodate for femoral condyle shape differences. Despite length variances, tension is present in both cruciates throughout the range. The anteromedial band of the PCL is under the most tension with full extension or hyperextension and is least taut in flexion.[1] The posterormedial band is taut in full extension and flexion, and the greatest amount of ten-

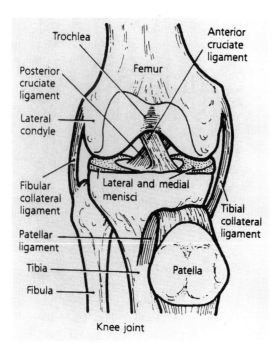

Fig. 15-1. Anatomy of the major ligaments and bones of the knee. The PCL is found immediately behind the ACL running in a lateral to medial direction. (From Ellison,[21] with permission.)

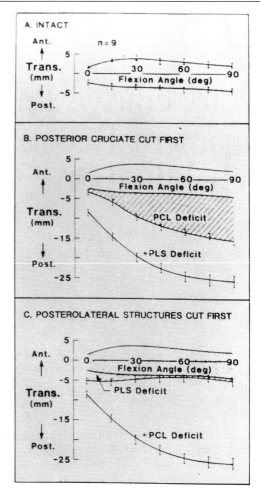

Fig. 15-2. Curves show the limits of anterior and posterior translation (vertical axis) when a 100-newton (N) anteroposterior force was applied. The neutral position (zero anteroposterior translation) was determined in the intact knee by allowing the tibia to hang vertically by its own weight. **(A)** Intact knees. The curves show the average limits of motion and the standard deviation for nine left knees. The range of total anteroposterior translation of the intact knee is shown shaded in panels **A, B,** and **C. (B)** PCL cut first (eight specimens). The increase in posterior translation after cutting the PCL is shown in the hatched area (PCL deficit). The limit of posterior translation and therefore the amount of increase is controlled by the remaining intact structures. The unshaded portion (+ PLS deficit) shows the added increase when the posterolateral structures were cut after the PCL had first been removed. A concurrent rotation took place with this cut. **(C)** Posterolateral structures cut first (seven specimens). There was only a small increase (PLS deficit) (hatched region) in the posterior limit near full extension when the posterolateral structural elements were cut first. A concurrent external rotation was also present. (From Grood et al.,[2] with permission.)

sion is in the midrange between 70 and 90 degrees. The ACL viewed as a whole demonstrates the least amount of tension between 70 and 90 degrees. Because of this tension relationship between the ACL and the PCL, ideal laxity testing for the PCL should occur between 70 and 90 degrees of knee flexion.

The PCL is responsible for controlling four motions of the knee, one translation and three rotations. The PCL serves as the primary restraint to posterior translation of the tibia on the femur as described by Grood et al.[2] The degree or amount of posterior translation in the PCL-deficient knee is dependent on the angle of knee flexion, with the greatest amount of translation demonstrated between 60 and 90 degrees.[2] Grood et al.[2] also describe an isolated cut of the posterolateral structures with an intact PCL. This reveals the greatest degree of laxity at 0 degrees with a progressive decrease in laxity as 90 degrees of knee flexion is approached (Fig. 15-2).

External tibial rotation at the knee is strongly coupled with anteroposterior translation. The degree of external rotation is dependent on the external load applied and the angle of knee flexion-extension. Isolated cutting of the PCL revealed no increase in external tibial rotation over the normal knee; however, when combined with insufficiency of the posterolateral structures, a significant increase in laxity is noted. This combined laxity of PCL and posterolateral structure deficits is greater than the laxity demonstrated by isolated insufficiency of the posterorlateral structures (Fig. 15-3).

Varus laxity on excessive tibial adduction is also associated with PCL insufficiency. In the intact knee varus laxity is slightly increased between 30 and 90 degrees of knee flexion over that demonstrated at 0 to 30 degrees. Isolated PCL deficit reveals a minimal increase in varus laxity over the intact knee. Isolated posterolateral deficit reveals a moderate increase in varus or adduction laxity, while combined PCL and posterolateral insufficiency reveals the greatest degree of varus laxity. The degree of this combined laxity is the same regardless of which structures are cut first (Fig. 15-4).

Grood et al.[2] showed that an average of 5.6 degrees of hyperextension occurs in the intact knee. This degree of hyperextension increased slightly with isolated PCL deficiency and to a greater extent when the posterolateral structures were also cut.

With deficiency of the PCL the biomechanics of both the tibiofemoral and patellofemoral joints are altered. PCL deficiency results in posterior translation of the tibiofemoral joint as described above. The altered tibial dropback is seen throughout the range of knee flexion and extension in addition to increased hyperextension.

Secondary to an increase in tibial dropback is the affect on the patellofemoral joint. Posterior tibial dropback alters the attachment of the patellar tendon on the tibial tubercle, creating a patella infera, reducing the quadriceps lever arm and increasing the patellofemoral joint reactive forces secondary to increased patellofemoral compressive forces.

PATHOMECHANICS

Injury to the PCL can result from three common mechanisms. PCL function is predominate for posterior tibial translation.[3] As previously described in the section on biomechanics, increasing the flexion increases the amount of posterior translation when the PCL is re-

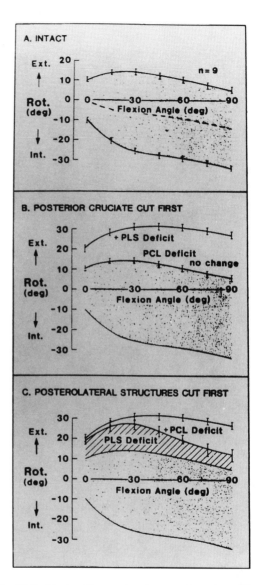

Fig. 15-3. Limits of internal and external rotation of the tibia when a 5-Nm torque was applied. The fully extended position, measured in the intact knee, was used as the zero-rotation reference. **(A)** Intact knee (nine specimens). The upper curve shows the limit of external rotation, and the lower curve shows the limit of internal rotation. The broken line shows the average position of the knee during passive flexion with the tibia hanging freely. The range of tibial rotation in the intact knee is shaded in panels **A, B,** and **C.** **(B)** PCL cut first (eight specimens). **(C)** Posterolateral structures cut first (seven specimens). (From Grood et al.,[2] with permission.)

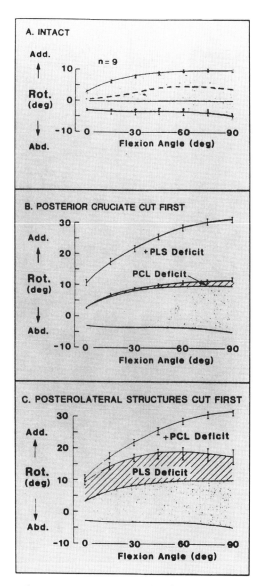

Fig. 15-4. Limits of adduction and abduction rotation when a 20-Nm moment was applied. The fully extended position, measured in the intact knee, was used as the zero-rotation reference. **(A)** Intact knees (nine specimens). The upper curve shows the limit of adduction rotation, and the lower curve shows the limit of abduction rotation. The broken line shows the amount of adduction when the knee is passively flexed with the tibia upside down to ensure tibiofemoral contact in both the medial and the lateral components. **(B)** PCL cut first (eight specimens). **(C)** Posterolateral structures cut first (seven specimens). (From Grood et al.,[2] with permission.)

moved. The most frequent mechanism of injury that is encountered is a direct blow to the tibial crest with the knee in flexion at 70 to 90 degrees. This occurs often in motor vehicle accidents or sports activities[3,4–7] (Fig. 15-5).

A second mechanism involves extreme rotation in the internal or external direction. Rotational injuries of this magnitude in many cases involve complete knee dislocations.[2,5] Clinically, this has been encountered five to six times annually. In injuries of this severity, popliteal artery damage and peroneal nerve damage are possible. In our clinical experience, peroneal nerve damage is a frequent occurrence and can delay the rehabilitation process. Internal rotation and varus forces are described more often than external rotation with valgus.

The third mechanism that may damage the PCL is hyperextension.[3,8] Since the PCL is in the posterior aspect of the knee, hyperextension will place tension on this structure as well as the posterior capsule. Patients whose injury results from hyperextension often

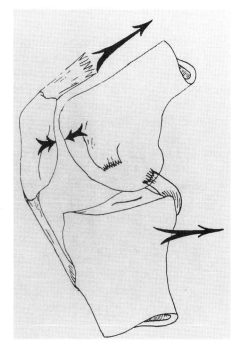

Fig. 15-5. Forces acting on the patellofemoral joint following rupture of the posterior cruciate ligament. (From Cross and Powell,[5] with permission.)

experience severe swelling and posterior capsular pain.

In the acute phase of injury, it may be difficult to assess the degree of injury. Often the patient is unable to remember the mechanism of injury and the clinician may have to rely on the physical examination to determine the extent of the injury. In many of these cases pain can be severe, especially if the peroneal nerve is involved.

In the chronic PCL patient, the physical examination is crucial. As previously stated, the injury often results from a severe mechanism in which other structural damage may have occurred. The evaluation in long-term deficiency centers on the primary and secondary stabilizers to posterior translation and posterolateral rotation. Secondary evaluation of the patella is also important since altered mechanics may involve the patella.

PHYSICAL EXAMINATION

Physical examination in the PCL-injured knee can often be difficult and confusing. It is not uncommon for PCL laxity to be confused with ACL laxity. Confusion stems from attempts by the clinician to establish the neutral point of the tibiofemoral position. For this reason, it is recommended that the clinician start with the antigravity test or dropback test. This examination is performed by placing the hip and the knee in a 90-degree flexed position. A straightedge is then laid across the anterior crest of the tibia to the inferior border on the patella. The superior patella is used as a reference point for the femur since it is located in the trochlear groove and has constant contact with the femur. By referencing the inferior border of the patella to the anterior tibial crack, a dropback of the plateaus of the tibia due to PCL insufficiency will be demonstrated by empty space at the proximal portion of the tibia. Once this reference point has been established, the clinician can assume that a dropback represents a deficiency in the PCL and that performing the allotment test will basically be relocating the posteriorly displaced tibia.

The primary function of the PCL is restraining posterior tibial translation. The second test which we perform is between 70 and 90 degrees of flexion in the traditional drawer position.[2] Grood et al.[2] have found this position to be effective in assessing PCL function and suggest this point for performing the drawer test in the posterior translation. This position is performed by placing the hip at approximately a 45-degree angle and flexing the knee between 70 and 90 degrees. The joint arthrometer test can also be performed in this position, with an increase in translation showing a PCL laxity. From this position, the clinician can assess total anterior and posterior displacement of both the medial and lateral compartments. A second portion of the evaluation would be the unilateral compartmental drawer test, which is described as a hand placement that will only effect a translation of either the medial or lateral compartment of the tibiofemoral joint. The clinician should note that in a PCL laxity, the posterior displacement of the lateral compartment will be greater than the posterior displacement of the medial compartment.[3,9] The secondary restraints in the medial side are better able to resist the PCL owing to the higher level of tension that is in these structures compared with the lateral side (Fig. 15-6).

The compartmental differences in translation will also result in an increase in external rotation by about 15 percent in the externally rotated position. Once again, this phenomenon is due to the fact that the lateral secondary restraints do not absorb tension at the same rate as the medial secondary restraints. Therefore, the lateral compartment has an increase in posterior translation about 15 percent greater than the medial compartment. This displays itself as an increase in rotational instability, which is simply defined as one compartment being able to translate either anteriorly or posteriorly more than the counter compartment.

For physical examination of the PCL to be effective, the clinician and the patient must accommodate each other. The clinician must also take into account the first-cycle effect or the first examination procedure whether a physical examination or mechanical testing, which often produces a false-negative test. PCL insufficiency will become easier to evaluate as the clinician becomes familiar with the tests that are associated with this laxity.

CONSERVATIVE MANAGEMENT

After the initial injury, the patient receives either conservative or surgical treatment. If the patient, surgeon, and rehabilitation specialist choose conservative man-

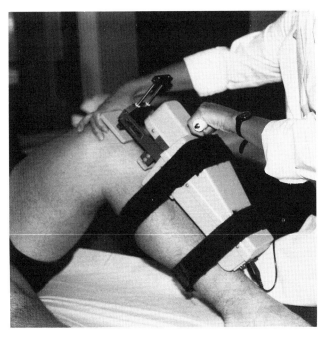

Fig. 15-6. A KT-1000 joint arthrometer can be useful in determining cruciate ligament function. For the PCL, the 70- and 90-degree angles for testing may be most accurate.

agement, it is important that key steps be taken in the treatment program.[10,11] The rehabilitation protocol itself very much parallels the postoperative course of exercise that starts at month 6 after surgery. Once this has been implemented and muscle strength, power, and endurance have been achieved to a functional level, then an ongoing maintenance program must be established with the patient and strongly emphasized.

The conservative approach has the following elements[4]:

1. Patella protection program because the increase in tibial dropback results in the increase of force.
2. Guarding the lateral structures of the knees that serve as the secondary stabilizer to posterior translation, for if the patient starts to compromise these tissues, then functional instability will increase.
3. Treatment of other associated pathology (mensicus repairs, other ligament laxities, capsular damage, or patellofemoral pathology). If at the time of the original injury other ligamentous trauma has occurred, then surgical intervention is the primary

treatment of choice. If at the time of the original injury meniscal damage has occurred, the meniscal damage should be repaired while a conservative approach to ligament insufficiency can be attempted.

4. Constant re-evaluation of the patient for joint articular surface deterioration. One of the most common deleterious side effects of ligament insufficiency is the progression of arthritic changes, which are found on the mediofemoral condyle or the patellofemoral joint. If progression occurs, surgical intervention should be attempted before the knee becomes unsalvageable.
5. Use of a brace for all recreational and sporting activity to provide some level of functional support. The most effective brace that we currently employ in our program is the DonJoy PCL or combined instability brace. If this unit is put on in the correct manner, it may aid the patient in increasing the functional level of activity.
6. Establishing proper levels of strength, power, and endurance to provide dynamic protection to the

joint. Once the appropriate levels have been established, the patient should be placed in a maintenance program.

If a conservative approach is attempted, the need for constant reassessment is crucial. Through the course of assessment any changes in the deleterious side effects of the insufficiency would result in surgical intervention.

SURGICAL INTERVENTION

Surgical intervention for the PCL-injured knee, whether it is an acute or chronic situation, is a area of diverse opinions.[8,12–18] Several investigators have expressed concern with the success rate of acute PCL reconstruction as well as demonstrated success at returning a patient with chronic PCL insufficiency to competitive athletics. Clancy et al.,[4] have demonstrated the need for acute repair or a replacement of the injured PCL. Their findings are based on deterioration of the patellofemoral joint and tibiofemoral joint that occurs over time. It is important for the clinician to be aware that the conservative approach should be defined early in the program so that surgical intervention can be implemented before deleterious side effects on the joint occur.

Changes that are often seen in chronic PCL insufficiency include compromise of the secondary stabilizers: iliotibial band, lateral/collateral ligament, and the arcuate complex.[19,20] Secondary changes to patellofemoral joint due to tibial dropback result from an increase in patellofemoral reaction force, development of a varus alignment during functional ambulation, and medial femoral condyle arthrosis and are associated with generative changes to the medial compartment.

While managing these patients in a conservative routine, if the side effects that are listed above start to present complications, surgical intervention should be implemented before the joint becomes unsalvageable.

Surgical intervention for PCL repair or reconstruction is a very complex and difficult procedure. Noyes has recently described an arthroscopic approach to PCL reconstruction that limits the deleterious side effects of arthrotomy. He has utilized this technique and demonstrated excellent results in his initial follow-up. The reconstruction itself is performed by placing a bone-patellar tendon-bone allograft through isometrically placed tibial and femoral attachment sites and securing with screw fixation (Figs. 15-7 and 15-8).

This type of repair and the variability of the isometric placement sites has led to the need to alter the postsurgical rehabilitation. This is described here in length. In association with PCL repairs, other surgical procedures are often performed. These include lateral meniscus repairs, medial meniscus repairs, or posterolateral reconstruction. If these associated repairs are performed at the time of the reconstructive procedures, careful implementation of the rehabilitation is crucial to avoid stretching the repaired tissue.

The surgical procedure will undoubtedly be further revised in the future. However, materials both biologic and synthetic that are currently available for implantation have not been as successful as they have been in ACL reconstructive procedures.

POSTSURGICAL REHABILITATION

Postsurgical management of PCL reconstruction gives physical therapists a greater challenge to apply their knowledge of basic science and clinical experience than other reconstructive procedures. The challenge of PCL reconstruction arises from the altered biomechanics and associated articular cartilage changes, pathomechanics of the injury, and difficulty of the reconstructive procedure.

The goals of the rehabilitation program include controlling postsurgical joint hemarthrosis; gradual controlled progression of range of motion; quadriceps strengthening; limiting hamstring (posterior translation) forces; progression of weight bearing; close monitoring of the patellofemoral joint to prevent patella infera; and gradual return to function. The progression of the rehabilitation program should be based on weekly evaluations, remembering that overly aggressive exercise programs can lead to forces not tolerated by the graft or the patellofemoral joint secondary to its altered biomechanics. The standard protocol as outlined in this chapter may require alteration based on the weekly evaluation.

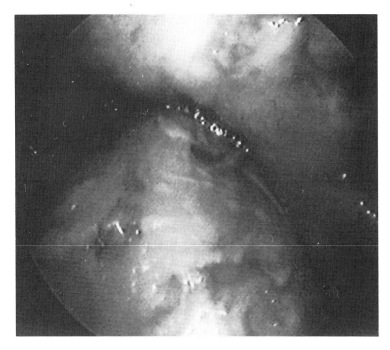

Fig. 15-7. Tension on a bone-tendon-bone allograft that is isometrically placed (Courtesy of F. R. Noyes, Cincinnati Sports Medicine and Orthopaedic Center.)

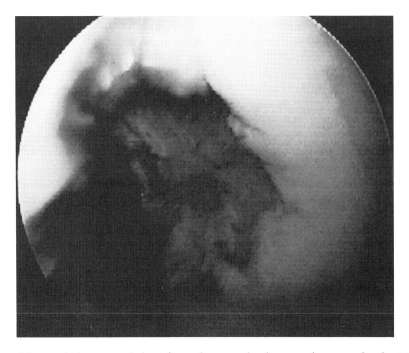

Fig. 15-8. Size of the notch that is needed to place a bone-tendon-bone replacement for the PCL. (Courtesy of F. R. Noyes, Cincinnati Sports Medicine and Orthopaedic Center.)

Protocol

Days 1 to 5

1. Compression dressing, continue until joint swelling is controlled.
2. Hemovac for 48 hours.
3. Continuous passive motion (CPM) of 30 to 70 degrees, six times per day for 10 to 15 minutes.
4. Quadriceps isometrics (isolated), rule of 10s, performed in the 70-degree flexed position. Avoid hamstring tension for the first 6 weeks isometrically and for the first 16 weeks for progressive resistive exercises (PREs) (Fig. 15-9).
5. Straight leg raises (SLR) in the supine position only.
6. Cryotherapy for hemarthrosis control; continue until hemarthrosis is under control and to reduce joint response to surgical procedure.
7. Electrical muscle stimulation to quadriceps to prevent shutdown.
8. Patellar mobilization; aggressive superior glides are important to avoid infrapatellar contracture (Fig. 15-10).

Weeks 1 to 4

1. CPM: remain at 30 to 70 degrees six times per day for 10 to 15 minutes. If restricted motion problems develop, increases to 90 degrees are recommended after 3 weeks.
2. SLR: initiate hip adduction at week 3 unless lateral or medial repairs are performed. Weight can be added in the supine position at week 4.
3. Cryotherapy is continued.
4. Toe-touch weight bearing is initiated at 2 weeks, being careful to emphasize a heel-to-toe gait pattern to promote proprioceptive re-education.

Weeks 5 to 16

1. Range of motion increased:
   Week 5: 15 to 90 degrees
   Week 6: 5 to 100 degrees
   Week 7: 0 to 115 degrees
   Week 8: 0 to 125 degrees
The therapist must realize that if a joint contracture develops, increases in motion must be accelerated.

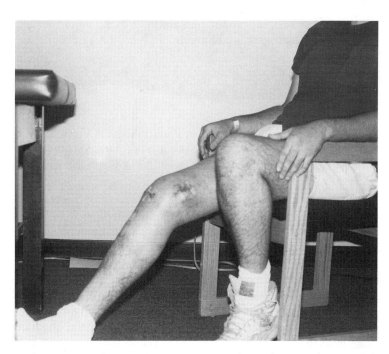

Fig. 15-9. Patient performing a 70-degree isometric exercise. This is the neutral point of the angle of the knee. In this position there should be minimal translation.

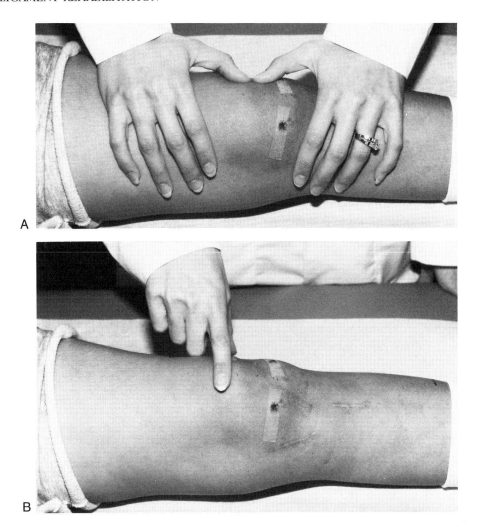

Fig. 15-10. (A) Medial patellar glides being performed on a postoperative PCL patient. The patient is instructed to perform this program four times a day. **(B)** If adequate quadriceps contraction can be performed, the patient will be providing an adequate superior glide. If they cannot sustain a 10-mm superior glide, then a home electrical stimulator is utilized.

This requires monitoring progress every 3 to 4 days to assess patient compliance and scar tissue formation.

2. Weight bearing: 25 percent at week 6, 50 percent at week 8, 75 percent at week 10, and 100 percent at weeks 12 to 16. Based on an arthrometer measurement showing total anteroposterior translation at 70 degrees either equal to or 2 mm greater in comparison to the opposite limb. If more than 2 mm anteroposterior translation is detected, then a careful examination of the exercise protocol and patient compliance must be performed. Arthrometer measurement should be repeated every other week for the first 16 weeks.

3. Exercise program:

Isometrics for the hamstrings at 70 degrees of knee flexion are initiated at 6 weeks after surgery on a submaximal basis.

Isometrics for the quadriceps are discontinued. Cycling is initiated at 8 to 10 weeks postsurgery, with the seat of the bicycle in a lower than normal position to reduce patellofemoral irritation.

PREs are initiated if certain criteria are met: the absence of joint swelling, objective weekly measurements of anteroposterior translation, minimal patellofemoral crepitus, and minimal pain symptoms. PREs are initiated between 90 and 60 degrees of extension and are gradually increased to 30 degrees. Flexion PREs are not initiated unless the arthrometer measurement shows that the reconstructed knee has a smaller amount of anteroposterior translation than the noninvolved knee.

Swimming can be initiated at week 12 after surgery. The criteria described for the PRE program are applied. The first phase consists of allowing the patient to ambulate in the water to build endurance.

Toe raises are begun when 50 percent weight bearing is achieved, progressing from flat standing to off-the-step exercises.

Wall sits (hold for 30 seconds), progressing by 10-second increments (Fig. 15-11).

Flexibility training for the hamstrings and gastrocnemius. If range of motion is excessive after removing the postoperative brace, avoid training.

Weeks 17 to 24

1. Continue above exercises, increasing weight and amount of time.
2. Endurance: initiate walking and gentle hip kicking in the pool or NordicTrac workouts. Upper extremity training can be accomplished via an airdyne or other ergometer system.

Weeks 24 to 48

1. Repeat arthrometer testing at 70 and 20 degrees of flexion and measure external rotation at 70 degrees of flexion. If measurements are within normal limits, proceed as described below.
2. Function: all activities are continued in the brace if there is a suggestion of lateral or PCL dysfunction. A PCL brace is used when the PCL is reconstructed alone; a DonJoy brace is used with combined instability or if the lateral compartment is involved.

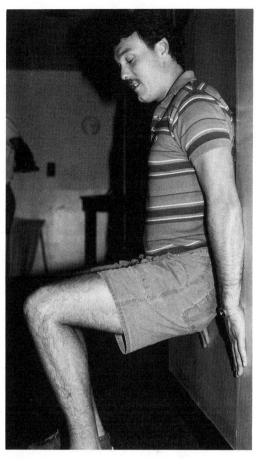

Fig. 15-11. Patient performing a wall sit in a 70-degree angle. This is a protective range to lower the anteroposterior translation.

3. Exercises:
    Isokinetics in the 300 to 450 degree/sec range if the patient does not have access to a pool. These exercises must be performed slowly, with constant evaluation for patellofemoral crepitus and graft healing.

    PREs are continued with increasing weight as symptoms of pain and swelling and KT-1000 measurements allow. Limit extension to 30 degrees, and patellofemoral crepitus must be minimal. Flexion PREs are initiated with light weight and limited range; the last 15 degrees of extension is avoided to protect the graft.

    Continue all other exercises, gradually increasing the amount of difficulty.

Weeks 48 to 60

Gradually increase function using all the above-mentioned criteria: patellofemoral crepitus, symptoms, arthrometer measurements. Use objective functional testing as a guide for safe return to activity.

REFERENCES

1. Girgis FG, Marshall JL, Monajem A: The cruciate ligaments of the knee joint. Clin Orthop Rel Res 106:216, 1975

2. Grood ES, Stowers SF, Noyes FR: Limits of movement in the human knee. J Bone Joint Surg 70A:88, 1988

3. Hughston JC, Bowden JA, Andrews JR, Norwood LA: Acute tears of the posterior cruciate ligament. J Bone Joint Surg 438, 1980

4. Clancy WG, Jr, Shelbourne KD, Zoellner GB et al: Treatment of knee joint instability secondary to rupture of the posterior cruicate ligament. J Bone Joint Surg 65A:310, 1983

5. Cross MJ, Powell JF: Long-term follow-up of posterior cruciate ligament rupture: a study of 116 cases. Am J Sports Med 12:292, 1984

6. Moore HA, Larson R: Posterior cruciate ligament injuries: results of early surgical repair. Am J Sports Med 8:68, 1980

7. Trickey EL: Injuries to the posterior cruciate ligament: diagnosis and treatment of early injuries and reconstruction of late instability. Clin Orthop Rel Res 147:76, 1980

8. Torg JS, Barton TM, Pavlov H, Stine R: Natural history of the posterior cruciate ligament-deficient knee. Clin Orthop Rel Res 246:208, 1989

9. Hughston JC: The absent posterior drawer test in some acute posterior cruciate ligament tears of the knee. Am J Sports Med 16:39, 1988

10. Jokl P, Stull PA, Lynch K, Vaughan V: Independent home versus supervised rehabilitation following arthroscopic knee surgery—a prospective randomized trail. Arthroscopy 5:298, 1989

11. Timm KE: Postsurgical knee rehabilitation: a five year study of four methods and 5381 patients. Am J Sports Med 16:463, 1988

12. Ogata K: Posterior cruciate reconstruction using iliotibial band. Trauma Surg 101:107, 1983

13. O'Meara CB, Tencer AF, Ivey FM, Jr, Woodard P: A comparison of various types of fixation devices for protection of the posterior cruciate ligament against a posterior drawer force. J Orthop Res 4:499, 1986

14. Parolie JM, Bergfeld JA: Long-term results of non-operative treatment of isolated posterior cruciate ligament injuries in the athlete. Am J Sports Med 14:35, 1986

15. Scott WN, Rubinstein M: Posterior stabilized knee arthroscopy: six years' experience. Clin Orthop Rel Res

16. Southmayd WW, Rubin BD: Reconstruction of the posterior cruciate ligament using the semimembranosus tendon. Clin Orthop Rel Res 15D:196, 1980

17. Tibone JE, Antich TJ, Perry J, Moynes D: Functional analysis of untreated and reconstructed posterior cruciate ligament injuries. Am J Sports Med 16:217, 1988

18. Wirth CJ, Jager M: Dynamic double tendon replacement of the posterior cruciate ligament. Am J Sports Med 12:39, 1984

19. Eriksson E, Haggmark T, Johnson RJ: Reconstruction of the posterior cruciate ligament. Orthopedics 9:217, 1986

20. Kochan A, Markolf KL, More RC: Anterior-posterior stiffness and laxity of the knee after major ligament reconstruction. J Bone Joint Surg 66A:1460, 1984

21. Ellison AE (ed): The knee. p. 236. In: Athletic Training and Sports Medicine. 1st Ed. American Academy of Orthopaedic Surgeons, Chicago, 1984

16

Patellofemoral Joint Considerations in Knee Ligament Rehabilitation

BYRON P. WILDERMUTH
ROBERT P. ENGLE

INTRODUCTION

Operative and nonoperative rehabilitation of knee ligament injuries is frequently complicated by patellofemoral dysfunction and pain, commonly referred to as patellofemoral pain syndrome (PPS).[1-3] Trauma to the knee can directly injure stabilizing peripatellar structures and articular cartilage. Patellofemoral symptoms can also develop later as the rehabilitation process unfolds. This is commonly secondary to a variety of problems including maltracking stresses, lost motion, increased contact shearing, stresses, and neuromuscular insufficiencies.[2,4,5]

Accounting for pre-existing or potential patellofemoral problems is critical to adequate patient management. Clinicians dealing with these patients must have a thorough understanding of the anatomy, biomechanics, diagnosis, examination, and treatment of the patellofemoral joint in addition to other structures involved in the rehabilitation process. This chapter reviews relevant information critical to this aspect of knee ligament rehabilitation.

ANATOMY AND BIOMECHANICS

Patellar anatomy and biomechanics have been presented in Chapter 1 and will not be repeated. How-

ever, several relevant aspects of this joint's unique function will be reviewed.

Articulating Surfaces

The articular cartilage of the patella's undersurface is among the thickest deposits found in the body. Softening, fissuring, and fibrillation are common with normal degradation associated with daily functional and sports activities. This process of degeneration can be further advanced by immobilization, excessive contact shearing forces associated with loss of joint stability (both anterior cruciate ligament (ACL)- and posterior cruciate ligament (PCL)-deficient knees) and recurrent synovitis.

Forces across the articular surface change depending on knee flexion-extension position. In full extension, patellar contact with its femoral counterpart is inferior and moves superiorly as the knee moves into flexion. Patellofemoral reactive forces are extremely high at the end range of knee extension in the open kinetic chain model.

Different patellar shapes have been described in the literature, emphasizing the need to appreciate patellar positioning in the femoral trochlear groove. The articular surface geometry can predispose the patella to instability or excessive compression syndrome. An example of this is the patellofemoral joint with a low lateral femoral condyle that provides poor restraint to lateral patellar subluxation.

Peripatellar Structures

The medial and lateral retinacula provide static support to lateral and medial stability, respectively. Lateral retinacular tightness is very common, predisposing the patient to further lateral patellar mobility. This is usually related to accompanying distal iliotibial band, biceps femoris, and fascial tightness. Disection through this area with ACL reconstructive procedures will lead to scarring and further tightening postoperatively. Stretching these structures early in the rehabilitation process is necessary to prevent further problems. Further lateral tracking influence is provided by the vastus lateralis, vastus intermedius, and rectus femoris force vector.

Medially, the retinaculum can be torn with traumatic knee injuries. If not recognized at initial examination and treated, it will heal poorly and lateral patellar instability will result. An intimate relationship between the retinaculum, medial capsular, and collateral ligaments and vastus medialis obliquus (VMO) exists medially.[6] Any atrophy, insufficiency, or dysplasia of the VMO leads to further lateral tracking.

The VMO, active throughout the full arc of knee motion, provides a very important "fine-tuning" qualitative function of patellar tracking and stabilization. Its functional loss through inhibition mechanisms can be devasting. Normal patellofemoral joint and, hence, normal knee function is not possible without normal VMO function.

Inferiorly, the patellar tendon and fat pads are very important structures clinically. Patellar tendon harvesting for cruciate ligament reconstruction has several potential devastating effects. During removal of a bone-tendon-bone strip the patella can fracture.

This sacrificing of a portion of the tendon leads to permanent quadriceps weakness in many cases. Postoperative scarring of the patellar tendon can lead to morphologic shortening or patella infera, in turn limiting superior patellar gliding and knee extension. This is a common, devastating complication of ligament surgery that is difficult to salvage with both conservative and surgical methods. Immediate mobilization is encouraged after ligament surgery for prevention.

Medial and lateral fat pad irritation is also frequently seen, especially with arthroscopic procedures. The medial synovial plica attaches to the medial fat pad. As a fold in the synovium it is affected by synovitis and is vulnerable to impingement between the medial femoral condyle and medial patellar facet. Other plicae are also recognized as a source of patellofemoral and related pain.

Other mechanical factors in the weight-bearing extremity that influence patellar tracking are lumbopelvic asymmetry, femoral neck anteversion, genu valgum or varum, and forefoot and rearfoot abnormalities. Compensation for a stiff, painful knee can accentuate these problems, repetitively stressing selective structures at the patellofemoral joint.

Diagnosis and Evaluation

Patellofemoral joint evaluation has been described by Beck and Wildermuth.[7] Common, subjective patient complaints include retropatellar pain, giving way, pain with stairs and inclines, snapping, popping, clicking, and occasional locking. An achy, burning pain associated with prolonged sitting can also be described. Malek and Mangine[4] call this "movie sign."

The examiner should note the onset, location, and behavior of patellofemoral symptoms and any past problems. In cases of trauma, forces directed toward the patellofemoral joint should be considered with the patient's pathomechanics of injury. For example, valgus-external rotation mechanisms that tear the medial collateral ligament can also include injuries to the medial retinaculum, VMO, and medial patellar facet.

Physical examination should include stability, mobility, palpation, and related neuromuscular and articular cartilage tests. After the clinician has made a thorough inspection of the patellofemoral joint, appropriate considerations should be made in the patient's treatment goals and plans.

CONSIDERATIONS IN SPECIFIC LIGAMENT INSTABILITIES

ACL reconstruction procedures can present a potential risk for patellofemoral problems. Several technical problems can lead to restricted knee extension, which in turn leads to patella infera. These include patellar tendon autograft harvesting, nonisometric graft placement, inadequate notchplasty, and inappropriate rehabilitation. Nonoperative management of ACL-deficient patients has also been associated with patellofemoral pain.[2]

PCL rehabilitation is highly dependent on the quadriceps for control of the posterior instability.[8] Parolie and Bergfeld[9] have shown patients with good quadriceps function returning to full sports activity following complete PCL tears. However, patellofemoral problems in both nonoperative and operative PCL patients have been shown. This is due, largely, to the grafts selected (bone-patellar tendon-bone), relatively high residual laxity accepted for good results in PCL reconstruction, and the resultant patellar contact shearing stresses through quadriceps compensation of this operative and nonoperative laxity.

Rehabilitation of the knee can affect the patella in a number of ways. Immobilization, by not allowing full knee extension, allows scarring and contracture of the posterior capsule and peripatellar structures, leading to abnormal functional stresses on the patella. Second, immobility of the knee has been shown to lead to negative cartilage changes and morphologic shortening of connective tissues such as the patellar tendon. Proprioception loss associated with ACL and PCL deficiency and joint instabilities has been demonstrated as well.[2,3,10–13]

Resistive exercises must also be considered a potential source for patellar problems. In an attempt to restore normal mechanical and neuromuscular (including proprioception) function, the knee can be cycled through arcs of motion that repetitively overstress the articular or peripatellar components. Before aggressive resisted quadriceps exercise can begin, good patellar tracking should be established by balancing medial and lateral quadriceps components. Weight-bearing techniques should be included whenever possible for joint stabilization (through compression), articular cartilage nourishment, and mechanoreceptor stimulation.

However, both individual patellar orientation and lower quarter examination must be considered in the weight-bearing model. Patellar type, size, mobility, and orientation should be assessed. Changes develop rapidly through the weight-bearing lower kinetic chain to compensate for the postoperative knee. If unaccounted for, these problems can magnify stresses at the patella. Patellar taping, orthotics, and lumbopelvic manual therapy and exercise procedures can help balance lower quarter function, thereby decreasing ab-

normal patellar stresses. Therapeutic exercise techniques for the quadriceps must be introspectively directed, keeping in mind the effect these exercises have on the patient's patella.

REHABILITATION

Our approach to the rehabilitation of patients involves the use of proprioceptive neuromuscular facilitation (PNF) as taught by Knott and Voss[14] for treatment of the dysfunctional knee extensor mechanism (primarily the VMO), tight shortened antagonists, and loss of proprioception. PNF, a manual approach to therapeutic exercise, uses the proprioceptors and mechanoreceptors found in muscles, tendons, ligaments, capsules, and fat pads to assist the patient in realizing full potential.

Neurophysiologic Basis

Wyke and others[15–20] have identified and described four mechanoreceptors, which have been delineated as types I, II, III, and IV.

Type I mechanoreceptors have a slow threshold of activation and are slow to adapt. Found in the superficial layers of the joint capsule, they have increased density in the proximal joints. Their primary function is to regulate joint pressure changes as well as the direction, amplitude, and velocity of joint movement.[15–21] These changes are measured through the variations in capsular tension created by altering the position of the knee.[20]

Type II mechanoreceptors lie in the deeper layers of the capsule and articular fat pads, have a low threshold of activation, and are rapid in adapting. The density of type II receptors is greater in the more distal joints.[15] One of their primary functions is to measure quick changes in movement, such as acceleration and deceleration. These receptors are therefore inactive in immobile joints.[15–21] Another important function of this type of receptor is to help initiate movement to overcome inertia.[19]

Type III receptors, on the other hand, are dynamic mechanoreceptors that have a high threshold and are slow adapting. They lie in the intrinsic and extrinsic ligaments of most joints and are sensitive to tension or stretch on the ligaments.[15–21] Their primary function is to monitor direction of movement, and they are particularly active at the end range of joint movement.[19,20] They act with a reflex effect to provide a braking mechanism against overstress of the joint.[20]

The last type of mechanoreceptors, type IV receptors, are high threshold, nonadapting pain receptors that are found in all joints. Activated only with extreme mechanical or chemical irritation, this type of receptor is found in the fibrous capsule, fat pads, intrinsic and extrinsic ligaments, walls of vessels, and the periosteum.[15–21] They are not found in the articular or intra-articular fibrocartilage and synovium.[19,20]

Muscle spindles are sensory organs that lie in the muscle and run parallel to the fibers. They are concentrated in the center of the muscle and are numerous in skill muscles. The overall function of the muscle spindles is to monitor length and velocity related to length. They do not, however, monitor changes in length. These parameters are reported on a moment-to-moment basis, with high sensitivity.[19,22,23]

The muscle spindle is supplied by a single large sensory neuron that attaches the spindle to the central nervous system. This primary afferent nerve fiber divides as it approaches the spindle and gives off to each intrafusal fiber.[22] These fibers are more numerous than the motor axons that innervate the same muscle.[24] The primary afferent fiber has a low threshold and is very sensitive to small stretches and velocity movement.[19,23] When stimulated by a passive stretch, the primary afferent fiber causes an excitation of itself, called autogenic facilitation. At the same time, it facilitates the synergist and inhibits the antagonists (direct inhibition).[22] This reflex to passive stretch is found in the flexor and extensor muscles of the limbs but not in the abductors and adductors.[19,21,23]

The secondary afferent fibers have a higher threshold than the primary fibers and have some differences in function as well. They monitor absolute muscle length and velocity of movement.[19,23] In general, the secondary afferents facilitate flexor muscles and inhibit extensors.[21,22] This is important where joint stabilization is necessary. If a single joint extensor is activated, it causes inhibition of itself and excitation of its antagonistic flexor. This inhibition is not enough to inactivate the extensor because the primary afferent is still functioning. This causes cocontraction about the joint, resulting in a stabilizing effect (especially at the proximal joints).[21,22]

The efferent innervation motor pathway from the spine to the muscle makes up 60 percent of the nerve fibers going to the muscle. These fibers are made up of larger alpha motor neurons that go to the contractile fibers of the muscle and small gamma motor fibers that go to the muscle spindle. The alpha motor neurons cause a direct contraction of the muscle, while the gamma fibers contract the polar ends of the spindle. This activates the sensory endings, causing the alpha motor neurons to be stimulated.[21,22] This gamma loop is responsible for registering the difference between the desired and actual contraction of the muscle. This error detection system is important in posture and fine motor control and may be the preferred pathway of activation of a muscle when there is adequate time.[21,22,25]

Golgi tendon organs are sensory organs that, unlike the muscle spindle, lie in series within the muscle at the musculotendinous junction.[22] Like the muscle spindle, the Golgi tendon organ resisters moment-to-moment changes in muscle tension.[22,23,26,27] Only a small fraction of the total number of fibers have tendon organs, yet the tension on a single fiber can have significant effect on the discharge rate of its afferent nerve.[28,29] These discharge rates give the central nervous system a good estimation of passive stretch of the total muscular force being developed.[30,31] This allows the monitoring of force generation and protects from overcontraction of the muscle. The inhibition of the same muscle and its synergists is termed autogenic inhibition. At the same time, the antagonist is excited to release the muscular tension.[23,30]

The muscle spindle and Golgi tendon organ are crucial to proprioception because they register and regulate the muscle tension. However, regulation of stress at the joints is also needed. This function is performed by the joint receptors.

Flexibility

Janda[32] states that tight, inflexible muscles act in an inhibitory way on their antagonists. Sachs et al.[2] state that a flexion contracture increases patellofemoral contact forces and contributes to quadriceps weakness. In their study group, 46 percent of patients who had no flexion contracture had no patellar irritability. Beck and Wildermuth[7] comment on the need for not only hamstring flexibility, but flexibility of the triceps surae as well.[7]

As stated previously, we prescribe to the concepts

of PNF and use these procedures and techniques to lengthen muscle.[14] In comparing the hold-relax (HR) procedure with passive mobilization, Tanigawa[33] found the HR procedure to be much more effective. He believes that tension on the Golgi tendon organ stimulates the muscles to relax reflexly. The Golgi tendon organ overrides the muscle spindle. To lengthen a muscle group using the HR technique, the extremity is brought to the limits of motion of the agonistic pattern. At this point, the clinician should tell the patient to "hold, do not let me move you." An isometric contraction of the antagonistic muscle group is done until the clinician commands the patient to "relax," and the extremity is moved to the newly gained range of motion. During the isometric contraction, the clinician should gradually increase resistance without breaking the hold to facilitate more muscle units. This should be done with both hip extension patterns to ensure optimal results.

In an electromyographic study, Moore and Hutton[34] compared ballistic stretch, slow movements, and static stretch with two PNF procedures: contract-relax (CR) and contract-relax with agonist contraction (CRAC). They concluded that CRAC was the preferred method for achieving maximum gain in flexibility. Wallin et al.[35] compared a modified CR to a ballistic stretch, concluding that CR is better for increasing flexibility than ballistic stretch. We think that their modified CR is really HR.

Osternig et al.[36] compared static stretch, CR, and agonist contract-relax (ACR) and found that ACR was the most effective for lengthening muscle.

To administer the CR technique, the patient actively flexes the hip to the limits of motion (knee extended). The clinician, with manual contact on the extensor surface, should tell the patient to "kick down and in, turn your heel in." The patient should then do an isotonic contraction into the extension-adduction-external rotation pattern. The clinician should resist this motion and only allow rotation to occur. Then the clinician should have the patient relax and should bring the limb into the new range of motion. In the CRAC, as mentioned by Moore and Hutton,[34] when the command "relax" is given, the patient does an agonist contraction of the hip flexors, moving into the newly gained range of motion.

The ACR technique that Osternig et al.[36] report on is performed by the patient actively contracting the quadriceps musculature to extend the knee. "After each contraction the subject relaxed with the attained knee position manually supported."[36]

Quadriceps Facilitation

Many investigators have noted the loss of quadriceps strength in ligament injuries of the knee.[1,2,9,37] In light of this, we do not feel that the ACR technique would be the optimal choice. Moreover, while the HR technique is used for pain modification, the other techniques (CR, CRAC, and ACR) are not. In addition, it is commonly agreed that there is quadriceps atrophy or weakness in ligament injuries.[1-3,5,9,37] If quadriceps weakness is one factor in PPS, then one should strengthen the quadriceps.

The tried and true method is quadriceps sets, or isometric contractions of the quadriceps. Wild et al.[38] say that: "quadriceps sets and straight leg raising exercises in full knee extension offer the best quadriceps rehabilitation program in the patient with a PPS and persistent symptoms." Beck and Wildermuth[7] also recommend starting with quadriceps isometrics, with particular attention paid to the VMOs. When instructing the patient in quadriceps setting, the clinician must emphasize contracting the VMO first. Failure to do so will exacerbate the PPS. As the quadriceps are set, the patient must look at the VMO and palpate it, so that the muscle contracts and the VMO tracks the patella medially.

Our approach is to start with the patient in supine and then resist the hip extension-adduction-external rotation pattern with the knee in full extension. One can approximate, compressing the joint surfaces in a close-pack position of both hip and knee, facilitating the type I, II, and III mechanoreceptors.[39] Afferent flow from the type I, II, and III receptors inhibits the type IV receptors (nociceptors).[39] Isolated knee pivots, with the patient seated at the end of the treatment table, are also effective in facilitating the quadriceps, particularly the VMO.

At full knee extension, the quadriceps exert one-fourth more effort than they do at 20 to 30 degrees of extension.[38] Knowing this, the clinician may want to start the patient at this range of motion. We have found, in some instances, that the patient has pain at 0 degrees of extension but not at 20 or 30 degrees. If that were the case, HR could begin at this point, again paying particular attention to the VMO. Patients who learn to contract the quadriceps and control the VMO could progress into full extension. The technique here is to use an HR technique, resisting dorsiflexion, inversion of the ankle, and extension and external tibial rotation of the knee. As the patient approaches 0 degrees of extension, the clinician should again approximate. As quadriceps function and VMO control improve, the emphasis would change from isometrics (HR) to short-arc repeated contractions (RC).[14] RC are isotonic movements repeated over and over again in a limited arc of motion (15 to 0 degrees) and increased in range of motion as function increases. As each increment of pain-free range of motion is completed, the next increase in range of motion should follow: if 10 to 0 degrees is pain-free, with good quadriceps and VMO function, then the clinician should progress to 45 to 0 degrees, 60 to 0 degrees, 90 to 0 degrees. Now the patient is moving through the full range of motion without pain, with good strength, function, and endurance. Slow reversals are now introduced to the program, alternating between flexion and extension, from a loose-pack to a close-pack joint position, stimulating the afferent discharge of the type I, II, and III mechanoreceptors.

Patients who progress from isometrics to isotonics and are pain-free with the above program should be progressed to more functional activities.

Pevsner et al.[40] suggest progressing to swimming, distance walking, bicycling, jogging, running, sprinting, and cutting. They feel that the major loss of muscles is the type II fibers, and these need retraining. Rose and Rothstein[41] state that: "muscle dysfunction may give rise to joint dysfunction, which may make muscle fiber type predominance important clinically." Making a sprint sport athlete do predominantly endurance work during the return to activity program may cause muscle fatigue and injury. As the patient continues to improve in strength, function and endurance, and if the patient has good flexibility and is pain-free, then other activities may be introduced into the rehabilitation program.

Facilitation of the proprioceptors is paramount to an optimal rehabilitation result. According to Ihara and Nakayama,[42] "there is a strong implication that simple muscle training does not increase the speed of muscle reaction, but dynamic joint control training has the potential to shorten the time lag of muscular reaction." Therefore, the clinician that feels that PPS has been resolved by doing straight leg raises, quadriceps sets,

or even knee pivots has not completed the patient's rehabilitation program. Only when the patient can return to his or her activity with strength, coordination, and little potential for injury or reinjury has the clinician completed the job.

Gray,[43] quoting Leach in his discussion of proprioception, emphasizes that the longer athletes are withheld from their sport or from beginning their rehabilitation, the more they lose their sense of proprioception. Gray also speaks of closed chain activities, activities with the extremity in a weight-bearing configuration, the lower extremity acting in a hip-knee-ankle synergy.[43] Straight leg raises, quadriceps sets and knee pivots are open chain activities and are necessary in the early rehabilitation phase of the ligament-injured patient with PPS, but the patient must be progressed to more functionally and sport-related activities.

Plyometrics

At our clinic, the progression from an open chain program to one utilizing closed chain activities is the use of plyometrics. Lundin,[44] quoting Atha, says that plyometrics refers to: "this principle as 'bounce-loading,' the nature of the exercise being a rhythmic hybrid of eccentric plus concentric activity which loads the elastic and contractile components of muscle." Lunden feels the proprioceptors most effected by plyometrics are the muscle spindle and Golgi tendon organ. We feel that the type I, II, and III mechanoreceptors are also facilitated.

Chu[45] lists innumerable plyometric exercises, from squat jumps to box drills. We start with horizontal movements, progressing to vertical movements, followed by a combination of the two.

The horizontal program starts with double-leg, forward hopping in a straight line (Fig. 16-1). The clinician must make sure the patient's weight bearing is equal bilaterally, both on takeoff and landing. A natural progression would be from forward hopping to hopping back and forth across a line, followed by hopping sideways. The next step would be hopping on the involved limb in a straight line, then hopping back and forth across a line (Fig. 16-2). Various height boxes (6, 12, 18, and 24 inches) are added to the program. At first the patient will jump off a 6-inch box, rebound, and hop, hop, hop down the floor (Fig. 16-3). The

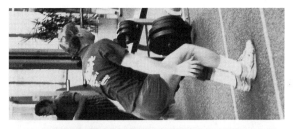
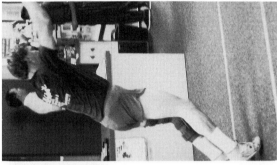
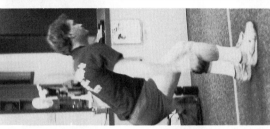
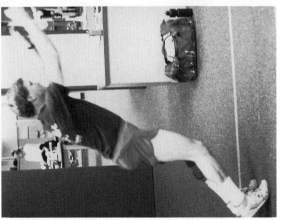
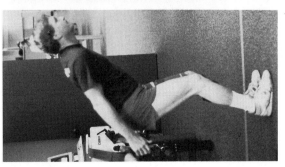

Fig. 16-1. Double-leg hopping in a straight line.

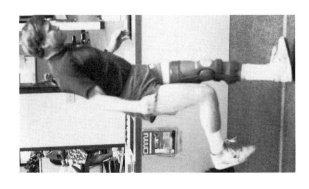

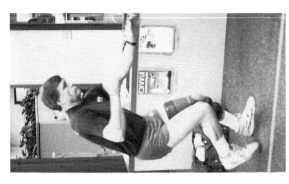

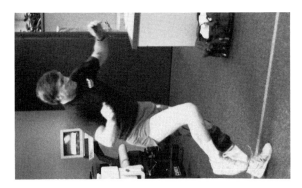

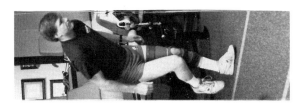

Fig. 16-2. Hopping back and forth across a line with the involved extremity.

184

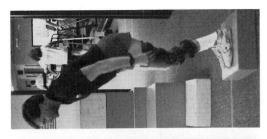
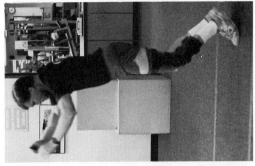
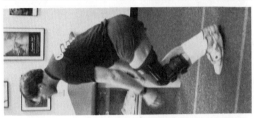
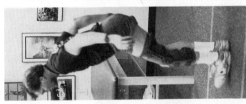
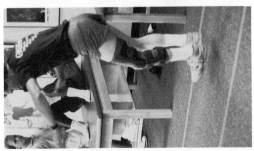
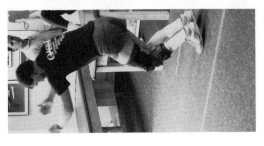

Fig. 16-3. Jumping off a 6-inch box and hop, hop, hop.

185

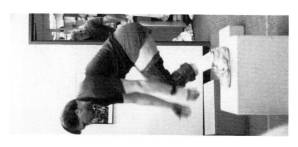

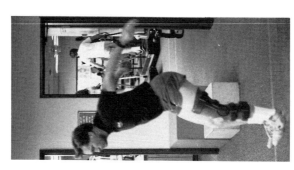

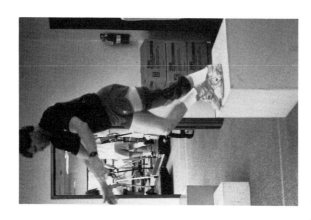

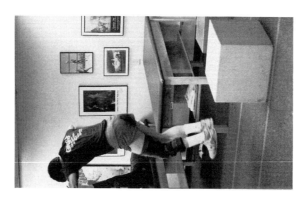

Fig. 16-4. Hopping off one box and onto another and jumping off that box.

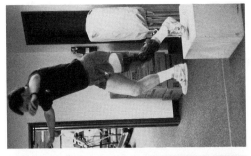
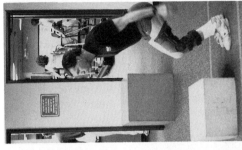
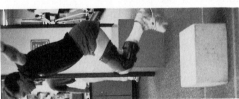
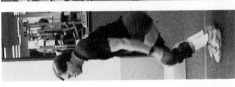
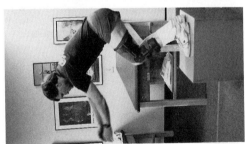
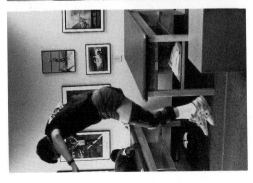

Fig. 16-5. Hopping off one box, over another, and onto a third, then hopping off.

187

patient may hop off one box and hop onto another (Fig. 16-4), or hop over the box and onto another (Fig. 16-5). The height of the boxes can be increased to put a greater demand on the patient. The variability of these exercises is only limited by the clinician's imagination.

Landing and jumping causes an eccentric force to be applied to the muscle, which prestretches the quadriceps and stimulates the muscle spindles. This causes a facilitation of the quadriceps and its synergists and inhibition of the antagonists. The type I and II mechanoreceptors are also stimulated by the change in joint pressure and the change in joint velocity and acceleration and deceleration. Type III mechanoreceptors are facilitated by the alternating tension and relaxation of the extrinsic and intrinsic ligaments.

For the ACL reconstruction patient, the above program usually starts about week 12 to 16, depending on the individual patient's progress (OASIS protocol, unpublished). With PCL-, medial collateral ligament- and lateral collateral ligament-injured patients, plyometrics may be started much earlier. To protect the reconstructed knee, the patient wears a protective brace. Johnson[46] has found that an off-the-shelf brace is capable of minimizing ACL strain.

As an adjunct to the above program, the patient may exercise with various types of equipment, such as the leg press, Kinetron, and Cybex (Ronkonkoma, NY) and any of the stepping devices.

Cycling has been reported by several investigators to be beneficial in taking stress off the patellofemoral joint and ACL as well as increasing quadriceps strength.[47–50]

For those patients who have difficulty gaining a proprioceptive awareness of the VMO, electrical stimulation may be a worthwhile adjunct to manual facilitory techniques. Several researchers have reported on the use of electrical stimulation to increase strength of the quadriceps femoris muscle group.[51–56] However, almost all the studies showed an increase in isometric strength. Dynamic, functional strength through the full range of motion, with coordination, is the clinician's goal.

If one accepts the premise that PPS is a result of quadriceps weakness, flexion contracture, and a loss of proprioception, then the treatment goal is obvious[2,3,12]: increase the extension range of motion, facilitate the proprioceptors, and increase quadriceps

femoris strength. The best tools the clinician can use are "his/her head and his/her hands" (A. McCleary, personal communication).

SUMMARY

Surgical procedures are now being developed to decrease patient rehabilitation time and complications. Patellofemoral complications secondary to intra-articular knee ligament surgery are very common. Most can be prevented by improved surgical technique, immediate restoration of motion, full restoration of quadriceps support, and return of normal lower quarter biomechanics. This must be accomplished without compromising the healing of surgically placed ligaments and grafts, articular cartilage, or menisci. This chapter reviews relevant concepts of anatomy, biomechanics, diagnosis, examination, and rehabilitation relevant to patellofemoral joint problems in knee ligament rehabilitation.

REFERENCES

1. Tibone JE, Antich TJ, Perry J, Moynes D: Functional analysis of untreated and reconstructed posterior cruciate ligament injuries. Am J Sports Med 16:217, 1988
2. Sachs RA, Daniel DM, Stone ML, Garfein RF: Patellofemoral problems after anterior cruciate ligament reconstruction. Am J Sports Med 17:760, 1989
3. LoPresi C, Kirkendall DT, Street GM, Alden AW: Quadriceps insufficiency following repair of the anterior cruciate ligament. J Orthop Sports Phys Ther 9:245, 1988
4. Malek M, Mangine RD: Patellofemoral pain syndromes: a comprehensive and conservative approach. J Orthop Sports Phys Ther 2:108, 1981
5. Baugher WH, Warren RF, Marshall JL, Joseph A: Quadriceps atrophy in the anterior cruciate insufficient knee. Am J Sports Med 12:192, 1984
6. Woo SLY, Iouye M, McGurk-Burlson E, Gomez MA: Treatment of the medial collateral ligament injury. Am J Sports Med 15:22, 1987
7. Beck JL, Wildermuth BP: The female athlete's knee. Clin Sports Med 4:345, 1985
8. Cross M, Powerll JF: Long-term followup of posterior cruciate ligament rupture: a study of 116 cases. Am J Sports Med 12:292, 1984
9. Parolie JM, Bergfeld JA: Long-term results of non-oper-

ative treatment of isolated posterior cruciate ligament injuries in the athlete. Am J Sports Med 19:35, 1986

10. Freeman WAR, Dean MRE, Hanaham IWF: The etiology and prevention of functional instability of the foot. J Bone Joint Surg 47B:678, 1965

11. Freeman WAR: Instability of the foot after injuries to the lateral ligament of the ankle. J Bone Joint Surg 47B:669, 1965

12. Barrack RL, Skinner HB, Buckley SL: Proprioception in the anterior cruciate deficient knee. Am J Sports Med 17:1, 1989

13. Dvir Z, Koren E, Halperin N: Knee joint position sense following reconstruction of the anterior cruciate ligament. J Orthop Sports Phys Ther 10:117, 1988

14. Knott M, Voss D: Proprioceptive Neuromuscular Facilitation/Patterns and Techniques. Harper & Row, New York, 1983

15. Wyke B: Articular neurology: a review. Physiotherapy 58:94, 1972

16. Wyke B: Neurology of Joints. Instructional Course at the 55th Annual Conference of the American Physical Therapist Association, Atlanta, GA, 1979

17. Wyke BD: The neurology of joints. Ann R Coll Surg Engl 41:25, 1967

18. Wyke BD, Polacek P: Articular neurology: the present position. J Bone Joint Surg 57B:401, 1975

19. Newton RA: Joint receptor contributions to reflexive and kinetic responses. Phys Ther 62:22, 1982

20. Kessler RM, Hertling D: Management of Common Musculoskeletal Disorders. Harper & Row, Philadelphia, 1983

21. Day RW, Wildermuth BP: Proprioceptive training in the rehabilitation of lower extremity injuries. Adv Sports Med Fitness 1:241, 1988

22. Gardner E: Reflex muscular responses to stimulation of articular nerves in the cat. Am J Physiol 161:133, 1950

23. Hasan Z, Enoka RM, Stuart RG: The interface between biomechanics and neurophysiology in the study of movement: some recent approaches. Exerc Sport Sci Rev 13:169, 1985

24. Mathews PBC: Mammalian Muscle Receptors and Their Central Actions. Arnold, London, 1972

25. Loeb GE: The control and responses of mammalian muscle spindles during normally executed motor tasks. Exerc Sports Sci Rev 12:157, 1984

26. Houk J, Henneman E: Responses of Golgi tendon organs to active contractions of the soleus muscle of the cat. J Neurophysiol 30:446, 1967

27. Prochazka A, Wand P: Tendon organ discharge during voluntary movements in cats. J Physiol (Lond) 303:385, 1980

28. Burke RE: Motor units: anatomy, physiology and functional organization. p. 345. In Books VB (ed): Handbook of Physiology. Section 1. Vol II. Part 1. American Physiology Society, Bethesda, MD, 1981

29. Fukami Y: Responses of isolated Golgi tendon organs of the cat to muscle contraction and stimulation. J Physiol (Lond) 318:429, 1981

30. Gardner EB: Contributions of proprioceptive reflexes to neuromuscular facilitation and inhibition. Monograph. Sargent College of Allied Health Professions, 1967

31. Stephens JA, Reinberg RM, Stuart DG: Tendon organs of cat medial gastrocnemius: responses to active and physic forces as a function of muscle length. J Neurophysiol 38:1217, 1975

32. Janda V: Treatment of Patients. International federation of Orthopaedic Manipulative Therapists, 4th Conference, Christ Church, New Zealand, 1980

33. Tanigawa MC: Comparison of the hold-relax procedure and passive mobilization of increasing muscle length. Phys Ther 52:725, 1972

34. Moore MA, Hutton RS: Electromyographic investigation of muscle stretching techniques. Med Sci Sports Exerc 12:322, 1980

35. Wallin D, Bjorn E, Grahn R, Nordenburg T: Improvement of muscle flexibility: a comparison between two techniques. Am J Sports Med 13:3263, 1985

36. Osternig LR, Robertson RN, Troxel RK, Hansen P: Differential responses to PNF stretch techniques. Med Sci Sports Exerc 32:106, 1987

37. Doxey G: Assessing quadriceps femoris muscle bulk with girth measurements in subjects with patellofemoral pain. J Orthop Sports Phys Ther 9:5:177, 1987

38. Wild JJ, Franklin TD, Woods GW: Patellar pain and quadriceps rehabilitation and EMG study. Am J Sports Med 10:12, 1982

39. Kennedy JC, Alexander IJ, Hayes KC: Nerve supply of the human knee and its functional importance. Am J Sports Med 10:329, 1982

40. Pevsner D, Johnson JRG, Blazina ME: The patellofemoral joint and its implications in the rehabilitation of the knee. Phys Ther 59:869, 1979

41. Rose SJ, Rothstein JM: Muscle mutability. Part I: General concepts and adaptions to altered patterns of use. Phys Ther 62:1773, 1982

42. Ihara H, Nakayama A: Dynamic joint control training for knee ligament injuries. Am J Sports Med 14:309, 1986

43. Gray GW: Rehabilitation of running injuries: biomechanics and proprioceptive considerations. Top Acute Care Trauma Rehab 1:67, 1986

44. Lunden P: A review of plyometric training. National Strength and Conditioning Journal 7:69, 1985

45. Chu DA: Plyometric exercise. National Strength and Conditioning Journal 6:56, 1984

46. Johnson RJ: The In Vivo Biomechanics of the Anterior Cruciate Ligament. First IOC World Congress on Sports Science, Colorado Springs, 1989

47. McLeod WD, Blackburn TA: Biomechanics of knee rehabilitation with cycling. Am J Sports Med 8:175, 1980

48. Ericson MO, Nisell R: Patellofemoral joint forces during ergometric cycling. Phys Ther 67:1365, 1987

49. Ericson MO, Nisell R: Tibiofemoral joint forces during ergometer cycling. J Orthop Sports Phys Ther 9:285, 1988

50. Ericson MO, Nisell R, Nemeth G: Joint motions of the lower limb during ergometer cycling. J Orthop Sports Phys Ther 14:285, 1986

51. Anderson AF, Lipscomb AB: Analysis of rehabilitation techniques after anterior cruciate reconstruction. Am J Sports Med 17:154, 1989

52. Boutelle D, Smith B, Malone T: A strength study utilizing the electro-stim 180. J Orthop Sports Phys Ther 7:50, 1985

53. Delitto A, Rose SJ, McKowen JM et al: Electrical stimulation versus voluntary exercise in lengthening thigh musculature after anterior cruciate ligament surgery. Phys Ther 69:661, 1988

54. Harsell HD: Electrical muscle stimulation and isometric exercise effects on selected quadriceps parameters. J Orthop Sports Phys Ther 8:203, 1987

55. Kubiak RJ, Whitman KM, Johnston RM: Changes in quadriceps femoris muscle strength using isometric exercise versus electrical stimulation. J Orthop Sports Phys Ther 8:537, 1987

56. Soo CL, Currier DP, Threlkeld AJ: Augmenting voluntary torque of healthy muscle by optimization of electrical stimulation. Phys Ther 68:333, 1988

17

Optimizing the Nonsurgical Treatment of Joint Contractures

ALEXANDER A. SAPEGA
LESLEY K. ROGAN

INTRODUCTION

Despite the use of early and/or continuous passive range of motion following trauma or surgery, joint contractures continue to occur. It is not uncommon for a patient to have difficulty attaining the last 5 or 10 degrees of extension and flexion following knee ligament reconstruction. Even greater difficulties in obtaining full motion are seen following elbow trauma. Traditionally, orthopaedists have attempted to resolve these difficulties through joint manipulation with the patient under anesthesia, either with or without surgical resection of adhesions or capsular release procedures. Physical therapists have also attempted to resolve these problems with a multitude of nonsurgical techniques, with varying degrees of success.

Basic research concerning the biophysical properties of connective tissue has recently been used to help devise more effective methods of nonsurgical treatment for these troublesome contractures. Resultant therapeutic protocols employing low-load, long-duration passive stretching have been shown to be superior to traditional higher-load and shorter-duration passive range of motion therapies. Low-load, long-duration stretching protocols have even proved successful in reducing residual joint contractures that may remain following surgical resection of joint adhesions and/or manipulation under anesthesia.[1] The recent availability of dynamic orthoses for large joints to allow for low-load, prolonged passive stretching now permits the continuation of this technique between supervised therapy sessions.

This chapter reviews the clinically relevant biophysical properties of connective tissue, discusses the application of this information to the treatment of extremity contractures, compares the reported results of prolonged, passive stretching protocols versus more traditional physical therapeutic measures, and reviews the implications of this information for warm-up and flexibility training in athletes.

CONNECTIVE TISSUE AND JOINT MOTION

Connective tissue is made up of collagen fibers of various densities and spatial arrangements, embedded in a protein-polysaccharide matrix referred to as ground substance. As a fibrous protein, collagen has a very high tensile strength. Collagenous tissue is organized into many different anatomic structures, including tendons, ligaments, joint capsules, aponeuroses, and fascia, among others. A joint's range of motion, in both normal and pathologic conditions, is limited primarily by one or more connective tissue structures. Clinical and laboratory studies have documented that the primary sources of passive resistance at the extremes of normal joint motion are ligamentous joint capsules, tendons, and muscles.[2,3] The relative contribution of each anatomic component to the total motion-limiting resistance varies with different body joints.

The inclusion of muscles as motion-limiting structures requires some clarification. Muscles, unlike joint capsules and tendons, are not primarily connective tissue structures. Even so, experimental evidence indicates that when a relaxed muscle is stretched, most of the physical resistance to that stretch is derived from the extensive connective tissue framework and sheathing within and around the muscle, rather than from the myofibrillar elements.[4–8]

Adhesions, scar tissue, and fibrotic contractures are types of pathologic connective tissue that often limit joint motion and that are commonly seen after trauma or surgery. These must be dealt with therapeutically.

Connective tissue is thus the common, primary target of range of motion (stretching) exercise, regardless of whether it is normal tissue or pathologic tissue. It is therefore essential that one understand the various factors that affect the mechanical behavior of connective tissue under tensile stress, to determine optimal methods for increasing range of motion.

DEFINITIONS

Certain definitions must be understood so that therapists and physicians appreciate, and make use of, the physical properties of connective tissue.

The term *viscoelastic* describes a substance that demonstrates both viscous and elastic material properties. *Viscous* properties are defined as those which permit *plastic or permanent deformation* of a material under load. Plastic stretching deformation results in a permanent or nonrecoverable elongation, that is, a putty-like behavior. *Elastic* properties permit *recoverable deformation.* Elastic stretching deformation results in temporary elongation, that is a rubber band-like behavior. Connective tissue is a viscoelastic material that demonstrates both viscous and elastic behavior when stretched.[9–12]

CONNECTIVE TISSUE MECHANICS

When connective tissue is stretched, some of the elongation occurs in the elastic tissue elements and some occurs in the viscous tissue elements. When stress is removed, elastic deformation recovers, but the plastic deformation remains. While the actual microstructural identity of the elastic and the viscous elements in connective tissue continues to be the subject of research

and debate, that uncertainty does not negate the clinical significance of its viscoelastic properties.

The relative proportion of elastic and plastic deformation that occurs when connective tissue is placed under tensile stress can vary considerably. The primary determinants are the *amount* and *duration* of the stretch and the *temperature* of the involved tissue at the time of stretch. The primary therapeutic goal of range of motion exercise should be to produce plastic, or permanent, connective tissue deformation. This goal, except in the case of adhesions, should be accomplished without physically tearing the connective tissue. If this occurs, pain, joint instability, and/or subsequent scar formation can combine to make the patient's condition worse.

RESEARCH FINDINGS

Laboratory research has demonstrated that high-force, short-duration stretching favors the elastic deformation of collagenous tissue, whereas low-force, long-duration stretching favors its plastic deformation.[9,13,14] When the initial elongation produced by each stretching method is held the same, the low-load, long-duration stretch results in a greater degree of permanent length change. Other studies have shown that when connective tissue structures are elongated, some degree of mechanical weakening occurs. This is the case even if outright rupture has not occurred.[9,13,15] The amount of structural tissue weakening depends on both the way the tissue was stretched, as well as how much it was stretched. For the same amount of lengthening, a high-force, short-duration stretching method causes more structural weakening than a slower, low-load method.[9,13]

Temperature has also been found to have a significant influence on the mechanical behavior of collagenous tissue under tensile stress. As connective tissue temperature rises, extensibility increases and stiffness decreases.[14–17] Raising the temperature of tendon samples above 103°F increases the amount of permanent elongation that occurs from a given amount of initial stretch.[14,16] There is a thermal transition that occurs in the microstructure of collagen at about 104°F. This transition significantly enhances stress relaxation of the viscous elements in collagen, allowing for a greater proportion of plastic deformation when the tissue is stretched.[15,17,18] While the mechanism behind this phenomenon is still uncertain, it is thought that the intermolecular bonding in collagen becomes partially destabilized, thus enhancing its viscous properties.[15,18]

The conditions under which heated, stretched collagenous tissue is allowed to cool can significantly affect the degree of plastic deformation that remains after the tensile stress is discontinued. The relative proportion of plastic deformation can be significantly increased by maintaining tensile stress on the tissue until it has cooled, rather than removing the stress while the tissue temperature is still elevated. This appears to allow the collagenous microstructure to restabilize more at its new stretched length.[16]

When stretching connective tissue at temperatures within the usual therapeutic range (102 to 110°F), the amount of structural weakening produced by a given amount of tissue elongation varies inversely with the temperature.[9,13] This is apparently related to the progressive increase in the viscous flow properties of the collagen as it is heated. The thermal destabilization of the intermolecular bonding most likely allows elongation to occur with less internal structural damage.

In summary, the elastic or recoverable deformation of connective tissue is most favored by high-load, short-duration stretches at normal or cooler temperatures. Plastic or permanent deformation is favored by low-load, long-duration stretches at elevated temperatures, and by cooling the tissue *before* releasing the stress. The structural weakening produced by permanent tissue deformation is minimized by the combination of high therapeutic temperatures and prolonged, low-load application.

CLINICAL APPLICATION OF IN VITRO DATA

In 1979, the Temple University Center for Sports Medicine and Science developed a comprehensive protocol for the nonsurgical treatment of joint contractures based on all the principles demonstrated in the previously discussed laboratory studies. Anecdotal success led to the publication of this protocol in 1981[19] and to clinical trials by other investigators.[20–22]

The Temple protocol was specifically designed to lengthen functional connective tissue structures (tight knee ligament substitutes and/or contracted joint capsules) without compromising their structural integrity. With that goal in mind, dynamic (spring-loaded) extension-flexion joint orthoses were later developed to extend the use of low-load, long-duration stretching outside of the therapist's office[23] (G. R. Hepburn, personal communication). The Temple protocol or variations thereof have since been successfully applied to contractures of the ankle,[20] elbow,[22,23] shoulder,[24] and knee.[1,21,24] Low-load, prolonged passive stretching has even been found to significantly reduce involuntary electromyographic activity in the hip adductor muscles of patients with spastic hip adduction contracture and to provide an increase in hip joint mobility.[25] The following section describes our currently preferred method of implementing the Temple protocol, using the knee as an example. Supplementary treatment with a dynamic orthosis[23] is used either for difficult cases or when regular outpatient therapy cannot be instituted on a consistent basis.

THE TEMPLE PROTOCOL

The entire knee joint is first evenly heated to the maximal tolerated degree using hydrocollator packs for 15 minutes. Care is taken to avoid thermal injury to the patient. Modest passive forces, created by hanging weights, are applied either directly (Fig. 17-1) or via traction cuffs (Fig. 17-2) for increasing extension or flexion, respectively. The amount of weight will vary considerably with the tolerance of the patient, but will rarely exceed 20 lbs. All efforts are made to apply the weights in a manner that creates force vectors that not only cause the knee to flex and extend but that will also gently distract the joint and enhance anterior and posterior glide of the tibia on the femur.

Such a complex combination of applied forces is not necessary to achieve positive results, but it is consistent with normal joint kinematics and may lessen abnormal patterns of articular cartilage compression during treatment. Passive stretching is generally applied for 20 to 60 minutes per session, depending on the patient's tolerance. The hydrocollator packs are changed as necessary to maintain tissue temperature elevation throughout the session.

The patient is encouraged to relax completely. If available, electromyographic biofeedback is used to

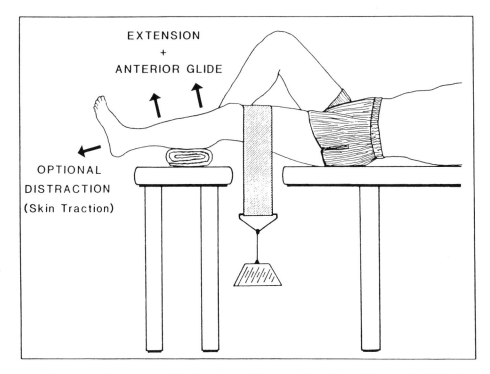

Fig. 17-1. Modest passive forces, created by hanging weights, are shown here being applied directly to increase knee extension.

promote local muscle relaxation. This helps to keep both the therapist and the patient aware of any tendency to actively resist the stretching forces.

Patients are allowed several 30-second breaks during the stretching period, when the weight is temporarily disconnected so they can move the extremity and relieve any discomfort caused by the continuous stretching. Transcutaneous electrical nerve stimulation (TENS) can also be used to decrease the discomfort during stretching.[24]

At the termination of treatment, the stretching force is maintained while the entire knee is chilled with bags of crushed ice for 15 minutes. The stretching force is always maintained until the end of the cooling period. This protocol should be followed daily if possible.

Stretching sessions should be scheduled to avoid circumstances in which heat is contraindicated. Tissue temperature elevation is not desirable when the knee is acutely irritated by physical trauma or excessive muscle-strengthening exercises.

When the clinical goal is to lengthen functional connective tissue structures in a safe, nontraumatic man-

ner, the above protocol is usually effective. If, however, adhesions are present, and the goal is to disrupt (tear) them, rather than stretch them, then theoretically they would be best dealt with in the opposite manner. The treatment of choice for adhesions would therefore appear to be high-force, short-duration manipulation at normal or depressed tissue temperatures. However, following reconstructive knee surgery, forceful joint manipulation often entails a risk of compromise to the structural integrity of the primary ligament graft or repair. In such cases, even if there is suspicion that adhesions are present, the safer, albeit slower, Temple protocol is generally our initial treatment method of choice.

CLINICAL INVESTIGATIONS

Rizk et al.[24] found that in the treatment of patients with adhesive capsulitis, prolonged pulley-traction (combined with TENS to minimize passive stretch discom-

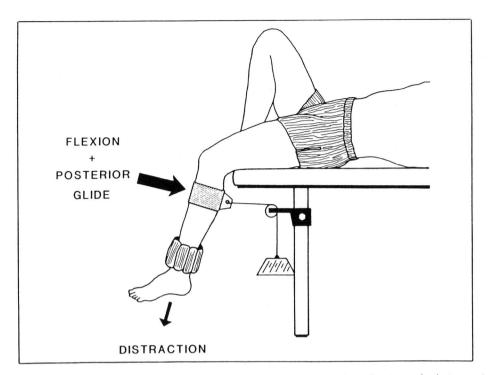

FLEXION
+
POSTERIOR
GLIDE

DISTRACTION

Fig. 17-2. Modest passive forces, created by hanging weights, are shown here being applied via traction cuffs to increase knee flexion.

fort) produced significantly ($P < .001$) greater gains in shoulder range of motion than did more traditional therapeutic methods (i.e., active exercise and rhythmic manipulation). Light et al.[26] demonstrated that low-load, prolonged stretching was significantly ($P < .05$) more effective than traditional high-load, brief stretching methods in reducing knee flexion contractures in chronically inactive patients. No investigations have yet evaluated the specific usefulness of the adjunctive tissue temperature modulation advocated in the Temple protocol, but Brodin and Tiensuu[27] have presented strong supportive evidence for the use of deep heating in combination with passive stretching. They compared four different methods of treating established knee joint contractures of 5 to 24 months' duration. Method I employed heat, passive stretching, and active resistive exercise; method II employed heat and passive stretching; method III employed heat and active resistive exercise; and method IV employed passive stretching and active resistive exercise. The methods involving the specific combination of tissue temperature elevation and passive stretching (I and II) produced approximately twice as much increase in range of motion per session as the other two methods.

STRETCHING EXERCISE AND THE ATHLETIC WARM-UP

Another topic worthy of discussion when talking about stretching is the place of stretching in the athletic warm-up. We have just discussed the benefit of stretching in conjunction with tissue temperature elevation. With this evidence in mind, it is logical to conclude that to derive maximal benefit with minimal tissue damage, athletes should stretch only *after* a period of light exercise, such as brisk walking or jogging, to increase peripheral circulation and raise extremity tissue temperature. Stretching that is done prior to such a tissue warm-up probably exposes the athlete to a greater risk of injury[28] and should provide lesser increases in range of motion. For maximum increases in muscle and joint flexibility, stretching should be repeated immediately after a workout, when tissue temperatures will be highest. In addition, stretching should always be done thoroughly and patiently, avoiding high-force, short-duration ballistic techniques.

SUMMARY

Connective tissue is the primary physical target of range of motion exercise, whether such exercise is employed in joint rehabilitation following injury or as part of an athletic warm-up performed by healthy individuals. Basic research has shown that prolonged, gentle stretching at elevated tissue temperatures maximizes the permanent lengthening of connective tissue while minimizing deterioration in its tensile strength. Treatment protocols for joint contracture devised in accordance with the above findings have thus far proved to be superior to more traditional therapeutic approaches involving active, active-assisted, and high-force, short-duration stretching techniques without tissue temperature modulation.

REFERENCES

1. Riddle D: Case study: a treatment approach for a resistant knee extension contracture. J Orthop Sports Phys Ther 7:159, 1986
2. Johns RJ, Wright V: Relative importance of various tissue in joint stiffness. J Appl Physiol 17:824, 1962
3. Wright V, Johns RJ: Quantitative and qualitive analysis of joint stiffness in normal subjects and in patients with connective tissue diseases. Ann Rheum Dis 20:36, 1961
4. Casella C: Tensile force in total striated muscle, isolated fibre and sarcolemma. Acta Physiol Scand 21:380, 1950
5. Banus MG, Zetlin AM: The relation of isometric tension to length in skeletal muscle. J Cell Comp Physiol 12:403, 1938
6. Ramsey R, Street S: The isometric length-tension diagram of isolated skeletal muscle fibers of the frog. J Cell Comp Physiol 15:11, 1940
7. Stolov W, Weilepp TG, Jr, Riddell WM: Passive length-tension relationship and hydroxyproline content of chronically denervated skeletal muscle. Arch Phys Med Rehabil 51:517, 1970
8. Stolov W, Weilepp TG, Jr: Passive length-tension relationship of intact muscle, epimysium, and tendon in normal and denervated gastrocnemius of the rat. Arch Phys Med Rehabil 47:612, 1966
9. Warren CG, Lehmann JF, Koblanski JN: Elongation of rat tail tendon: effect of load and temperature. Arch Phys Med Rehabil 52:465, 1971
10. Abrahams M: Mechanical behavior of tendon in vitro: a preliminary report. Med Biol Eng 5:433, 1967
11. Stromberg D, Weiderhielm CA: Viscoelastic description of a collagenous tissue in simple elongation. J Appl Physiol 26:857, 1969
12. VanBrocklin JD, Ellis DG: A study of the mechanical behavior of toe extensor tendons under applied stress. Arch Phys Med Rehabil 46:369, 1965
13. Warren CG, Lehmann JF, Koblanski JN: Heat and stretch procedures: an evaluation using rat tail tendon. Arch Phys Med Rehabil 57:122, 1976
14. LaBan MM: Collagen tissue: Implications of its response to stress in vitro. Arch Phys Med Rehabil 43:461, 1962
15. Rigby BJ, Hirai N, Spikes JD et al: The mechanical properties of rat tail tendon. J Gen Physiol 43:265, 1959
16. Lehmann JF, Masock AJ, Warren CG et al: Effect of therapeutic temperatures on tendon extensibility. Arch Phys Med Rehabil 51:481, 1970
17. Rigby B: The effect of mechanical extension on the thermal stability of collagen. Biochim Biophys Acta 79:634, 1964
18. Mason T, Rigby BJ: Thermal transitions in collagen. Biochim Biophys Acta 66:448, 1963
19. Sapega AA, Quendenfeld TC, Moyer RA et al: Biophysical factors in range-of-motion exercise. Physician Sportsmed 9:57, 1981
20. Bouche RT, Kuwada GT: Equinus deformity in the athlete. Physician Sportsmed 12:81, 1984
21. Bohannon RW, Chavis D, Larkin P et al: Effectiveness of repeated prolonged loading for increasing flexion in knees demonstrating post-operative stiffness. Phys Ther 65:494, 1985
22. Gibson KR: Effect of manual traction on elbow flexion contractures. Phys Ther 64:749, 1984
23. Hepburn GR: Case studies: contracture and stiff joint management with Dynasplint. J Orthop Sports Phys Ther 8:498, 1987
24. Rizk TE, Christopher RP, Pinals RS et al: Adhesive capsulitis (frozen shoulder): a new approach to its management. Arch Phys Med Rehabil 64:29, 1983
25. Odeen D: Reduction of muscular hypertonus by long-term muscle stretch. Scand J Rehabil Med 13:93, 1981
26. Light KE, Nuzik S, Personius W, et al: Low-load prolonged stretch versus high-load brief stretch in treating contractures. Phys Ther 64:330, 1984
27. Brodin H, Tiensuu A: Evaluation of contracture treatment. Europa Med Phys 11:1, 1975
28. Strickler T, Malone T, Garrett WE: The effects of passive warming on muscle injury. Am J Sports Med 18:141, 1990

18

The Problem Knee: Soft Tissue Considerations

ANDREW R. EINHORN
MICHAEL SAWYER

INTRODUCTION AND RATIONALE

The problem knee is a recognized area of disability secondary to many complications, such as knee trauma, extensive surgical procedures, sepsis, psychogenic factors, and poor patient compliance during rehabilitation. This chapter focuses on soft tissue considerations related to decreased motion, increased instability, and proprioceptive loss following injury, surgery, or long immobilization. Rehabilitation and treatment techniques, as related to the above areas, are discussed.

PHYSIOLOGY OF CONNECTIVE TISSUE

Connective tissue has both a primary and secondary organization in the body. The primary organization is made up of various densities and arrangements of collagen fibers embedded in a gelatinous matrix. This protein-polysaccharide matrix reduces friction between fibers, especially during movement, and is commonly referred to as the ground substance.

The secondary organization of connective tissue includes many higher-order structures, such as tendons, ligaments, joint capsules, aponeuroses, skin, and fascial sheaths.[1] The structural orientation of these tissues is suited to their particular function. Collagen fibers of tendons show a parallel alignment, which allows them to withstand high tensile loads. Ligament fibers contain both parallel and wavy orientations, which contribute to their high tensile strength and their abil-

ity to store energy. Fibers of the skin are intermeshed and contain no predominant orientation but allow the skin extensibility in all directions. Collectively, these tissues are composed of a network containing three types of fibers: Collagen fibers, elastic fibers, and reticulin fibers. Collagen fibers provide strength and stiffness to the tissue; elastic fibers give extensibility under load; and the reticulin fibers provide bulk.[2] These elements appear to be randomly oriented fibers that attach to one another at specific intervals. The overall length between the points of attachment ultimately determines the degree of motion that occurs during joint kinematics. The longer the distance between points of attachments, the greater the range; as the distance shortens, conversely, the range also shortens.

JOINT STIFFNESS: BIOCHEMICAL OBSERVATION IN FIBROUS CONNECTIVE TISSUE

Most studies on joint stiffness have been conducted using animal models.[3–6] The information obtained has been useful in the mobilization and remobilization of human soft tissue injury. The effect of immobilization on the bone-ligament-bone complex of primates immobilized in body casts for 8 weeks has been studied by Noyes.[7] When compared with ligaments from the control group of animals, the anterior cruciate ligaments (ACLs) showed a 40 percent decrease in maximum load to failure and a significant decrease in energy storage.

Various biochemical changes in fibrous connective tissue have also been carefully studied in tissue that has undergone periods of stress deprivation. Changes in the connective tissue matrix include decreased water content and total glycoasminoglycans (GAGs). The obvious implication of the GAG and water losses is a significant diminution of spacing and lubrication efficiency of the matrix.[8]

Changes in the collagen tissue also occur secondary to immoblization.[3,9,10] Decreased intermittent stretching of the tissue significantly alters its nutritional state. The collagen tissue itself shows reduced mass and increased turnover rate. At the same time, stress-generated electrical potentials in the connective tissue decrease, which is a signal interpreted by the fibroblasts to undertake an active contraction process involving degradation of old "longer" collagen molecules and synthesis of new "shorter" collagen molecules.[8,9]

The potential effects of such changes in soft tissue mechanics are considerable. The extensibility of the periarticular structures and the critical distance between collagen fibers is hampered, thus decreasing the normal collagen gliding mechanism that is necessary during arthrokinematic movement.[8,9,11]

RESTRICTED KNEE MOTION

Arthrofibrosis about the knee can involve combinations of knee flexion-extension range of motion (ROM) restrictions. Rarely does the patient present decreased ROM limited only to flexion or extension. However, flexion loss is better tolerated functionally and appears to be easier to treat than extension loss.[12]

Immobilization of the knee in the presence of a hemarthrosis usually leads to proliferation of intra-articular connective tissue adhesions and joint fibrosis. This occurs when the ACL and knee capsule are injured. The hemarthrosis that develops from the ACL injury then extravasates into the mediolateral knee gutters. If the knee is then immobilized without controlled movement, the patient usually develops fibrosis about the knee. In this situation, if surgery is indicated, return of motion prior to surgery is a priority, thus avoiding further arthrofibrosis or a captured knee joint.

Knee flexion loss can occur for many reasons. Intra-articular fibrosis, adaptive shortening of the periarticular tissues, and restricted patellofemoral motion are the most common factors. Lengthy immobilization or untimely progression of the rehabilitation program are other considerations.

A common complication that follows injury and/or surgery that is preventable and treatable is loss of extension ROM. The long-term effects of delayed return of extension can cause permanent knee disability or other abnormalities in the kinetic chain. Altered gait secondary to lack of extension ROM can lead to a painful extensor mechanism. Initially, a tendonitis condition may develop, leading to a joint chondrosis. Extension loss about the knee can also alter gait,[13] which could lead to dysfunctions about the hip or lumbar spine.

The pathogenesis of extension loss following ACL surgery has been debated.[14] Jackson and Schaefer[12] recognized that extension loss following intra-articular ACL reconstruction constitutes an unacceptable result in the high-performance knee. They also stated that residual loss of extension can be more disabling than the preoperative instability. The causes of extension loss include intercondylar adhesions about the cruciate ligaments, tibiofemoral adhesions,[15] and proliferation of intercondylar rather than the suprapatellar pouch.[16,17] Posterior compartment adhesions or capsular contractures could also contribute to extension loss.[16,17] Inappropriate tensioning or nonisometric positioning of the ACL graft is a surgical cause of extension loss. Bony impingement of graft in the area of the femoral notch could also be another related factor in extension loss. The surgical management of this functional disability has included several procedures, with limited success. Surgical procedures include posterior releases or lengthenings involving the posterior capsule, hamstrings, or posterior cruciate ligament (PCL).[18–22] Jackson and Schaefer[12] reported other findings from a study involving 13 patients following intra-articular ACL surgery, using patella tendon autograft. They found that in addition to postoperative loss of full extension, this group of patients presented an audible and palpable "clunk" during active terminal extension.[12] Arthroscopic findings showed a fibrous nodule anterolateral to the tibial tunnel. this nodule was also attached to the soft tissue overlying the tibia and the anterior surface of the ACL graft. This soft tissue proliferation in the intracondylar notch was excised, improving knee extension.

Adaptive shortening of the extensor mechanism or infrapatellar contracture syndrome[23] is another cause of decreased extension ROM. Early patella mobilization will help reduce this potential problem (Fig. 18-1).

MANAGING SOFT TISSUE CONTRACTURES

Managing soft tissue contractures depends on the maturity of the scar tissue. Cummings[24] has divided scar tissue into two main groups, adaptable and unadaptable. Adaptable scar tissue is highly vascular and reactive tissue. This tissue contains a dense population of cells that supply nutrients and help remove wastes. The fibroblastic cells are also present and function to shorten and contract the scar.

Clinically, adaptable scar tissue will remodel during the first 7 to 8 weeks after injury or surgery.[24] Between 7 and 14 weeks, scar vascularity decreases and its ability to remodel into flexible tissue diminishes. By 14 weeks, the tissue is considered unadaptable.

Adaptable scar tissue is very fragile and strength levels are low. The tissue has about 10 percent of its maximum strength at 5 days, 40 percent at 40 days, 70 percent at 60 days, and 100 percent at 1 year. Early trauma during the first 1 to 2 weeks causes an increase in the size of the scar secondary to increased fibroplasia. Minor trauma can lead to chronic inflammation and signals the fibroplastic cells to accelerate their rate of contraction, thus shortening scar length. Repeated trauma will eventually lead to fibrotic adhesions and further restricted movement.

THERMAL INFLUENCE OF HEAT AND COLD

Sapega and co-workers[1,25] have studied both the forces and temperature-related factors that affect the behavior of connective tissue. Principles of treatment presented here are based on these factors. As heat is applied to the soft tissue around the knee, temperature rises, stiffness decreases, and extensibility increases. Temperatures around 104°F have caused a change in

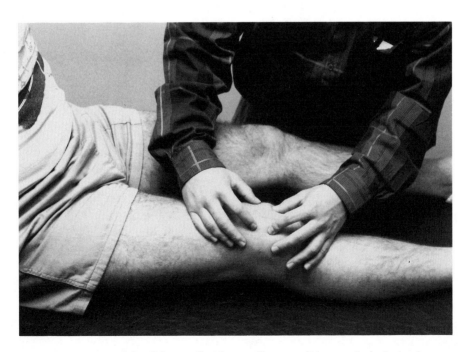

Fig. 18-1. Inferior to superior glide of the patella. The patella must glide superiorly during knee extension and inferiorly during knee flexion.

the thermal transition of the collagenous microstructure. This enhances the viscous stress relaxation of the collagen tissue, allowing greater plastic deformation as stretching occurs. Elevated temperatures applied with lower forces also cause less structural weakening of the tissue when compared with higher forces and lower temperatures. After heating and the application of low stretching force, the tissue is cooled before releasing the stretching forces. This enables the collagenous microstructure to restabilize in its newly stretched length.

Principles in Treating Adaptable Scar Tissue

The physiologic basis of treating adaptable scar tissue is early controlled motion. This will help stimulate remodeling of the tissue and avoid excessive stress. Early controlled motion is the most effective method in preventing arthrofibrosis about the knee. Most knee rehabilitation protocols include controlled ROM exercises or the use of a continuous passive motion machine (CPM). The CPM works effectively to gain flexion ROM.

Early dynamic splinting and serial casting can both be used to help reduce contracture in cases involving immature scar tissue. When using either method, the therapist should evaluate the patient for signs of ischemic trauma and/or abnormal sensation. The therapist should also observe the patient's subjective reaction to the treatment. The Dynasplint (Dynasplint Systems, Inc., Baltimore, MD) is a dynamic splint used at night and provides prolonged-duration stretching with low forces.[26] This device provides a constant low loading force over an extended period of time. Slow deformation of the soft tissue, or creep, takes place especially during the first 6 to 8 hours of loading. Initial usage of the Dynasplint begins at low tension during continuous awake hours of the day. Treatment time is extended as patient tolerance permits. Treatment time is progressed to 4, 6, and 8 continuous hours of awake usage before overnight wear is attempted. The patient should be able to sleep all night without pain before increasing tension on the device. Dynasplint works best in reducing knee flexion contractures.

Initial clinical treatment of scar tissue contractures should provide mild forces of short duration. Increase intensity with each treatment and observe for signs of over treatment. For example, if pain lasts 1 to 2 hours beyond the clinical treatment, the therapist is causing trauma to the affected tissues and pushing well beyond the maximum comfortable position.

The forces used during early motion are very important. Generally, the greater the force, the shorter the time it will be administered.[26–28] The smaller the force, the longer it can be tolerated. A balance of forces is needed in treatment. Too much force causes trauma to the scar. This will promote increased throbbing, aching, and tenderness as well as increased temperature and swelling. All of these are signs of overtreatment. Chemical components of inflammation may accelerate the rate of fibroblastic contraction and scar retraction, decreasing ROM. If this occurs, a systematic backtracking of the patient's activities and clinical treatment is indicated. Did the treatment cause this setback in ROM? How much pain was present when the patient left the clinic? Did the pain last more than 1 to 2 hours? Was the patient involved in too much activity at home? Did the patient wake up in the morning with this problem? Did the patient twist and turn at night? Was the Dynasplint treatment increased too much? Did the patient develop "mall syndrome," or increased pain and swelling secondary to walking at the local shopping mall? These are all important questions to discuss with the patient who returns with exacerbated pain and decreased ROM.

Various factors may affect the treatment process. Psychogenic problems, low tolerance toward pain, and work-related injuries have shown a slower rate of functional return.

Precautions are needed during passive ROM. Techniques that are overly aggressive can create many problems, such as increased patellofemoral joint compression forces, articular cartilage loading, rupture of the extensor mechanism, and meniscus entrapment. Current protocols following ACL surgery that utilizes bone-patella tendon-bone grafts encourage early motion. Care should be taken to avoid rupture of the already weakened extensor mechanism.

Various contraindications may apply to specific rehabilitation conditions. The physician-therapist team may need to discuss both active and passive ROM precautions when dealing with capsuloligament repairs or fractures about the tibiofemoral joint. In these cases, ROM will be delayed until necessary soft tissue or bony healing occurs. Figures 18-2 through 18-5 show ROM

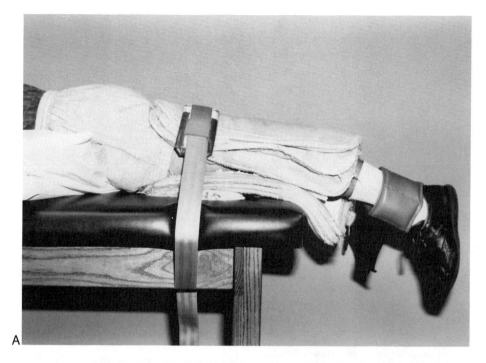

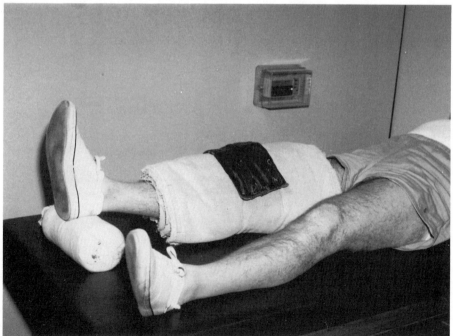

Fig. 18-2. (A) Prone lying; Heat is applied as the patient is strapped to the table. Lumbar spine problems may prohibit this technique for knee extension. **(B)** Alternative technique would place the patient in a supine position. A towel roll is placed under the ankle as heat is applied to the knee. The ankle roll is high enough to permit low-load knee extension.

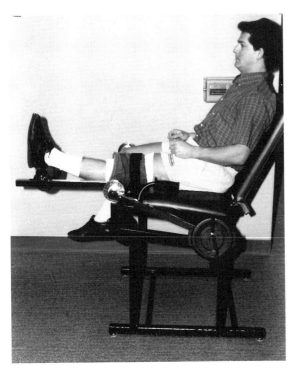

Fig. 18-3. Passive ROM on the N/K Table (N/K Products, Soquel, CA). Heat is applied around the knee during this extension technique, followed by ice.

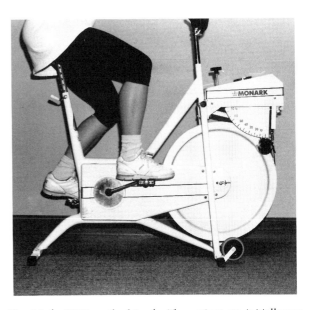

Fig. 18-4. ROM on the bicycle. The patient can initially use the bicycle in a limited range, halfway backwards and halfway forwards. Progress to riding in the backwards direction and, as ROM improves, riding in the forwards direction. Avoid excessive hip hiking and plantar flexion of the ankle during bicycling techniques.

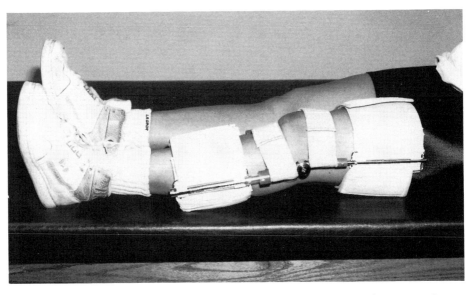

Fig. 18-5. The Dynasplint is used during sleeping hours to promote knee extension.

exercises that are commonly used in treating adaptable scar tissue.

PRINCIPLES IN TREATING MATURE SCAR TISSUE

Characteristics of mature scar tissue include a reduction in cellularity and vascularity. After 14 weeks, the metabolic rate of scar tissue is slow, hence the rate of remodeling is slow; 2 to 3 degrees of increased ROM is considered good progress. Strong molecular bonding of collagen cross-linking creates a contracture that provides considerable difficulty for the treatment team.

Treatment of mature scar tissue includes extended positioning at least 12 hours per day. This requires a considerable effort by the patient, but without this necessary dedication, a major change in lifestyle could develop. The patient could use necessary modalities, exercise, and still have time to do activities of daily living.

If the patient is not progressing with ROM, a lysis and manipulation may be indicated. A premanipulation plan should be discussed with the treatment team. If flexion ROM is the main problem, then a CPM should be used following surgery. Extension loss is a much more difficult problem to solve. Expectations following a lysis-manipulation are usually about a 50 percent reduction in the flexion contracture, although many patients do achieve better results. The patient will either use a Dynasplint or receive a bivalved extension cast following this procedure. The CPM is not used for the patient with an extension problem. The use of serial casting may be indicated in the more difficult case of mature scar tissue in the captured knee. Treatment includes ranging the limb to the maximum point of limitation, then backing off a few degrees as the bivalve cast is drying. Serial castings should not be changed more than once a week.

Arthrofibrosis of the knee is the most difficult problem presented to the treatment team. This usually involves loss in flexion-extension ROM and the normal roll-gliding mechanism that accompanies arthrokinematic movement (Fig. 18-6 and 18-7). Treatment of the extension problem involves extended positioning (Fig. 18-8). Both a distraction and a gliding force are

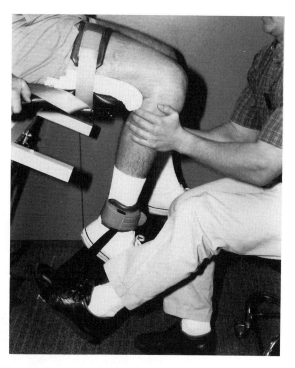

Fig. 18-6. Passive flexion ROM, posterior glide, and distraction force are used to gain knee flexion.

provided during this treatment, first using heat for 15 to 30 minutes, followed by another 15 to 30 minutes using ice. Patient setup includes placement of a towel roll under the dorsoproximal aspect of the tibia and the distal ankle region. A padded counter strap placed two finger widths above the patella is placed over the knee and provides a posterior force. A second padded strap is placed around the mediolateral malleolar regions, distracting the tibia. Heat is then applied around the entire knee. *Two towels* are placed under the knee, protecting the skin and neurovascular structures from the thermal effects of heat. The femoral strap is tightened, pulling the femur posteriorly. This, in conjunction with the posterior-positioned towel rolls, causes the tibia to glide anteriorly. A distraction force of 20 to 35 lbs is then fastened to the ankle strap. The therapist must observe the patient for ischemic trauma and pain tolerance. The treatment is then followed by the same protocol using ice to the anterior and posterior knee regions (Fig. 18-8B). *Always* cover the posteriorly positioned ice bag with a towel for additional protection of the skin and neurovascular structures. Observe

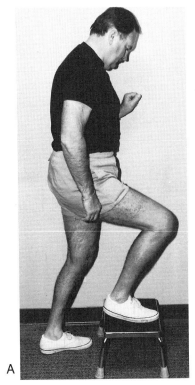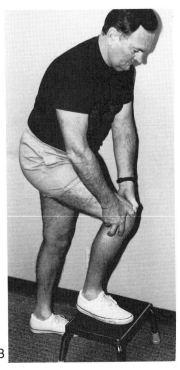

Fig. 18-7. (A) Self-mobilization technique for flexion ROM. The patient provides controlled body weight and leans forward on a step stool. **(B)** Self-mobilization of the patellofemoral joint is added during the exercise. Patient is pushing the patella inferiorly as hip and knee flexion occur simultaneously.

the patient for ischemia trauma. A 5-minute break between hot-cold sessions is recommended.

REHABILITATION OF THE KNEE WITH INCREASED INSTABILITY

Rehabilitation of the knee with increased instability poses a unique challenge to the physical therapist. All forces that are applied to the surrounding musculature are simultaneously applied to the joint in the form of joint reaction forces. It is imperative that practitioners have a clear understanding of the forces they may be applying to the joint and which anatomic structures are being stressed with each exercise or mobilization technique.

Increased instability in the knee may occur for a number of reasons. After knee ligamentous surgery, the desired result may not have been achieved. This may be due to poor surgical technique, postsurgical trauma resulting in a disrupted repair, or multidirectional instability in which part of the instability can be addressed surgically. In some cases a nonsurgical treatment may result in the rehabilitation of a knee that has a residual instability. In any case, the practitioner must be aware of the forces placed on the ligamentous structures via muscle strengthening and mobilization techniques. Each major muscle group in the lower extremity has an effect on specific ligaments in the knee. Of greatest concern are the effects on the ACL and PCL with knee flexion and extension. The vast amount of knee rehabilitation exercises currently employed involves isolated contractions of these muscle groups at some stage of the rehabilitation program.[29–33]

Rehabilitation of the ACL requires certain precautions. Isolated contraction of the quadriceps in isometric, isotonic, and isokinetic exercise places a great

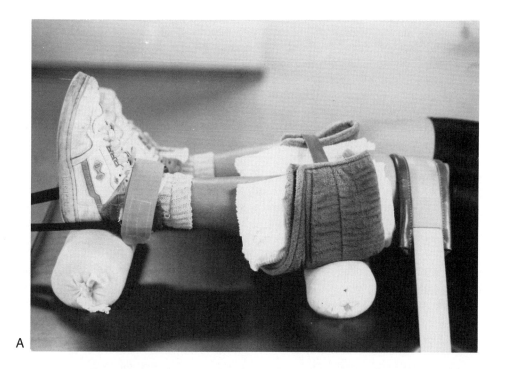

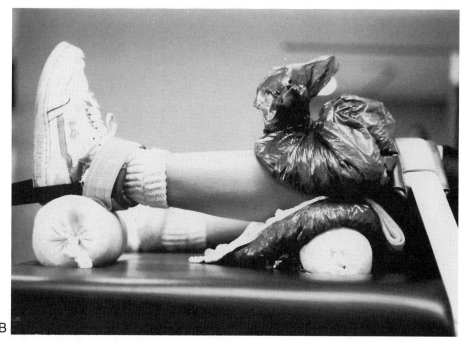

Fig. 18-8. Extended positioning technique with heat and ice (see text for description).

deal of anterior shear force on the ACL.[31,34] The quadriceps, with the aid of its fulcrum, the patella, and the vector pull of the patellar tendon, causes strong anterior shear forces as the knee approaches full extension. The straight leg raise exercise has tremendous effects on the ACL.[31] During this exercise, the hamstrings remain parallel to the long axis of the femur and are unable to resist the anterior pull of the quadriceps. These forces can further traumatize healing tissues or cause premature loading of the postsurgical repair.[31,35]

Posterior shearing forces need to be controlled in PCL rehabilitation. Isolated open chain hamstring exercises cause increased loading of the PCL. Hip extension exercises with the foot fixed and the knee in a near-extended position reduce the shearing forces on the PCL.

Residual instabilities, if not properly addressed during the rehabilitative phases, may lead to increased instability or damage to other structures in the knee.[31,36] In chronic instabilities, not only are the primary restraints compromised, but the secondary restraints become lax and further degeneration of the stabilizing mechanisms occurs.

Manifestations in the knee with chronic instability are numerous. Articular cartilage damage occurs with a disruption of normal arthrokinematics. Meniscal problems including tears and degeneration have been reported.[37] Altered gait patterns place increased stresses in the kinetic chain, with resulting changes in the adjacent joints. Back pain commonly develops secondary to compensatory movements of the lumbar spine.

Techniques

The goal of any rehabilitation program is to increase the function of the extremity involved to normal values and beyond. This always involves a return of strength. The key to a successful rehabilitation program is to strengthen the muscles around the knee, thus aiding in dynamic stability. Care must be taken not to add to the instability or cause further injury to the compromised structures.

Devices have been developed to limit the anterior shearing forces on the knee that occur while performing high-velocity quadriceps exercises.[35,36,38] Attempts to document decreased anterior tibial displacement via radiographs have also been studied. The question arises whether or not decreased movement translates to decreased loading of the ACL during isolated leg extension.[39]

Other means of limiting anterior shearing during quadriceps exercise have been to work the extremity in a limited ROM. By limiting the knee to no less than 45 degrees of extension while performing resisted knee extension exercises, excessive forces on the ACL can be avoided.[32,34] This method has limits secondary to the patellofemoral compression forces.[14] This type of strengthening fails to provide functional carryover to movements commonly used in the kinetic chain or sporting activities.

Teaching cocontractions of opposing muscle groups has merit in dealing with increased instability in both the anterior and posterior directions (Fig. 18-9). By teaching quadriceps exercises with simultaneous contraction of the hamstrings, anterior translation of the tibia can be avoided. It is difficult to teach cocontractions of antagonistic muscle groups because neurologic organs in the opposing tendons limit the force of the contraction.[32] Attempts at training the muscles using electrical stimulation or biofeedback techniques have become popular among clinicians.[31,33,40,41] The functional applications have yet to be investigated as to their effectiveness in decreasing tibial translation. In addition, most cocontraction exercises are completed in the early phases of rehabilitation in nonfunctional positions. This method may have greater merit when used as an intermediate step to progress the patient to more advanced exercises in the standing position.

There have been studies that investigate the use of proximal weighting of the tibia during leg extension exercises to reduce anterior shear. It has been found that this technique will limit the amount of tibial translation.[42] The amount of resistance for larger values of distal loading has not been determined. This technique has limited clinical application because of cumbersome methods in applying proximal resistance.

The use of orthotic devices during rehabilitation has been a common practice for many years.[29] Timing of implementation, ROM settings, and activity selection are debates that continue among clinicians. Functional and rehabilitative braces have their limit on the amount of tibial translation and rotation they control. The American Academy of Orthopaedic Surgeons has

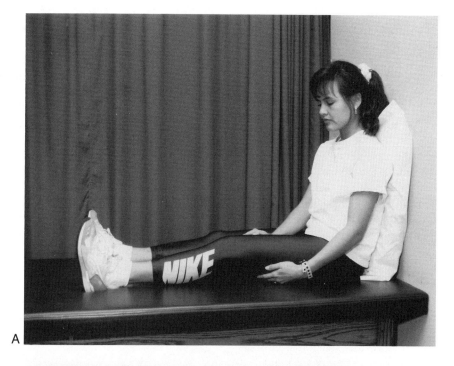

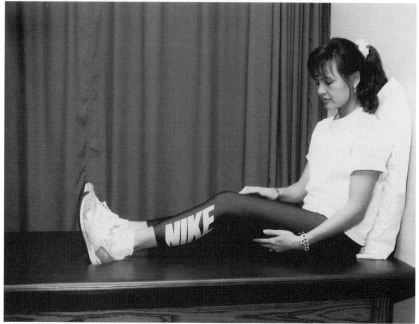

Fig. 18-9. **(A)** Starting position for quadriceps and hamstring cocontraction. **(B)** Contraction with the patient palpating the VMO and hamstring muscles.

reviewed a wide variety of knee braces. The Academy's 1987 Position Statement[43] and the work of others[44–46] have shown that the use of knee braces currently available provides little or no protection against knee instability.

Role of Closed Chain Rehabilitation in Limiting Shear Forces about the Knee

Closed chain rehabilitation provides exercises in which the end segment (the foot in the lower extremity) is in a stationary (fixed) position. With muscle contraction around the joint, the body moves in relation to the fixed end segment. By contrast, open chain exercises are exercises in which the end segment (the foot) is free in space. Muscular contraction affecting the joint causes a movement of the end segment in space. Closed chain exercises stress the musculature around the knee in a functional manner, both in movement patterns and with synergistic muscle contractions.[47] In contrast to isolated muscle contractions, agonist muscle groups work against antagonist muscles groups to limit shearing forces at the knee joint.

Lower extremity closed chain exercises allow strengthening of the muscles around the knee joint without the deleterious effects of increased shear forces.[48–50] Shear forces are controlled by a number of mechanisms. During a squatting maneuver, antagonistic contraction of the hamstring and quadriceps muscles limits anterior shear. The quadriceps contract to extend the knee at the same time that the hamstrings contract to stabilize and extend the hip.[50] In addition, hip adductors and abductors contract to stabilize the hip, and those that cross the knee act to provide further stability to the joint. Shear forces are reduced secondary to the axial loading of the femur on the tibia. As increased long-axis compression occurs, this reduces the effects of surrounding musculature, thus limiting shearing forces.

Closed chain exercises for rehabilitative purposes range from the simple knee dip (shallow standing knee bends) to maneuvers utilizing exercise devices. Examples include leg squat machines and stair stepping devices such as the Stairmaster 4000PT (Randal Sports Medical Products, Kirkland, WA).

Closed chain exercises provide an ideal method for rehabilitation of the knee with increased instability. With proper progression of exercise, strengthening can be performed without causing increased laxity of the joint. Additional benefits occur in stimulating proprioception and kinesthetic responses, thereby reducing delayed return to activity.[40,51,52]

Progression of Closed Chain Exercises in Treatment of Increased Instability

With any method of rehabilitation, timely progression of the rehabilitation process is critical to the outcome. Since new goals must include activity modification as a lifetime program, the progression of the rehabili-

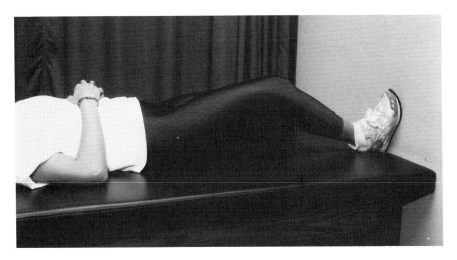

Fig. 18-10. Non-weight-bearing isometric wall push.

tation may be much slower than in a stable joint. Protection of the remaining functioning ligamentous structures must be paramount, as well as preservation of the secondary stabilizers.

Closed chain exercises can begin as non-weight-bearing exercises in the form of the wall push (Fig. 18-10). As quadriceps and vastus medialis oblique (VMO) strength improves, closed chain exercises can be progressed to the standing position. The normal sequela is from the two-leg partial weight-bearing position to the one-leg knee dip (partial squatting exercise) (Figs. 18-11 and 18-12). As quadriceps and VMO control is mastered, step-up exercises progressing to

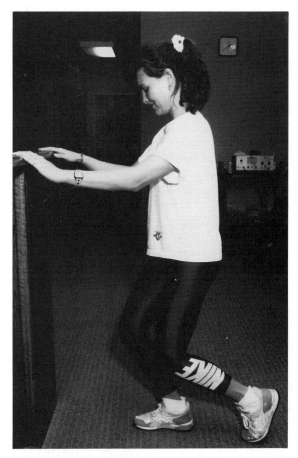

Fig. 18-12. Single-leg knee dips provide a basis for the progression of closed chain exercises.

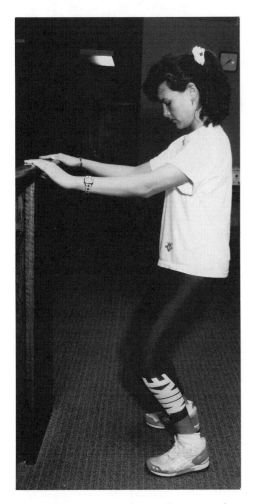

Fig. 18-11. Patient is seen during short-range knee dips. Patient squats down slowly to a maximum depth of 65 degrees of knee flexion.

step-down exercises can be implemented. As strength increases, weight can be added to increase resistance. Although these exercises appear to be exclusively quadriceps exercises, the hamstrings as well as hip extensors are being strengthened in this functional position.[47] Long-term studies have shown that the return to functional activity has a direct relationship to the amount of quadriceps return.[37]

Advanced exercises may include exercise apparatus such as hydraulic or pneumatic squatting machines (Fig. 18-13). Stair-stepping devices have been used to increase strength at higher speeds without jeopardizing the integrity of the knee joint (Fig. 18-14).

Functional exercise devices such as the BAPS board, the Fitter board, or the skier's edge allow exercise with directional changes in a safe and predictable manner and do not cause undue stress on the knee joint.

Progression of Treatment Modalities

To successfully treat the knee with increased or residual instability, a cookbook method cannot be employed. The first step in treating these problems is to correctly identify the direction and magnitude of instability.

Depending on the direction and severity of knee instability, rehabilitation goals must be reconsidered and altered appropriately. Return to preinjury activities for the individual may not be a reasonable goal. Recreational activities may have to be modified. As an example, cycling and swimming activities may be taken up in lieu of tennis and skiing.

Progression of the strengthening program needs to be monitored. Close attention to the reaction of the joint to each modality and tolerance to each technique

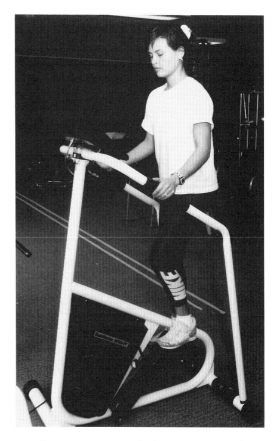

Fig. 18-14. Patient uses small choppy steps on the Stairmaster 4000PT.

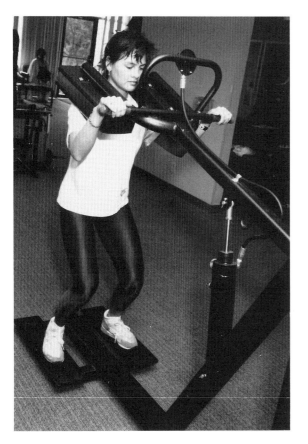

Fig. 18-13. Patient is seen using a closed chain squatting apparatus.

must be noted. Each joint with increased instability presents a different clinical picture, and the reactions to exercises are not as predictable as those in the stable joint.

Exercise progression must always be considered on the basis of tolerance to that activity and the volitional control of the musculature of the lower extremity. The VMO is an important patellar stabilizer and indicates the condition of the extensor mechanism. This muscle must be functioning for safe progression of the exercise program to proceed.

One technique, whether orthotic devices, range-limiting exercise, or closed chain exercise, does not necessarily hold the answer to success in treating unstable joints. The clinician must use an eclectic approach in selecting modalities for the rehabilitation process.

REFERENCES

1. Sapega AA, Quendenfeld TC, Moyer RA, Butler RA: Biophysical factors in range of motion exercise. Physician Sportsmed 9:57, 1981

2. Frankel VH, Nordin M: Basic Biomechanics of the Skeletal System. p. 87. Lea & Febiger, Philadelphia, 1987

3. Akeson WH, Woo LY: The connective tissue response to immobility: biochemical changes in periarticular connective tissue of the immobilized rabbit knee. Clin Orthop Rel Res 93:356, 1973

4. Akeson WH, Woo LY: Rapid recovery from contracture in rabbit hindlimb. Clin Orthop Rel Res 122:359, 1977

5. Frank C, Woo SLY: Medial collateral ligament healing. Am J Sports Med 11:379, 1983

6. Woo SLY, Inoue M, McGurk-Burleson E et al: Treatment of the medial collateral ligament injury. II: Structure and function of canine knees in response to differing treatment regimes. Am J Sports Med 15:22, 1987

7. Noyes FR: Functional properties of knee ligaments and alterations induced by immobilization. Clin Orthop 123:210, 1977

8. Akeson WH: Effects of immobilization on joints. Clin Orthop Rel Res 219:28, 1987

9. Andriacchi T, Sabiston P, Dallaven K et al: Ligament injury and repair. p. 103. In Woo S, Buckwalter J (eds): Injury and Repair of the Musculoskeletal Soft Tissues. American Academy of Orthopaedic Surgeons, Park Ridge, Illinois, 1987

10. Booth FWA: Physiologic and biochemical effects of immobilization on muscle. Clin Orthop Rel Res 219:15, 1987

11. Donatelli R: Mobilization of the shoulder. p. 244. In Donatelli R (ed): Physical Therapy of the Shoulder. Churchill Livingstone, New York 1987

12. Jackson DJ, Schaefer RK: Cyclops syndrome: loss of extension following intra-articular ACL reconstruction. Arthroscopy 6:171, 1990

13. Perry J: Contractures. Clin Orthop Rel Res 219:8, 1987

14. Sachs RA, Daniel DM, Stone ML, Garfein RF: Patellofemoral problems after anterior cruciate ligament reconstruction. Am J Sports Med 17:760, 1989

15. Enneking WF, Marshall H: The intra-articular effects of immobilization on the human knee. J Bone Joint Surg 54A:973, 1972

16. Sprague NF, O'Connor RL: Arthroscopic treatment of postoperative fibroarthrosis. Clin Orthop Rel Res 166:165, 1982

17. Sprague NF: Motion-limiting arthrofibrosis of the knee: the role of arthroscopic management. Clin Sports Med 6:537, 1987

18. Bennett GE: Lengthening of the quadriceps tendon. J Bone Joint Surg 4:279, 1922

19. Conner AN: The treatment of flexion contractures of the knee in poliomyelitis. J Bone Joint Surg 52B:138, 1970

20. Heydorian K, Akbarnia B, Jabalameli M et al: Posterior capsulectomy for the treatment of severe flexion contractures of the knee. J Pediatr Orthop 4:700, 1984

21. Nicell EA: Quadricepsplasty. J Bone Joint Surg 45B:483, 1963

22. Thompson TC: Quadricepsplasty to improve knee function. J Bone Joint Surg 26:366, 1963

23. Paulos LE, Rosenberg TD: Infrapatellar contracture syndrome: an unrecognized cause of knee stiffness with patella entrapment and patella infera. Am J Sports Med 15:331, 1987

24. Cummings GS: Selection of Treatment of Soft Tissue Contractures. Vol. 2. Stokesville Publishing, Atlanta, GA, 1982

25. Sapega AA: Advances in the nonsurgical treatment of joint contracture: a biophysical perspective. Presented at the Postgraduate Advances in Sports Medicine, sponsored by the University of Pennsylvania School of Medicine, 1988

26. Hepburn GR: The Dynasplint LPS Treatment Device and Therapeutic Stretching of Connective Tissue. Dynasplint Systems, Inc. 1984

27. Fullerton LR: Knee flexion device: a device for gaining and maintaining knee flexion after manipulation. Am J Sports Med 9:326, 1981

28. Light KE: Low-load prolonged stretch vs. high-load brief stretch in treating knee contractures. Phys Ther 64:330, 1984

29. Brewster CE, Moynes DR, Jobe FW: Rehabilitation for anterior cruciate reconstruction. J Orthop Sports Phys Ther 5:121, 1983

30. Jones AL: Rehabilitation for anterior instability of the knee: preliminary report. J Orthop Sports Phys Ther 3:121, 1982

31. Paulos LE, Payne FC, Rosenberg TD: Rehabilitation after anterior cruciate ligament surgery. p. 291. In Jackson DW, Drez D, Jr (eds): The Anterior Cruciate Deficient Knee—New concepts in Ligament Repair. CV Mosby, St. Louis, 1987

32. Seto JL, Brewster CE, Lombardo SJ, Tibone JE: Rehabilitation of the knee after anterior cruciate ligament reconstruction. J Orthop Sports Phys Ther 10:8, 1989

33. Steadman JR, Forster RS, Silferskiold JP: Rehabilitation of the knee. Office Practice of Sports Medicine. Clin Sports Med 8:605, 1989

34. Jonsson H, Karrholm J, Elmqvist L: Kinematics of active knee extension after tear of the anterior cruciate ligament. Am J Sports Med 17:796, 1989

35. Nisell R, Ericson MO, Nemeth G, Ekholm J: Tibial femoral joint forces during isokinetic knee extension. Am J Sports Med 17:49, 1989

36. Timm KE: Validation of the Johnson anti-shear accessory as an accurate and effective clinical isokinetic instrument. J Orthop Sports Phys Ther 7:298, 1986

37. Clancy WG, Ray JM, Zoltan DJ: Acute tears of the anterior cruciate ligament. J Bone Joint Surg 70A:1483, 1988

38. Malone T: Clinical use of the Johnson anti-shear device: how and why to use it. J Orthop Sports Phys Ther 7:6, 1986

39. Peppard A, Dehaven K, Bush M: Anterior tibial displacement during quadriceps exercise with and without the Johnson anti-shear accessory. Athl Train 24:117, 1989

40. Dvir Z, Koren E, Halperin N: Knee joint position sense following reconstruction of the anterior cruciate ligament. J Orthop Sports Phys Ther 10:117, 1988

41. Kain CC, McCarthy JA, Arms S et al: An in-vivo analysis of the effect of trancutaneous electrical stimulation of the quadriceps and hamstrings on anterior cruciate ligament deformation. Am J Sports Med 16:147, 1988

42. Maltry JA, Nobel PC, Woods GW et al: External stabilization of the anterior cruciate ligament deficient knee during rehabilitation. Am J Sports Med 17:550, 1989

43. American Academy of Orthopaedic Surgeons Position Statement: The Use of Knee Braces. October 1987

44. Baker BE, Van Hanswyk E, Bogosian S et al: A biomechanical study of the static stabilizing effect of knee braces on medial stability. Am J Sports Med 15:566, 1987

45. France PE, Paulos LE, Jayaraman G, Rosenberg TD: The biomechanics of lateral knee bracing. Part II: Impact response of the braced knee. Am J Sports Med 15:430, 1987

46. Garrick JG, Requa RK: Prophylactic knee bracing. Am J Sports Med 15:471, 1987

47. Porche E: Orthopaedic application of the Kinetron II. J Orthop Sports Phys Ther 9:315, 1988

48. Collins C, Yack J, Whieldon T: A case for using closed kinetic chain activities in the rehabilitation of ACL deficient knees. Athl Train 24:120, 1989

49. Delsman PA, Loosse GM: Isokinetic shear and their effect on the quadriceps active drawer. Med Sci Sports Exerc 16:151, 1984

50. Ohkoshi Y, Yasuda K: Biomechanical analysis of shear force exerted on anterior cruciate ligament during half squat exercise. Presented at the 35th Annual Meeting of the Orthopaedic Research Society, February 6–9, 1989, Las Vegas, NV

51. Harter RA: Knee joint proprioception following anterior cruciate ligament reconstructive surgery. Athl Train 24:119, 1989

52. Schutte MJ, Dabezies EJ, Zimny ML, Hapel LT: Neural anatomy of the human anterior cruciate ligament. J Bone Joint Surg 69A:243, 1987

19
Knee Bracing

PATRICK W. CAWLEY

INTRODUCTION

Commercial knee bracing is a relatively recent phenomenon in this country, emerging roughly about the time the Lenox Hill Derotation Brace was introduced in the early 1970s. In the fall of 1984, the Sports Medicine Committee of American Academy of Orthopaedic Surgeons convened a symposium to evaluate the state of current research on knee bracing and to categorize the types of braces commercially available. They developed three primary classifications for commercially available knee braces: prophylactic braces, designed to prevent or reduce the severity of injury in the athletic setting; rehabilitative braces, designed to be used immediately following injury or surgery; and functional braces, designed to provide mechanical stability in the knee with ligament deficits.

The number of manufacturers and variety of products on the market testifies to the current popularity of all types of knee bracing. The sheer volume of brace types, the lack of adequate documentation by many manufacturers and the scarcity of quantitative research have all led to confusion and controversy regarding optimum brace design and function. This chapter reviews available research on all types of commercially available knee braces and discusses the biomechanical factors that affect the function of each brace type.

PROPHYLACTIC KNEE BRACING

No category of knee bracing has stimulated as much debate as has the most recent entry into the knee brace market, the prophylactic knee brace. The first commercially available prophylactic brace, the Anderson Knee Stabler, was introduced in 1978 to prevent knee injuries to football players. This concept was almost universally applauded, and consequently, the growth of this market was rapid, with at least eight different manufacturers entering the market within 5 years. Unfortunately, the manufacturers provided no quantitative data to validate this bracing concept, and there were no independent studies of prophylactic brace efficacy.

In 1984, the American Orthopaedic Society for Sports Medicine called for research into the efficacy of prophylactic bracing, resulting in a frenzy of research activity (K. R. Moser, unpublished data).[1–8,60–62] This flurry of activity only created greater confusion, however, as some studies found reductions in injuries while others found no change or even increases in injury rates. Regrettably, two studies that might have deflected much of the controversy were never published (R. D. Curran and D. S. Linquist, unpublished data; Moser, unpublished data). As a result of this confusion, the American Academy of Orthopaedic Surgeons issued a position statement, cautioning clinicians regarding recommending the use of prophylactic braces. Subsequent evaluation of these published studies revealed that there were some significant problems with all of them, including injury classification and terminology, assignment of subjects to test categories and controls, treatment protocols, and classification of exposures. Perhaps the greatest difficulty for the clinician was that there was no biomechanical correlation for this clinical work.

The persistence of the controversy stimulated additional research, both biomechanical and well-controlled clinical work. In 1987, France et al.[1] initiated a biomechanical investigation of prophylactic brace function using an instrumented mechanical surrogate. These investigators concluded that some prophylactic braces do provide increased mechanical knee stability. They encouraged further well-controlled biomechanical and clinical investigation and indicated that prophylactic bracing appeared to be a viable concept, provided additional work was done.

Subsequent unpublished clinical data also appears to support the continued development of prophylactic braces. A well-controlled prospective clinical study (M. Sittler et al., personal communication) has shown that at least one prophylactic brace does offer protection to the knee in football. Additional biomechanical work[9] also indicates that some prophylactic knee braces may provide significant protection to the anterior cruciate ligament under load. Even with this new data, the debate about prophylactic braces will probably continue. The decision to use these braces should be based on an understanding of their function and limitations, and each patient must understand the inherent risks associated with sport, whether braces are used or not.

POSTOPERATIVE KNEE BRACES

There appears to be little controversy regarding the use of postoperative or rehabilitative braces. There has been little biomechanical or clinical investigation of their function, but the *fact* that more postoperative braces are used than both prophylactic and functional braces combined indicates their popularity. The lack of research seems odd considering that these orthoses are applied during the most critical period following injury or surgery.

In 1981, Krackow and Vetter[10] showed that even tightly applied cylinder casts with little or no padding permitted significant amounts of varus-valgus rotation, anteroposterior tibial translation, and rotatory motion at the knee. This study, as well as a changing and more aggressive approach to knee rehabilitation,[11-16] stimulated interest in finding alternatives to this more traditional method of immobilization following injury or surgery. When compared to serial casting, postoperative braces had several advantages. They were more cost-effective, were lighter in weight and therefore more comfortable, and could be adjusted for optimum fit throughout the rehabilitation process. Moreover, postoperative braces allowed access to the wound, could be removed and reapplied for passive or manual therapy, and permitted controlled motion through

preselected arcs. These factors all contributed to the increased use of postoperative braces.

In 1983, Gerber et al.[17] investigated the use of a cast brace following anterior cruciate ligament surgery. They were disappointed with its function compared with a traditional cylinder cast and a modified Lenox Hill Brace; however, these investigators did encourage further development, stating that they felt that postoperative bracing was a viable alternative. In 1984, Hoffman et al.[18] investigated the function of several commercially available postoperative braces. These investigators found that all the braces tested improved valgus, anterior, and rotatory stability in knees with sectioned ligaments. However, these investigators did not discuss in detail the mechanical factors that influenced brace function.

In 1989, Cawley et al.[19] utilized a mechanical surrogate to do a comparative study on several commercially available postoperative braces. This study was aimed at defining the mechanical factors that influence brace function. These investigators defined the primary role of the postoperative brace as range of motion control rather than control of abnormal translation at the knee. They felt that control of abnormal translations was of only secondary importance because most patients are generally on only a partial weight-bearing status; therefore, shearing forces from the quadriceps mechanism were likely to be small during the initial stages of brace use. (Note that this observation is probably accurate for most current applications but is likely to change as rehabilitation becomes more aggressive and encourages full weight bearing more early.)

These investigators identified several factors that affect the ultimate function of the brace, including the number and arrangement of straps, the means of interfacing straps and bars with the underwraps and limb, and the design and alignment of hinge bars. The main conclusion of this study was that braces that most efficiently integrated individual components were more effective at controlling limb range of motion. The presence or absence of shells attached to the hinge bars was not found to be a significant factor affecting ultimate function of the brace.

Unlike functional bracing, in which different brace designs may address different pathologic conditions, it is likely that one postoperative brace design can meet most of the potential demands in the postoperative setting. While factors such as cost-effectiveness, ease of application, patient comfort, and esthetic value will all influence the ultimate decision, the choice of a postoperative brace should be based on sound mechanical principles. The material properties and basic design should be analyzed to determine suitability for all potential applications.

All braces, whether functional, prophylactic, or postoperative, utilize leverage as their principal mode of function. In a postoperative brace, brace length must be adequate to provide positive control of limb motion, and brace composite material properties should provide adequate stiffness to resist all potential active and passive bending moments. Of particular interest is that the postoperative brace provides sufficient stiffness to resist accidental passive bending moments, such as when the patient slips and catches himself with the braced limb. The hinge on the postoperative brace should be easy to adjust and permit a wide range of settings for both flexion and extension control.

The postoperative brace should also be versatile enough to allow easy adjustment for the rapid girth changes that occur following injury or surgery and during rehabilitation. As most rehabilitation programs now encourage both active and passive motion earlier in the protocol, the postoperative brace should permit easy removal and reapplication as a single unit. Moreover, this brace should be adaptable to accommodate a range of limb contours and girths. One feature that may become more attractive as cost containment becomes more of an issue is convertibility to an interim range of motion control brace. In the future, truly modular bracing systems will become available that will accommodate anything from rigid immobilization through athletic participation.

One caution should always be observed with postoperative braces. Following severe injury or surgery, the involved limb enters a period of trophic crisis in which active muscular contraction is limited by pain, and blood tends to pool in the dependent limb. With application of a brace, circulation to the dependent limb can be further compromised due to a tourniquet effect or hoop compression of the brace straps. To avoid this, the postoperative brace should incorporate sufficient strapping to distribute loads over a wide area. Care must be taken not to fasten individual straps too tightly. In older patients, those with very low tissue compliance, or those with pre-existing clotting disorders or neurovascular compromise, particular care must be taken not to interfere with circulation. In these patients, a brace with large shells might significantly reduce the chance of brace-induced problems.

FUNCTIONAL BRACES

Although there is less controversy concerning the use of functional knee braces than that surrounding prophylactic braces, a review of the literature[20-57] shows that there is still a great deal of confusion regarding the function and efficacy of this category of braces. While a good deal of research has been done, many of the basic questions regarding functional knee brace biomechanics have yet to be answered. Unfortunately, most manufacturers still have not provided scientifically sound, quantitative data on brace function, and much of the existing research is contradictory or limited in scope.

The existing literature on functional knee bracing can be divided into four categories based on subject, approach or technique: overview, review of specific brace type, measurement of tibial translation, and biomechanical investigations other than tibial translation. The first two categories of work are largely anecdotal and contain a good deal of the authors' own opinions. These papers can provide a valuable insight into the development of individual brace designs and can provide the clinician a general overview of what is available.

A number of different methods have been used in studies of functional braces measuring tibial translation. Several of these studies used the cadaveric model. While the cadaveric model does offer the advantages of being able to directly measure ligament strain, and the specimen can be tested in the true physiologic loading range, there is one major disadvantage to this method. Soft tissue serves as the principal mechanical interface between brace and limb, and once the brace is applied, brace and limb form a composite structure whose behavior is dependent on the mechanical and material properties of both structures. In the cadaveric model, axial tissues on the limb are nondynamized, significantly altering composite response. While studies using the cadaveric model have contributed significantly to our understanding of the biomechanics of functional knee bracing, one must be very cautious in applying these results to the in vivo situation.

Most perplexing in this category were the nine studies that utilized the knee ligament arthrometer as the principal tool of investigation. Through personal communication, I am aware of at least four similar studies currently under way. While the arthrometer is unquestionably a valuable diagnostic tool in the clinical setting, its applicability for functional brace testing is questionable for several reasons: it is an examiner-dependent device; it must be modified to accurately measure limb translation and not brace translation; loads applied are far below the physiologic norm; and testing cannot be performed on the axially loaded limb. With so much data from the arthrometer already available, it would appear that any further study using this device is repetitive and nonproductive.

Several of the studies in this category have also utilized subjective response as one tool of brace evaluation. There is no question that this is a valid approach as these braces are intended to be used by living individuals. I would caution that subjective response alone is not enough and that subjective findings must always be correlated biomechanically when possible. The fact that most of the subjective responses in the literature do not correlate with the biomechanical findings in these studies would lead one to ask whether or not the appropriate biomechanical tests are being employed to study brace function.

Perhaps the data of most potential use to the clinician are contained in those studies[35,37-40,56,58,59] that evaluated factors other than tibial translation. The characteristic that sets this category apart is that all the work was done in vivo and, in most cases, attempted to duplicate normal physiologic loading conditions. Most studies in this category utilized sophisticated and costly instrumentation and data acquisition systems and consequently were generally limited in scope. The majority of the data presented in this category of study has definite clinical applications. For true clinical relevance, study in these areas should be expanded and an attempt made to correlate with existing data.

Despite the volume of data referenced above, there is little there to assist the clinician in selecting the appropriate brace for a given application. Fortunately, there are some general guidelines that can help in this selection. The most important factor to consider with functional braces is that a single brace design will probably not meet all the patient's potential needs. Rather, the clinician should be selective and fit the brace design to the application. Part of the controversy about functional knee bracing involves custom versus off-the-shelf orthoses. The method of manufacture should be of only secondary importance and the emphasis when selecting a brace should be on whether or not the material properties and functional design meet the individual patient's needs in terms of weight, durability, and functional control.

As noted previously, all knee orthoses function using the leverage of the long axis of the limb. Since the principle mechanical interface for the brace is soft tissue, it is unlikely that functional knee orthoses can provide true rotational limb stability under physiologic loading conditions. Therefore, the knee orthosis can address only planar translations or angular displacements and not axial rotation. When selecting a functional orthosis, determine whether the leverage applied by the brace is appropriate to the instability(ies) present and whether the main leverage points are opposed to provide optimum resistance.

Length has an obvious effect on the function of the orthosis, but in the case of the functional knee brace, length is one of the necessary trade-offs. With additional length comes improved leverage, but at the sacrifice of weight and agility. The functional braces currently marketed are all of approximately the same length because this is the maximum length patients can reasonably tolerate. Another factor affecting the function of the brace is the type of straps or restraint used. An orthosis that employs elastic restraints at the principal leverage points is obviously less effective in transferring loads than one that employs nonelastic restraints.

One area about which there exists a great deal of controversy concerns hinge systems on functional knee braces. Many manufacturers claim to incorporate truly kinematic hinge designs in the braces, and others claim a wide range of kinematic effects due to a particular hinge design. None of these manufacturers have quantified these claims with validated research data. In a truly kinematic design, medial and lateral components would exhibit different patterns of motion to accommodate *normal* automatic rotation at the knee. I know of no brace hinge system currently on the market that accomplishes this. In fact, due to the lack of a firm mechanical interface with bone, it is unlikely that any external hinge system would have significant effect on knee kinematics under physiologic loading conditions.[58,59] The main requirement for the hinge system on the functional knee brace is to transfer loads between tibial and femoral portions of the brace and preserve the leverage relationship. Secondarily, hinge systems should probably also incorporate range of motion controls so that they can be employed earlier in the rehabilitation protocol.

Before selecting an orthosis, the clinician should also determine whether the instability is mechanical or functional in origin. A mechanical instability is the result of disruption of one or more of the primary soft tissue stabilizers of the knee, while a functional instability is generally the result of a muscular deficit. The mechanical instability can be served well by a functional knee brace, whereas the functional instability requires additional strengthening and will not be affected significantly by an orthosis. It is also important to determine whether the principal application of the orthosis is primarily for control of an instability or for prophylaxis. A majority of the functional braces in use have been applied to repaired or reconstructed knees. If the repair was competent and rehabilitation completed, this patient would be considered to have a stable knee and, consequently, the brace is being used primarily for prophylaxis. For control of instability, the braces must address specific pathologic motions, whereas in a prophylactic application, the brace must address the specific demands of the sport.

A number of patient factors also influence brace choice. Patient age, compliance, activity level, and expectations should all be considered when selecting the appropriate brace. Bracing requirements for a more sedentary individual who plays weekend tennis and those for a young college football player would be quite different, even though both individuals had the same pathology. Undesirable behaviors such as brace dependence and risk taking can also occur because the patient does not understand the limitations imposed by the injury and does not understand the limitations of the brace. It is incumbent upon the clinician to inform the patient of all risks and limitations so that the patient can make informed decisions regarding brace use.

SUMMARY

Knee bracing is a complex issue, and many of the questions regarding efficacy and function remain unresolved. However, the clinician will be better prepared to make informed choices by becoming familiar with the relatively simple mechanics of brace function, while bearing in mind the physiologic and psychologic implications of brace use. The clinician is also well served by having an accurate picture of what is available in the marketplace. Brace choice should always be individualized based on both mechanical and patient factors. In many cases, the appropriate orthosis may not be commercially available and the orthotist should be considered for special custom applications.

REFERENCES

Prophylactic Bracing

1. France EP, Paulos LE, Jayaraman G, Rosenberg TD: The biomechanics of lateral knee bracing. Part II: Impact response of the braced knee. Am J Sports Med 15:430, 1987
2. Gaynes Testing Laboratories Inc.: Impact testing of knee braces: MKG and Anderson Knee Stabler models. Clarendon Test Report 1/1984–1/1985. McDavid Knee Guard, Inc., Clarendon Hills, IL, 1985
3. Grace TG, Skipper BJ, et al: Prophylatic knee braces and injury to the lower extremity. J Bone Joint Surg 70A:422, 1988
4. Hewson GF, Mendini RA, Wang JB: Prophylactic knee bracing in college football. Am J Sports Med 14:262, 1986
5. Rovere GD, Haupt HA, Yates CS: Prophylactic knee bracing in college football. Am J Sports Med 15:111, 1987
6. Schriner JL, Schriner DK: The Effectiveness of Knee Bracing in Preventing Knee Injuries in High-School athletes. American Orthopaedic Society for Sports Medicine Annual Meeting, Nashville, May, 1985
7. Taft TN, Hunter S, Funderburk CH: Preventive Lateral Knee Bracing in football. American Orthopaedic Society for Sports Medicine Annual Meeting, Nashville, May, 1985
8. Teitz CC, Hermanson BK, Kronmal RA, Diehr PH: Evaluation of the use of braces to prevent injury to the knee

in collegiate football players. J Bone Joint Surg 69A:2, 1987

9. Paulos LE, France EP, Cawley PW: Impact biomechanics of lateral knee bracing: The anterior cruciate ligament. Trans 35th Annu Meet Orthop Res Soc 14:202, 1989

Postoperative Braces

10. Krackow KA, Vetter WL: Knee motion in a long-leg cast. Am J Sports Med 9:233, 1981
11. Bilko TE, Paulos LE, et al: Current trends in repair and rehabilitation of complete (acute) anterior cruciate ligament injuries. Am J Sports Med 14:143, 1986
12. Blackburn TA, Jr: Rehabilitation of anterior cruciate ligament injuries. Orthop Clin North Am 16:241, 1985
13. Holden DL, Jackson DW: Treatment selection in acute anterior cruciate ligament tears. Orthop Clin North Am 16:99, 1985
14. Huegel M, Indelicato PA: Trends in rehabilitation following anterior cruciate ligament reconstruction. Clin Sports Med 7:801, 1988
15. Müller W: The Knee: Form, Function, and Ligament Reconstruction. p. 266. Springer-Verlag, New York, 1982
16. Paulos LE, Payne FC III, Rosenberg TD: Rehabilitation after anterior cruciate ligament surgery. p. 291. In Jackson DW, Drez D (eds): The Anterior Cruciate Deficient Knee: New Concepts in Ligament Repair. CV Mosby, St. Louis, 1987
17. Gerber G, Jacob RP, Ganz R: Observations concerning a limited mobilization cast after anterior cruciate ligament surgery. Arch Orthop Trauma Surg 101:291, 1983
18. Hoffman AA, Wyatt RWB, Bourne MH, Daniels AU: Knee stability in orthotic knee braces. Am J Sports Med 12:371, 1984
19. Cawley PW, France EP, Paulos LE: Comparison of rehabilitative knee braces: a biomechanical investigation. Am J Sports Med 17:141, 1989

Functional Braces

20. Baker BE, Van Hanswyck E et al: A biomechanical study of the static stabilizing effect of knee braces on medial stability. Am J Sports Med 15:566, 1987
21. Barrack RL, Skinner HB, Buckley SL: Proprioception in the anterior cruciate deficient knee. Am J Sports Med 17:1, 1989
22. Bassett GS, Fleming BW: The Lenox Hill Brace in anterolateral rotatory instability. Am J Sports Med 11:345, 1983
23. Beck C, Drez D, et al: Instrumented testing of functional knee braces. Am J Sports Med 14:253, 1986
24. Branch T, Hunter R, Reynolds P: Controlling anterior tibial displacement under static load: a comparison of two braces. Orthopedics 11:1249, 1988

25. Branch TP, Hunter R, Donath M: Dynamic EMG analysis of anterior cruciate deficient legs with and without bracing during cutting. Am J Sports Med 17:35, 1989
26. Butler PB, Evans GA, Rose GK, Patrick JH: A review of selected knee orthoses. Br J Rheumatol 22:109, 1983
27. Cawley PW: Functional knee bracing for skiing: a review of factors affecting brace choice. Top Acute Care Trauma Rehabil 3:73, 1988
28. Colville MR, Lee CL, Ciullo JV: The Lenox Hill Brace: an evaluation of effectiveness in treating knee instability. Am J Sports Med 14:257, 1986
29. Coughlin L, Oliver J, Berretta G: Knee bracing and anterolateral rotatory instability. Am J Sports Med 15:161, 1987
30. D'Ambrosia R, Solomonow M: A viscoelastic knee brace for anterior cruciate ligament deficient patients. Orthopedics 8:478, 1985
31. D'Ambrosia R: Knee braces (editorial). Orthopedics 11:1247, 1988
32. Faso DR, Montgomery JB: The dynamic rotating functional knee orthosis concept. Orthotics Prosthet 41:32, 1987
33. Flint J: A comparative study of the effectiveness of the Lenox Hill Knee Brace, the Omni TS-7 1 Knee Brace, and the Omni TS-7 2 Knee Brace in controlling anterior displacement of the tibia of six ACL injured knees. Omni Scientific, Inc., Martinez, CA, 1988
34. Helfet AJ, Manley MT, Vaughn CL: The holicoid knee brace: A lightweight but effective support for the damaged knee. Injury 15:189, 1983
35. Houston ME, Goemans PH: Leg muscle performance of athletes with and without knee support devices. Arch Phys Med 63:431, 1982
36. Hunter LY: Braces and taping. Clin Sports Med 4:439, 1985
37. Inglehart TK: Strength and Motor Task Performance as Affected by the Carbon Titanium Knee Brace in Normal Healthy Males. Innovation Sports, Irvine, CA, 1985
38. Knutzen KM, Bates BT, Hamill J: Electrogoniometry of post-surgical knee bracing in running. Am J Phys Med 62:172, 1983
39. Knutzen KM, Bates BT, Hamill J: Knee brace influences on the tibial rotation and torque patterns of the surgical limb. J Orthop Sports Phys Ther 6:116, 1984
40. Knutzen KM, Bates BT, Schot P, Hamill J: A biomechanical analysis of two functional knee braces. Med Sci Sports Exerc 19:303, 1987
41. Lewis JL, Lew WD, et al: A new concept in orthotics—the Northwestern University Knee Orthosis System. Part II: The complete orthosis. Orthotics Prosthet 38:13, 1984
42. Millett C, Drez D: Knee braces. Orthopedics 10:1777, 1987

43. Mishra DK, Daniel DM, Stone ML: The use of functional knee braces in the control of pathologic anterior knee laxity. Clin Orthop Rel Res 241:213, 1989

44. Mortenson WW, Foreman K, et al: An in vivo study of functional knee orthoses in the ACL disrupted knee. Trans 34th Annu Meet Orthop Res Soc 13:520, 1988

45. Nicholas JA: Bracing the anterior cruciate deficient knee using the Lenox Hill Derotation Brace. Clin Orthop Rel Res 172:137, 1983

46. Rebaman LW: Letter to the Editor. Orthopedics 12:354, 1989

47. Rink PC, Scott RA, Lupo RL, Guest SJ: A comparative study of functional bracing in the anterior cruciate deficient knee. Orthop Rev 18:719, 1989

48. Scott E, Mita H: Comparing the Paths of Motion of Orthotic Knee Joints and Normal Human Knees. Omni Scientific, Martinez, CA, 1989

49. Skyhar MJ, Cawley PW: Clinical Evaluation of the 4-Point ACL Brace: A Preliminary Report of Phase One. DonJoy Orthopedic, Carlsbad, CA, 1984

50. Smith EM, Juvinal RC, et al: Bracing the unstable arthritic knee. Arch Phys Med Rehabil 51:22, 1970

51. Tegner Y, Pettersson G, Lysholm J, Gilquist J: The effect of derotation braces on knee motion. Acta Orthop Scand 59:284, 1988

52. Tippett SR: A case study: Lenox Hill bracing for postoperative total knee replacement. J Orthop Sports Phys Ther 5:265, 1984

53. Van Hanswyck EP, Baker BE: Orthotic Management of Knee Injuries in Athletes With the Lenox Hill Orthosis. Lenox Hill Brace Co., NY, 1987

54. Wellington P, Stother IG: The Lenox Hill Derotation Brace in chronic post-traumatic instability of the knee. Injury 16:242, 1983

55. Wojtys EM, Goldstein SA, et al: A biomechanical evaluation of the Lenox Hill Knee Brace. Clin Orthop Rel Res 220:179, 1987

56. Zetterlund AE, Serfass RC, Hunter RE: The effect of wearing the Lenox Hill Derotation Brace on energy expenditure during horizontal treadmill running at 161 metres per minute. Am J Sports Med 14:73, 1986

57. Zogby RG, Baker BE, et al: A biomechanical evaluation of the effect of functional braces on anterior cruciate ligament instability using the Genucom knee analysis system. Trans 35th Annu Meet Orthop Res Soc 212, 1989

58. Regalbuto MA, Rovick JS, Walker PS: The forces in a knee brace as a function of hinge design and placement. Am J Sports Med 17:535, 1989

59. Walker PS, Rovick JS, Robertson DD: The effects of knee brace hinge design and placement on joint mechanics. J Biomech 21:965, 1988

60. Colwell HR: College Football: To brace or not to brace. Editorial, J Bone Joint Surg 69A(1):1, 1987

61. Curran RD, Linquist DS: Statistical analysis of the effectiveness of prophylactic knee braces. Unpublished paper, Dept. of Mechanical Engineering, Duke University, 1986

62. Paulos LE, France EP, et al: The biomechanics of lateral knee bracing part I: Response of the valgus restraints to loading. Am J Sports Med 15(5):419, 1987

Index

Page numbers followed by f *indicate figures; page numbers followed by* t *indicate tables.*

221